The Meaning of Spirituality and Spiritual Care Within Nursing and Health Care Practice

Note

Health care practice and knowledge are constantly changing and developing as new research and treatments, changes in procedures, drugs and equipment become available.

The author and publishers have, as far as is possible, taken care to confirm that the information complies with the latest standards of practice and legislation.

The Meaning of Spirituality and Spiritual Care Within Nursing and Health Care Practice

A study of the perceptions of health care professionals, patients and the public

Wilfred McSherry

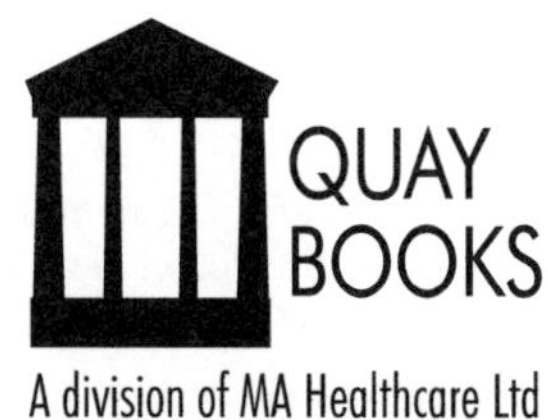

A division of MA Healthcare Ltd

Quay Books Division, MA Healthcare Ltd, St Jude's Church, Dulwich Road, London
SE24 0PB

British Library Cataloguing-in-Publication Data
A catalogue record is available for this book

ISBN-10: 1 85642 341 7
ISBN-13: 978 1 85642 341 0

Printed by Athenæum Press Ltd, Dukesway, Team Valley, Gateshead, SE11 0PZ

Contents

Foreword – John Swinton

Wilf McSherry has been and continues to be one of the leading lights in the development of spiritual care within the United Kingdom and beyond. Consistently, over an extended period of time and often in the face of opposition, he has pushed the boundaries with his determination to allow all of us to see more clearly the importance of recognising the centrality of spirituality for health care practices. Time and again he has reminded us that health care has a heart, and at the centre of that heart is a spiritual core. Recognising and responding to that spiritual core is vital for the development of forms of caring which remember the fullness of human persons. In this book McSherry takes us yet another step down the road of spiritual discovery and urges us to move even further into this mysterious yet vital realm of contemporary health care practice.

I like this book. I like it because it is honest, rigorous, thoughtful and potentially transformative. With a fine eye for detail and the importance of method for the development of practical knowledge, McSherry opens up the field of spirituality and health care to new understandings and perspectives. He is not prepared simply to deal with pat answers or slogans: 'spirituality is good for your health'. Whilst recognising the significance of the essence of spirituality for peaceful living and healing practices, he at the same time takes seriously the lack of clarity surrounding precisely what spirituality is and what it is intended to do within the practice of health care. His approach is theoretically thorough and practically grounded and his conclusions are challenging and at times, surprising. My sense is that this piece of work will fill a gap in the literature which very much requires to be filled. Within these pages the reader will find the fruits of many years of thought, reflection and practice. They will encounter a health-oriented model based on practical wisdom that focuses on the role of spirituality in defining modes of care which truly respect what it means to be human and to practice humanely.

Books are meant to do something. They are meant to take us into new worlds and open up fresh horizons which change the way we see the world. When we begin to see the world differently, so also we begin to practice differently. I look forward to seeing what difference this book will make as, through its pages, it allows us to see some things just that little bit more clearly, and in so doing helps us to act in ways that are a little more compassionate and a little more caring.

John Swinton
Centre for Spirituality, Health and Disability
(http://www.abdn.ac.uk/cshad/)
University of Aberdeen
Scotland
UK

Foreword – Peter Draper

I first met Wilf McSherry when he was an undergraduate student nurse at the University of Hull, in the academic department in which we both now work as Senior Lecturers. I was one of the supervisors for Wilf's MPhil dissertation, and I examined his PhD thesis. I have thus been privileged to observe Wilf's academic and professional development, and also to observe his commitment to the development of spirituality research and spiritually informed practice in nursing. That spirituality is now recognised as an important dimension to health care practice is in no small part due to Wilf's persistence and determination.

This book, which is Wilf's latest contribution to the literature, is based on his PhD thesis. The book addresses some fundamentally important questions. It is easy to assume, given the volume of current literature, that the meaning of spirituality is agreed by all, but in this book Wilf uncovers some important and unexpected differences in understanding, and his work represents an important contribution to scholarship in this area.

The book will be of interest, first of all, to those who are interested in the spirituality in nursing and health care practice more widely. Secondly, however, it will be of considerable interest to anyone who is interested in grounded theory methodology, and it represents an excellent example of rigorous research using a qualitative approach.

If this is the first book you have read on spirituality and health it will give you an excellent overview of scholarship in the field. If you have already read many books on this topic, then you will find things here to surprise and challenge you.

I recommend this volume to you most warmly.

Peter Draper
Department of Applied Health Studies
Faculty of Health and Social Care
University of Hull
HU6 7RX
UK

Preface

This book presents the findings of my PhD (Doctor of Philosophy) thesis investigating the meaning of spirituality within health care. In effect the book is a culmination of 12 years' thinking and researching into this area. The pages reveal my thoughts and various questions that I have engaged and at times struggled with as I delved deeper into the spiritual dimension. The completion of this thesis was in itself a spiritual journey and the obstacles and hardships I faced are described and documented within.

Every step has been taken to remain true to the original submission (thesis). Therefore I have not tampered with the structure and content. I am very conscious that a great deal of 'new material' has been published since the submission of my work (August 2004). However, I have made negligible alterations to the original literature and text only to add clarity or to be more inclusive for a wider health care audience.

My initial proposal was to investigate 'only' nurses' and patients' perceptions of spirituality. However, as the research unfolded it became apparent that I would need to include a wider group of health care professions. The factors that led to this are presented. This point needs to be raised because it explains why the book in parts does have a nursing focus.

The book reveals my commitment to delivering holistic care and improving the quality of 'spiritual care' that we as practitioners provide to our patients or clients by ensuring that our care is research-based. With this point in mind every step has been taken to handle sensitively the issues arising from the participants' transcripts and involvement in the investigation.

Finally, I hope that this book will shed a little more light on how the concepts of spirituality and spiritual care are understood by health care professionals and patients. This understanding is essential if we are to provide spiritual and health care that is relevant and appropriate to all in a society that is ethnically, religiously, and culturally diverse.

Wilfred McSherry
May 2007

Acknowledgements

I would like to thank Professor Keith Cash for his patience and support throughout this research study, especially when times were difficult and the going was tough. His motivation and encouragement were very much appreciated. Gratitude is also extended to my supervisors, Professor Alan White and Dr Linda Ross, for their support and the constructive feedback they provided during this research study. Again, their inspirational guidance provided encouragement throughout the project.

I thank all the managers and charge nurses who assisted in the distribution and collection of questionnaires, allowing me access to and use of their facilities. A special thank you must also be extended to all of the participants, who provided me with a rich insight into the meaning of spirituality. This insight was the most humbling of experiences and I feel privileged to have shared their understanding. Without their generosity this study would never have been possible.

List of abbreviations

DOH	Department of Health
GT	Grounded Theory
HCPs	Health Care Professionals
HDL	Health Department Letter
LREC	Local Research Ethics Committee
NAHAT	National Association of Health Authorities and Trusts
NMC	Nursing and Midwifery Council
QAA	Quality Assurance Agency
SEHD	Scottish Executive Health Department
SSCRS	Spirituality and Spiritual Care Rating Scale
UK	United Kingdom
UKCC	United Kingdom Central Council for Nurses, Midwives and Health Visitors
USA	United States of America

Introduction

Historically, it is recognised that nursing and indeed health care have held a strong association with religious traditions, predominantly Christianity. Tracing the antecedents of the nursing and health care professions reveals how they possessed a rich religious and (it could be said) spiritual heritage (Swaffield, 1988; Bradshaw, 1994; Cobb and Robshaw, 1998; Narayanasamy, 1999; McSherry, 2001; Koenig, 2002; Cook, 2004). Koenig (2002, p. 15) writes:

> Although addressing spiritual needs of patients as part of medical care is seen today as something new and different, this practice is actually a very old one.... Indeed, throughout most of recorded human history, religion and medicine walked quite closely together.

Koening *et al.* (2001) suggest that in the past a variety of religious orders of monks, brothers, priests and nuns, whilst caring for the 'soul', ministered to the physical and psychological needs of the sick. The idea of vocation and service of God through self-sacrifice and performing works of charity and mercy resulted in integrated care being provided to the marginalised, vulnerable and destitute within communities.

There was a realisation that ministry and caring were harmonious and that the sick required holistic care. There was an innate consciousness of the importance of balance while attending to the physical, psychological, social and spiritual needs of those in receipt of care. Spirituality infiltrated and permeated every aspect of the caring relationship. It was not isolated or fragmented since it was the force that motivated the religious in their desire to fulfil the Christian beatitudes, which emphasised service. Carson (1989), Bradshaw (1994, 1996) and Narayanasamy (1999) inform us that this approach to the organisation of care existed until the 19th century, when economic and political change resulted in the separation of religious communities from state-controlled welfare and health care systems. Bradshaw (1994) describes this in terms of secularisation, which manifested itself as a loss of the vocational aspect of care and the institution of a contractual model of care. These factors, in conjunction with the technological and scientific advances that have occurred during the 20th century, have led to a preoccupation with the physical and medical aspects of care. Koenig *et al.* (2001) indicate that due to the dominance of scientific thought and practice a schism occurred between religion and science.

Therefore, insidiously and unconsciously, 'integrated care' has been replaced with a reductionism that has marginalised and eroded the spiritual and humanistic elements from caring.

The erosion of spirituality from nursing and the wider health care agenda prevailed until the middle of the 20th century, when interest in and the significance of spirituality and religious practice were once again rediscovered. It was realised that attending to the religious and spiritual needs of patients may help to promote health and enhance one's quality of life (Simsen, 1985, 1986; Ross, 1995; Koenig *et al.*, 2001). This reawakening was initially instigated by nurse theorists (for example Hubert, 1963; Henderson, 1966) and some physicians (for example Tournier, 1954). This interest has now spread and gained momentum, resulting in the concept of spirituality within health care being debated internationally, with almost every professional group contributing.

Bradshaw (1994) is cautious in her review of contemporary nursing theory pertaining to the spiritual dimension indicating that many early theorists focused upon the functional aspects of spirituality in terms of religious practices and cultural influences. Bradshaw (1994) also argues that nursing theory lacks epistemological analysis, which leads to the construction and perpetuation of incoherent underdeveloped discourses.

A review of the nursing and wider health care literature revealed that spirituality is now being explored and debated within diverse care settings and with almost every professional group engaging. There is also a noticeable shift in the way that the concept is being presented and applied to health care. From the literature it appears that the exegesis and subsequent application of spirituality as a concept was initially at a 'macro' level. That is, the literature implied that spirituality is relevant to all and therefore applied generally to health care. A definition of spirituality that is commonly cited in nursing and health care literature is the one developed by Murray and Zentner (1989, p. 259)

> A quality that goes beyond religious affiliation, that strives for inspirations, reverence, awe, meaning and purpose, even in those who do not believe in any good. The spiritual dimension tries to be in harmony with the universe, and strives for answers about the infinite, and comes into focus when the person faces emotional stress, physical illness or death.

This definition supports the premise that spirituality is located in all people. It highlights that spirituality is deeply subjective, emphasising how for some people it may be associated with religious, theistic, and existential elements. The quotation legitimises the importance of the spiritual dimension for health care contexts, stressing that illness and death are the occasions when there may be a refocusing upon spiritual matters. Much of the early work assumed that everyone possessed spirituality and was therefore in need of spiritual care

(Shelly and Fish, 1988; Carson, 1989; McGilloway and Myco, 1985; Narayanasamy, 1991).

Within contemporary society there is still some unease and misconception associated with the use of the term *spirituality*. Allen (1991) informs us that this may be due to the fact that many individuals still view spirituality synonymously with a religious belief or faith. Hollins (2005) suggests that this apprehension still exists reflected by the reluctance of some nurses to enquire about patients' religious beliefs, either on the basis that they either do not see it as being important or are too embarrassed to enquire.

Despite all the conceptual and theoretical debate surrounding the use of the term there is no single authoritative definition of what constitutes spirituality (Narayanasmay, 1991, 2001). There seems to be a growing acceptance within health care that such a definition is not required in order to advance understanding and practice in this area. It is now established that spirituality is multifaceted in nature, pertaining to individuals with a theistic belief (believers) and non-theistic belief (non-believers). Yet health care seems to make the assumption that the definitions of spirituality constructed within nursing and health care while attempting to be all encompassing will have significance and meaning for all people. Bash (2004, p. 12) terms this universal approach as 'The via media' – the middle road – which he describes as a secular form of spirituality that uses religious and transcendent language while denying that the transcendent may have anything to do with the question or answer. This sentiment is shared by Hollins (2005, p. 23) when she uses the phrase 'believing without belonging'.

Despite some of the growing criticisms, the early pioneering work was instrumental in again highlighting and, to a lesser degree, establishing spirituality at the heart of nursing and health care by reinforcing that the spiritual dimension was central to the human condition. The concept of spirituality is now said to exist in all people, whether individuals possess a conscious or unconscious awareness of the importance of this dimension within their lives.

A noticeable omission of the early work was that it appeared very descriptive and prescriptive, in that it stated that nurses should be meeting the spiritual needs of their patients without giving guidance on how this could be achieved (Narayanasamy, 1991; Waugh, 1992; McSherry, 1997). Furthermore, this approach to care assumes that spiritual care may be different from other fundamental care that is provided by Health Care Professionals (HCPs). This separatist view does not seem to accommodate the idea that spiritual care may be provided during the daily interactions and tasks performed by nurses and other HCPs, such as bathing, dressing and feeding. In essence, this perspective accommodates the view that everything that HCPs do to and with patients has a spiritual significance and meaning. With reference to practice issues, HCPs are now starting to explore the practical implications of addressing the spiritual dimension: for example, spiritual assessment (Johnson, 2001; McSherry and Ross, 2002; Ledger, 2005). This may be because there is a growing awareness that theory will not be of any use unless it is transferred into the reality of practice (Oldnall, 1995, 1996).

Perhaps the necessity to transfer theory into practice is in part due to a number of political and professional drivers that are asking HCPs to attend to the spiritual needs of their patients. For example since the early 1990s the *Patient's Charter* (DOH, 1991) and the *Code of Professional Conduct* (UKCC, 1992) have made implicit reference to spirituality, drawing nurses' and indeed all HCPs' attention to the importance of spirituality for consumers of health care.

These political and professional publications have continued to be revised and thrust upon practitioners without any explanatory guidance on how to achieve competency in this area (NMC, 2000, 2004). The concept of spirituality is now very explicit in both the political and professional arenas, placing a tremendous amount of pressure and expectation upon service providers. This is especially evident in Scotland, where National Health Service Trusts have been asked to produce and monitor spiritual care policies (SEHD, 2002). In reality, these political innovations are creating a culture of managed spiritual health care where every aspect of the consumer's life has to be accounted for and documented through a series of systematic processes. The danger is that spiritual care, rather than being perceived as something integral to the caring relationship, becomes another dimension to be managed, irrespective of whether this is what consumers want and what service providers can realistically achieve.

This book presents the findings from a research study exploring the above assumptions and limitations in the nursing and health care literature pertaining to patients' and the general public's perceptions and expectations regarding spirituality and the provision of spiritual care. This type of insight is required so that the language of spirituality (McSherry and Cash, 2004; Hollins, 2005) created in health care reflects the needs and wants of consumers and service providers. These insights must also reflect the cultural, ethnic and religious diversity that now exists throughout the UK. At present the language of spirituality seems to reflect the majority white and Christian ethnic group's meaning that the approach adopted is very much Anglo-American and Judeo-Christian (Markham, 1998). This view needs to be revised and broadened, so that contemporary definitions of spirituality reflect the changes in the social composition of modern society, where this is appropriate.

In addition, this research aimed to broaden and extend the professional and practical knowledge base associated with spirituality by testing some of the epistemological arguments. As indicated by Bradshaw (1994), this type of epistemological analysis is required so that contemporary theory can be validated and refined preventing the perpetuation of incoherent, weak theories that have no real direct relevance when applied to practice. This aim was achieved in part by including both professional and public perspectives within the study, allowing comparisons to be made. These comparative and analytical processes will provide a fuller and richer understanding of spirituality that reflects the perspectives of key stakeholders, ensuring that all voices of the health care community are heard and hopefully incorporated in future political, professional, and practice development.

Outline plan of research conducted

In order to gain access to perceptions of spirituality held by HCPs, patients and the general public, and to information about the extent to which they expect to either provide or receive spiritual care, I used a qualitative research method. A grounded theory (GT) investigation was undertaken, using semi-structured interviews (a fuller definition and exploration of GT is provided in Chapter 4). These were conducted with a sample of HCPs, patients and members of the public who were neither patients nor HCPs, but came from particular faith communities. The investigation took place between September 1998 and August 2003. This time frame included theoretical and methodological preparation, prior to data collection, as well as data collection and analysis.

The investigation was undertaken in three areas:

- Area I (A hospice)
- Area II (A large Acute National Health Service Trust)
- Area III (A large Acute National Health Service Trust)

Areas I and III were situated in the same city in the North of England. Area II was in another city in the same geographical region. Using two different regions allowed me to capture the ethnic and religious diversity that existed. Area II was specifically selected because from the last national census (Office for National Statistics, 2001) the region contained a greater diversity of ethnic groups than the region in which Areas I and III were situated.

Ethical approval

Before data collection commenced ethical approval was obtained from the relevant Local Research Ethics Committee (LREC).

Data collection

Initial approval to start data collection was made with the first of the areas in July 2000, followed by data collection, analysis and the writing of the merging theory. In line with the grounded theory approach adopted, all these activities were undertaken throughout the project in a cyclical manner throughout the duration of the investigation.

The interviews (semi-structured) were conducted in three phases.

■ Phase 1

Phase 1 explored participants' perceptions and understandings of the term *spirituality*. It was conducted principally with patients and nurses from the hospice, who identified their willingness to participate by responding positively to a question on the questionnaire about their views of spirituality. This phase suggested that there might be major differences in the way that (as groups of individuals) patients and nurses understood the word 'spirituality'. Several patients had no real understanding about what the word meant; indeed, some had never even heard of the word. More surprisingly some of the representatives from a number of the major religions also seemed to have difficulty understanding it. This finding resulted in the need to conduct Phase 2.

■ Phase 2

Phase 2 was carried out with nurses and patients in the two acute Trusts. In this phase a number of questions were asked in order to determine whether patients and nurses would recognise the constituents of spirituality as expressed in the health care literature. For example, participants were asked to comment upon what provided their life with meaning, purpose and fulfilment. They were also asked whether they considered that these aspects of their lives were part of spirituality. This phase helped to develop further insights into how participants viewed spirituality. In addition, it revealed that spiritual care was provided by a number of health care professions; interestingly, it also suggested that nurses feel that no single professional group has a monopoly regarding this area of practice. These findings led to the development of Phase 3.

■ Phase 3

In Phase 3, the findings from Phases 1 and 2 were explored with a number of health care professionals, including a social worker, two physiotherapists and seven chaplains, who were recruited from Areas I and III. These groups were perceived by participants in the previous phases as being responsible for the provision of spiritual care.

In this phase several aspects of the theory that had begun to be developed in the previous phases were tested out and substantiated. These were that the word 'spirituality' was not recognised by all participants; that not all the constituents of spirituality were recognised as such by all participants; and that not all patients or members of the public had an expectation that spiritual care would be provided as part of health care.

During this phase it was noticed that not all the major world religions had been represented. As a result, a member of the Jewish community was recruited (from the Orthodox tradition).

The three phases of the investigation led to the creation of the theory titled 'assumption versus expectation' and the creation of a model for advancing the understanding of spirituality and spiritual care within health care.

Overview of the book

The book comprises six chapters, each outlining a different stage within the research process in an attempt to disentangle what is meant by the word 'spirituality' and why health care professionals may have become interested in this area of practice. The danger with publishing any academic work is ensuring that the academic style is not offputting to its target audience. With this in mind I have tired to write in a style that is both scholarly and accessible. In order to engage the reader with the material a number of reflective questions and activities are provided where these are considered appropriate.

Chapter 1 offers some insights into why we need to investigate this area, justifying this need on the basis of evidence derived from personal, professional, conceptual and empirical sources.

Chapter 2 explores some of the literature on the subject highlighting what we know about spirituality. This chapter is split into three parts. Part I looks at issues surrounding the meaning of spirituality, presenting a philosophical, conceptual analysis of the word 'spirituality' and how this word is understood within health care. Part II explores key issues such as impact of religion on spirituality; culture and diversity; holism and holistic care; science versus holistic practice; spiritual care being morally relative; and the managerial and political agendas that have shaped the spirituality agenda. Part III provides an overview of the international empirical studies that have been undertaken with regard to the spiritual dimension. This examination of the literature will inform our understanding of the contemporary debates associated with spirituality in nursing and health care practice.

Chapter 3 – 'Identifying the issues' – presents the aim and objectives of the investigation.

The research methods used in this investigation are presented in Chapter 4. This chapter is structured in two parts. In Part I there is an overview of why grounded theory was chosen and how it assisted in meeting the aim of the investigation. Part II explains the methodological processes such as selection of the sample, research setting, data collection, data analysis, and a review of the ethical issues that impacted on the study. The chapter concludes with an exploration of the concept of reflexivity, indicating its epistemological importance for this investigation. This section contains a personal account of the forces and life experiences that have influenced either consciously or subconsciously my understanding of spirituality. This declaration is provided so that the reader and the researcher (I) are theoretically sensitised to issues that may have influenced this investigation

The findings of this investigation are presented in Chapter 5. The chapter commences with a discussion of the core category titled 'assumption versus expectation' and its associated properties. This is followed first by a description of the findings from Phase I, detailing the five subcategories constructed, which have been labelled definitions of spirituality, diverse perceptions of spirituality, provision of spiritual care, socialisation of the spirit, and drivers. Secondly, Phase II illuminates how the categories in Phase I were validated. This phase also explored some of the components considered to be important aspects of spirituality, such as relationships, forgiveness and creativity. Phase II resulted in the creation of two further categories: spiritual narratives and subconscious awareness of spirituality, which expanded the emerging theory. Finally, the Principal Component Model derived from the data is illustrated in Phase III, suggesting how this may advance understanding of spirituality and spiritual care within health care practice.

The book concludes in Chapter 6 by summarising some of the significant findings. In terms of recommendations, six propositions are made targeting health care theory, practice and education. Appendices are provided containing relevant supplementary documentation.

Activity 1 What constitutes spiritual things

Before proceeding any further it would be helpful for you to reflect and record your response to the following question.

People seem to have different ideas about spiritual things. What do you think of as spiritual matters/things?

As you read through the remainder of the text the rationale for asking this question will become clearer.

References

Allen, C. (1991) The inner light. *Nursing Standard*, **5**(20), 52–3.

Bash, A. (2004) Spirituality: the emperor's new clothes. *Journal of Clinical Nursing*, **13**(1), 11–16.

Bradshaw, A. (1994) *Lighting the Lamp: The spiritual Dimension of Nursing Care*. Scutaria Press, London.

Bradshaw, A. (1996) The legacy of Nightingale. *Nursing Times*, **92**(6), 42–3.

Carson, V. B. (1989) *Spiritual Dimensions of Nursing Practice*. W. B. Saunders, Philadelphia.

Cobb, M. and Robshaw, V. (1998) *The Spiritual Challenge of Health Care*. Churchill Livingstone, Edinburgh.

Cook, C. C. H. (2004) Addiction and spirituality. *Addiction*, **99**, 539–51.

Department of Health (1991) *Patient's Charter*. HMSO, London.

Henderson, V. (1966) *Nature of Nursing*. Macmillan, New York.

Hollins, S. (2005) Spirituality and religion: exploring the relationship. *Nursing Management*, **12**(6), 22–6.

Hubert, S. M. (1963) Spiritual care for every patient. *Journal of Nurse Education*, **2**(6), 9–11.

Johnson, C. P. (2001) Assessment tools: are they an effective approach to implementing spiritual health care within the NHS? *Accident and Emergency Nursing*, **9**, 177–86.

Koenig, H. G. (2002) *Spirituality in Patient Care: Why, How, When and What?* Templeton Foundation Press, Pennsylvania.

Koenig, H. G., McCullough, M. E. and Larson, D. B. (2001) *Handbook of Religion and Health*. Oxford University Press, Oxford.

Ledger, S. D. (2005) The duty of nurses to meet patients' spiritual and/or religious needs. *British Journal of Nursing*, **14**(4), 220–5.

Markham, I. (1998) Spirituality and the world faiths. In: *The Spiritual Challenge of Health Care* (eds. M. Cobb and V. Robshaw), Chapter 6. Churchill Livingstone, Edinburgh

McGilloway, O. and Myco, F. (1985) *Nursing and Spiritual Care*. Harper and Row, London

McSherry, W. (1997) A descriptive survey of nurses' perceptions of spirituality and spiritual care. *Unpublished Master of Philosophy Thesis*, University of Hull, England.

McSherry, W. (2001) Spirituality and learning disabilities: are they compatible? *Learning Disability Practice*, **3**(5), 35–8.

McSherry, W. and Cash, K. (2004) The language of spirituality: an emerging taxonomy. *International Journal of Nursing Studies*, **41**, 151–61.

McSherry, W. and Ross, L. (2002) Dilemmas of spiritual assessment: considerations for nursing practice. *Journal of Advanced Nursing*, **38**(5), 479–88.

Murray, R. B. and Zentner, J. B. (1989) *Nursing Concepts for Health Promotion*. Prentice Hall, London.

Narayanasamy, A. (1991) *Spiritual Care: a Practical Guide for Nurses*. Quay, Lancaster.

Narayanasamy, A. (1999) Learning spiritual dimensions of care from a historical perspective. *Nurse Education Today*, **19**, 386–95.

Narayanasamy, A. (2001) *Spiritual Care: a Practical Guide for Nurses and Health Care Practitioners*, 2nd edn. Quay, Wiltshire.

Nursing and Midwifery Council (2002) *Requirements for Pre-registration Nursing Programmes*. NMC, London.

Nursing and Midwifery Council (2004) *The NMC Code of Professional Conduct: Standards for Conduct, Performance and Ethics*. NMC, London.

Office for National Statistics (2002) *Census 2001*. HMSO, London. http://www.statistics.gov.uk/census2001/census2001.asp

Oldnall, A. S. (1995) On the absence of spirituality in nursing theories and models. *Journal of Advanced Nursing*, **21**, 417–18.

Oldnall, A. (1996) A critical analysis of nursing: meeting the spiritual needs of patients. *Journal of Advanced Nursing*, **23**, 138–44.

Ross, L. (1995) The spiritual dimension: its importance to patients' health, well-being and quality of life and its implication for nursing practice. *International Journal of Nursing Studies*, **32**(5), 457–68.

Scottish Executive Health Department (2002) *Guidelines on Chaplaincy and Spiritual Care in the NHS Scotland (NHS HDL (2002) 76)*. Scottish Executive, Edinburgh.

Shelly, J. A. and Fish, S. (1988) *Spiritual Care: The Nurses Role*, 3rd edn. Inter Varsity Press, Illinois.

Simsen, B. (1985) Spiritual Needs and Resources in Illness and Hospitalisation. *Unpublished Masters Thesis*, University of Manchester, England.

Simsen, B. (1986) The spiritual dimension. *Nursing Times*, **82**, 41–2.

Swaffield, L. (1988) Religious roots. *Nursing Times*, **84**, 28–30.

Tournier, P. (1954) *A Doctor's Case Book In The Light of The Bible*. SCM Press Ltd, London.

United Kingdom Central Council for Nursing, Midwifery and Health Visiting (1992) *Code of Professional Conduct*. UKCC, London.

Waugh, L. A. (1992) Spiritual Aspects of Nursing: a Descriptive Study of Nurses' Perceptions. *Unpublished PhD Thesis*. Queen Margaret College, Edinburgh.

CHAPTER 1

Why do we need to investigate this area?

Introduction

This chapter provides a backdrop for the investigation, justifying it on the basis of limitations and omissions within the existing knowledge base that surrounds spirituality and spiritual care.

Activity 1.1

What constitutes evidence?
There is a growing debate within health care as to precisely what constitutes the best evidence. In relation to developing the areas of spirituality and spiritual care what types of evidence might we use?

You might want to reflect upon the following domains outlined in this chapter:

Personal, Professional/Political, Conceptual and Empirical

A review of the existing literature (presented in the next chapter) in conjunction with the process of reflexivity authenticates the need for this[1] investigation within the following domains: personal, professional/political, conceptual and empirical. These domains reflect the different types of evidence that may be used to develop practice through; necessitating the need to explore an area of practice; giving rise to research questions.

1 In qualitative research this is a process whereby the researcher attempts to maintain the rigour and trustworthiness of the study through reflection. This process is described in more detail within Chapter 4.

- **Personal**: encounters or incidents (critical) within one's own area of specialism may reveal practice or care is deficient in a particular area.
- **Professional/Political**: guidelines published by government or professional regulatory bodies alert practitioners to focus upon a particular area of practice. They may also reveal the types of behaviour a practitioner may need to adopt within their practice.
- **Conceptual**: in this instance refers to the language and discourses that have been established within health care pertaining to the construct of spirituality.
- **Empirical**: refers to published and unpublished research studies investigating the spiritual dimension.

With reference to the movement towards evidence-based practice, these domains will be presented using a ranking system, commencing with a discussion of personal evidence (which is considered the weakest form of evidence) and concluding with a discussion of the empirical evidence (deemed to be the strongest form of evidence; McSherry *et al.*, 2002).

Personal

A clear statement is provided in the section termed *personal account* of spirituality (Chapter 4) that I have had first hand experience of providing spiritual care to patients, in a health care system that Swinton and McSherry (2006, p. 802) state is 'spirituality bereft'. These personal experiences demonstrate that despite all the conceptual and theoretical attention accredited, the concept of spirituality and the provision of spiritual care are still poorly understood and neglected within health care practice. The critical incident recalled is only one example taken from a repertoire of scenarios that could have been used to support my concerns (McSherry, 1996, 2006). In addition, there is a growing amount of personal, anecdotal evidence published within the nursing and health care literature affirming that my experiences are not isolated cases (Simsen, 1986; Speck, 1992; Salvage, 1997; Wright, 1997). Although this evidence is circumstantial and anecdotal, it is still an important form of evidence that cannot be discounted reinforcing the need for this investigation.

The personal and anecdotal evidence supports the proposition that for some individuals the spiritual dimension is an important aspect of their humanity and existence. Several of the anecdotal accounts demonstrate that spirituality is perceived as integral and central to health and well-being in that it provides the person with a sense of self and purpose, whether this is expressed and achieved through adherence to a formal religious framework or as more secular, humanistic pursuits (Stoll, 1979; Ryan, 1984; Dobmeier, 1990; McSherry, 1996; Highfield, 1997).

Another form of personal evidence is the findings of a survey I undertook investigating nurses' perceptions of spirituality and spiritual care as a part of a Master of Philosophy Degree (McSherry, 1997). A questionnaire incorporating 'The Spirituality and Spiritual Care Rating Scale' was distributed to 1029 ward-based nurses working in a large NHS Trust. A response rate of 55.3% (n = 549) was obtained. The research found that nurses had very diverse perceptions and understanding of spirituality. The questionnaires were analysed using a range of statistical procedures. The results suggested that an individual's approach to spirituality could be accommodated by one of three broad groups: those trying to find meaning, purpose and fulfilment in life (Existentialism); those for whom spirituality was something that was present in all people (Universal); and a final group who suggested that nurses' understanding of spirituality was very individual, in that people's understanding and awareness of spirituality was influenced by many factors, such as their own beliefs and values. The study established that 'spirituality' applied to all nurses: those professing a religious belief and those who did not.

A major limitation of this study was that I did not have the opportunity to ask nurses to qualify or explain some of their responses. I was not afforded the opportunity to ask 'why' they provided or selected a particular response to the questions or items used in the questionnaire. Therefore this study was not really able to establish or reveal the individual's own deep understanding of spirituality. It only scratched the surface. This inability to gain a deep insight into participants' understanding indicated to me that there was a need to conduct a qualitative piece of research. This type of research would generate a deeper and fuller understanding of nurses' and patients' perceptions of spirituality and spiritual care.

Professional/political

As the literature review highlights, implicit and explicit in some of the professional regulatory bodies' publications is the notion of the nurse achieving competence and being professionally accountable in terms of providing spiritual care to patients (UKCC, 1992, 2000; QAA, 2001; NMC, 2002). Yet it would appear that there are few guidelines on how this should be achieved. In light of this emerging trend, not just for nurses but indeed for all HCPs, to attend to the spiritual dimension of their patients, there is an urgent need to establish the views of both service users and service providers in terms of their perceptions of spirituality and expectation in terms of receiving and providing spiritual care.

The notion of professional competence needs to be considered against the backdrop of the evolving bureaucratic and political climate that locates responsibility for spiritual care firmly at the feet of HCPs (DOH, 1991, 2001, 2003; SEHD 2002). The expectation that HCPs will provide spiritual care is based upon an erroneous set of assumptions in terms of what consumers want in relation to spiritual care and what can be realistically accommodated by service providers. This shortfall and mismatch between political and professional expectation warrants closer scrutiny to establish the feasibility of providing spiritual care to all service users.

Conceptual

The conceptual evidence could be categorised as one of the strongest in terms of its ranking. The issues identifiable within Parts 1 and 2 of the literature review suggest an urgent need to evaluate existing theory associated with spirituality and spiritual care. This review revealed spirituality to be:

1. A very amorphous, subjective and complex phenomenon in that it may have a different 'meaning' for individuals depending upon their own worldview or personal philosophy (Martsolf and Mickley, 1998); a meaning that may have been shaped or derived from social, cultural or religious influences.
2. Perceived differently by patients and HCPs. Analysis of the literature reveals that nursing and health care may have unwittingly manufactured a definition of spirituality that reflects a professional discourse (Rumbold, 2002); a discourse in which HCPs make assumptions regarding people's needs in this area and where there appears to be an 'imposed terminology' (Rumbold, 2002, p. 227) regarding people's understandings with regards to what constitutes spirituality.

These two significant findings suggest a need for health care professionals to evaluate and clarify the language and definitions they have constructed. This type of review may lead to the creation of a language and discourse that reflects the voice and concerns of all groups involved in health care. Narayanasamy (2004, p. 463) indicates that resolution to the above discrepancies may be found 'through more open inquiry to capture the lived experiences of the phenomenon of spirituality in health and illness'. Embedded in this recommendation is a need for qualitative investigations. This standpoint is echoed by McGrath (2002, p. 189), who writes:

> The hope and expectation is that the findings from well-constructed projects using innovative qualitative methodologies will go some way to protecting the compassionate hospice vision and will place spirituality firmly on the healthcare agenda.

It is hypothesised that an exploration and comparison of patients' and the public's perspectives with that of HCPs using qualitative methods will prevent the perpetuation of professional assumption and lead to the formulation of a more balanced understanding of spirituality and subsequently the delivery of spiritual care.

Empirical

It could be argued that the strongest form of evidence which substantiates the need for this investigation originates from the findings of previous empirical research.

> **Reflective questions**
>
> - What are your thoughts about conducting systematic reviews and randomised controlled trials into the area of spirituality?
> - Would this type of research assist in the advancement of spiritual care?

A review and critique of the empirical literature (Chapter 2, Part III) revealed that there are some major drawbacks with adopting a purely quantitative approach when investigating the spiritual dimension. It is apparent that those quantitative studies:

1. Provide only a glimpse, a superficial insight into the issue under investigation.
2. Are unable to explore the complexity of the area or portray and convey the meaning, feeling and emotion that an individual or group may have regarding the issue(s) under investigation.

There also exists a notable omission within the existing empirical knowledge base, because very few comparative studies have been undertaken contrasting simultaneously the perceptions of diverse groups such as nurses, patients, chaplains and HCPs. The studies that have been undertaken are predominantly quantitative. It seems that no comparative studies have been undertaken that have just utilised qualitative methodologies. This type of detailed, comparative exploration is required so that the perceptions and experiences of diverse groups can be established.

Optimistically, the empirical evidence (quantitative and qualitative) reveals that a great deal of conceptual and theoretical work has been undertaken into a wide range of issues pertaining to spirituality. Yet a limitation of the studies is that their samples are often homogeneous. Participants reflected one particular group; for example, in terms of religious affiliation a large proportion were derived from the Judeo-Christian traditions. In addition, the purposes of the studies reviewed are sometimes specialised, meaning that the studies include individuals living with a specific condition or illness residing in a particular area or working in certain situations. These limitations mean that generalisations cannot be made and the findings may not be representative, or indeed reflect the views, of a wider audience or population.

Key points

- The voice of academics and practitioners expressed in the conceptual and empirical evidence recommends that qualitative methodologies may be the most appropriate when investigating the spiritual dimension.
- Contrasting the shortfalls in the existing knowledge base regarding perceptions of spirituality and spiritual care with the personal and professional evidence justifies the need for this investigation.

References

Department of Health (1991) *Patient's Charter*. HMSO, London.

Department of Health (1992) *Meeting the Spiritual Needs of Patients and Staff* (HSG (92)). HMSO, London.

Department of Health (2001) *Your Guide to the NHS*. Department of Health, London.

Department of Health (2003) *NHS Chaplaincy Meeting the Religious and Spiritual Needs of Patients and Staff*. Department of Health, London.

Dobmeier, T. (1990) Professionalizing spiritual care *Journal of Christian Nursing*, **7**(1), 32.

Highfield, M. F. (1997) Spiritual assessment across the cancer trajectory: methods and reflections. *Seminars in Oncology Nursing*, **13**(4), 237–41.

Martsolf, D. S. and Mickley, J. R. (1998) The concept of spirituality in nursing theories: differing world-views and extent of focus. *Journal of Advanced Nursing*, **27**, 294–303.

McGrath, P. (2002) New horizons in spirituality research. In: *Spirituality and Palliative Care* (ed. B. Rumbold), Chapter 12. Oxford University Press, Australia.

McSherry, W. (1996) Raising the spirits. *Nursing Times*, **92**(3), 48–9.

McSherry, W. (1997) A descriptive survey of nurses' perceptions of spirituality and spiritual care. *Unpublished Master of Philosophy Thesis*, University of Hull, England.

McSherry, W. (2006) *Making Sense of Spirituality in Nursing and Health Care Practice: An Interactive Approach*. Jessica Kingsley, London and Edinburgh.

McSherry, R., Simmons, M. and Pearce, P. (2002) An introduction to evidenced-informed nursing. In: *Evidenced-Informed Nursing a Guide for Clinical Nurses* (R. McSherry, M. Simmons and P. Abbott), Chapter 1. Routledge, London.

Narayanasamy, A. (2004) Commentary on MacLaren, J. (2004) A kaleidoscope of understandings: spiritual nursing in a multi-faith society. *Journal of Advanced Nursing*, **45**(5), 457–62. *Journal of Advanced Nursing*, **45**(5), 462–4.

Nursing and Midwifery Council (2002) *Requirements for Pre-registration Nursing Programmes*. NMC, London.

Nursing and Midwifery Council (2004) *Code of Professional Conduct*. NMC, London.

Quality Assurance Agency for Higher Education (2001) *Nursing Benchmark Statements: Health Care Programmes*. Quality Assurance Agency for Higher Education, Gloucester.

Rumbold, B. (2002) *Spirituality and Palliative Care*. Oxford University Press, Australia.

Ryan, J. (1984) The neglected crisis. *American Journal of Nursing*, October, 1257–8.

Salvage, J. (1997) Journey to the centre. *Nursing Times*, **93**(17), 28–30.

Scottish Executive Health Department (2002) *Guidelines on Chaplaincy and Spiritual Care in the NHS Scotland (NHS HDL (2002) 76)*. Scottish Executive, Edinburgh.

Simsen, B. (1986) The spiritual dimension. *Nursing Times*, **82**, 41–2.

Speck, P. (1992) Nursing the soul. *Nursing Times*, **88**(23), 22.

Stoll, R. I. (1979) Guidelines for spiritual assessment. *American Journal of Nursing*, September, **79**(9), 1574–7.

Swinton, J. and McSherry, W. (2006) Editorial: Critical reflections on the current state of spirituality-in-nursing. *Journal of Clinical Nursing*, **15**(7), 801–2.

United Kingdom Central Council for Nursing, Midwifery and Health Visiting (1992) *Code of Professional Conduct*. UKCC, London.

United Kingdom Central Council for Nursing, Midwifery and Health Visiting (2000) *Requirements for Pre-registration Nursing Programmes*. UKCC, London.

Wright, S. (1997) Free the spirit. *Nursing Times*, **93**(17), 31–2.

CHAPTER 2

What we know about spirituality

Overview

This chapter presents the literature review and it has been structured and presented in three discrete but interconnecting parts. Part I conceptualises spirituality, focusing specifically upon the language and meaning associated with its use in nursing and health care. Part II is an analysis of the nursing and health care literature, focusing upon key issues that may have resulted in the emergence, and subsequent development, of the concept of spirituality and the provision of spiritual care. This section presents a framework, a set of ideas that have been tested throughout the course of this grounded theory investigation. Part 3 provides a brief overview of selected empirical research surrounding spirituality and spiritual care.

> **Ask yourself the following:**
>
> - Is the language of spirituality universal?
> - What are your patients' or clients' expectations with regard receiving spiritual care?
> - In your experience, do HCPs support patients/clients with their spiritual needs?

Part I: Issues surrounding the meaning of spirituality[1]

Part I explores the relationships that exist between the language used to describe spirituality within nursing and the appropriateness of constructing a

1 Aspects of this section are reprinted from McSherry, W. and Cash, K. T. (2004) The language of spirituality: an emerging taxonomy. *International Journal of Nursing Studies*, **41**(2), 151–61. Copyright 2004, with permission from Elsevier.

universal definition acceptable to *all* individuals. 'Spirituality' is a term that is increasingly used in nursing, but there may be problems surrounding exactly what the term means and how it is interpreted and understood by both nurses and patients. The aim of the section is to explore some of the commonly cited definitions to establish whether the concept of spirituality could be termed 'universal'. The section presents a discussion, based upon a limited literature review, of the nursing and health care databases, combined with manual searches. The review demonstrates how the term 'spirituality' is being constructed within nursing, suggesting that there are numerous definitions, each with several layers of meaning.

From the review a *spiritual taxonomy* was developed that may explain and accommodate the different layers of meaning found within nursing and health care definitions. At the extreme left there is a spirituality based on religious and theist ideals, while at the extreme right there is a spirituality based upon secular, humanistic, existential elements. A middle way is explained, containing elements from both the left and right but not as fundamental or radical.

Part I concludes that as there are so many definitions with different layers of meanings, spirituality can imply different things depending upon an individual's personal interpretation or worldview. The results of the review suggest that health care professionals are constructing a 'blanket' definition of spirituality which has a broad, almost inexhaustible, set of defining characteristics. If this approach continues then there is a danger that the word may become so broad in meaning that it loses any real significance.

Contextualisation

It is evident that the term 'spirituality' has become fashionable within nursing. Books and articles regularly appear exploring this subject. The increased interest may be due to the notion of holistic care. However, reference to spirituality is often anecdotal or rhetorical (Turner, 1996; Emdon, 1997; Hall, 1997; Wright, 1997; McSherry, 2006). The emerging literature is rather prescriptive, suggesting that nurses should be providing spiritual care without really defining what is meant by the term (Narayanasamy, 1993; McSherry, 1996; Emdon, 1997; Hall, 1997; Ross, 1997b; Wright, 1997). This activity signals an attempt to educate HCPs about spiritual matters. However, the definitions and recommendations, rather than bringing clarity, add to the confusion that surrounds the term 'spirituality'. This may originate from the fact that definitions are often based on individual interpretation and understanding rather than on empirical evidence. There is also an assumption that nurses and patients understand what is meant by the word when the contrary may be true (McSherry,

1997; Markham, 1998). A review of contemporary definitions suggests that there may be no common understanding of the concept of spirituality. It seems that we could have a term – 'spirituality' – but no common set of defining characteristics of the term that are universally transferable or recognised.

Background

Spirituality has become a highly salient term, not only in relation to nursing and health care, but within society at large (MacQuarrie, 1972a; McSherry, 2000). Within health care attention has turned to the provision of holistic care, that is, care for the individual's physical, psychological, social and spiritual dimensions (Buckle, 1993; Woods, 1998; Narayanasamy, 2001). As a result several documents have been published, educationally (UKCC, 1986; NMC, 2002, 2004; QAA 2001) and clinically (DOH, 2001, 2003a; SEHD, 2002), which emphasise this notion of holistic health care. These publications reinforce the need for health care workers to pay attention to the spiritual dimension of care. Implicit in these publications is recognition that the United Kingdom is no longer a monocultural society but multicultural and ethnically diverse. Therefore, if health care workers are to respond to this transition in society, attention must be paid to the different factors that are fundamental and specific to particular cultures, such as religious customs (Gerrish, 1997; Henley and Schott, 1999; Holland and Hogg, 2001). For some individuals spirituality will be expressed and shaped by religious customs and practices that provide a meaning to their existence. Nurses require the correct education and information about these customs and practices if they are to offer culturally sensitive religious and spiritual care, avoiding stereotypical assumptions (Gilliat-Ray, 2001).

With reference to nurse education, there is a growing debate as to how best to proceed with teaching spirituality within the nursing profession (Ross, 1996; McSherry and Draper, 1998; Bradshaw, 1997; Greenstreet, 1999; McSherry, 2000). In analysing the emerging position as to whether spirituality should or should not be taught it becomes evident that ambiguity in meaning is a source of contention.

Database searches

A search of the electronic databases CINHAL, MEDLINE and EMBASE was undertaken spanning the period of 1985–2003. The terms 'spirituality', 'spiritual care', and 'spiritual dimension' were used to identify literature in English. Some seminal works that did not satisfy the following search criteria were included. Due to the vast amount of literature available, the following search criteria were set: only those works that provided an abstract, contributed to the growing conceptual or theoretical debate and provided a definition were included.

Manual searching of the literature was also undertaken. Because of my previous interest and research in the area I had collected a wide range of resources in the form of published research articles, journal articles, edited books and theses spanning a wide range of disciplines. These were catalogued and made a substantial contribution to the review. I must stress that the literature search and review were not an isolated, single activity that occurred at the outset of the investigation. Literature searches and reviews were continually performed to ensure that emerging theory reflected and was substantiated by current material.

Activity 2.1 Searching the databases

If you have access to any of the electronic databases mentioned earlier you might want to replicate the search that I undertook using the following key words:

- spirituality (and your own professional group)
- spiritual care
- spiritual needs

What does all the activity say about the concept of spirituality and health care? Do you notice anything else about the activity that has been undertaken? For example types of study?

Literature reviews and qualitative research

Within qualitative research there is some uncertainty about conducting literature reviews. It is thought that by reviewing technical literature (for example research reports and academic publications) and non-technical literature (for example diaries and manuscripts) (Strauss and Corbin, 1998) prior to undertaking the investigation may result in the researcher entering the field with a set of preconceived ideas. However, my interpretation of this debate is that the question as to when, and indeed whether, a literature review be conducted be determined by one main variable – the research question. The type and nature of the research question should guide the scope and extent of the review and fundamentally how the literature should be used. It is the research question that decides the level of theoretical sensitivity to be achieved prior to undertaking any investigation.

The role of the literature review in grounded theory investigations

It would be a grave misconception, and indeed a fallacy, to legislate suggesting that a literature review should only be undertaken at the end of data collection. The origins of this view stem from a misguided fear of instilling bias or prejudice that may influence or distort data analysis and ultimately lead to limited or restricted theory development. However, this type of generalisation would not accommodate the research questions developed for this investigation, which seek to test existing conceptual theoretical arguments surrounding the nature of spirituality. In this instance, there is a need for me to be theoretically sensitive to the literature and aware of existing conceptual and theoretical arguments throughout the entire research process. This broadening of horizons ensured that I was aware of and conversed with the issues emerging within the health care and nursing literature.

Religion: its historical influence

When undertaking a philosophical analysis of the word 'spirituality' it is useful to trace its origins (Narayanasmay, 1999a; McSherry, 2000). It is recognised that the Judeo-Christian heritage and influence in the UK and other parts of the world has been an important factor in shaping cultural and attitudinal norms (Smart, 1969). By plotting nursing's heritage one can recognise that this has been influenced by principles from the Judeo-Christian tradition. This is evident in Florence Nightingale's philosophy of care, which Macrae (1995) and Bradshaw (1996) would argue is founded on the divine by advocating that Nightingale's work operated around the principle of vocation, that is selfless giving and love of one's neighbour. Proceeding from this historical perspective, then, the term 'spirituality', as used in the UK, derived its meaning from its association with religion and a belief in a God. If one subscribes to this view, the religious and theistic components inherent in the historical heritage of nursing must be acknowledged when considering the origins of the word 'spirituality'.

Cupitt (1997) suggests that the creation of the word 'god' and subsequent religious worship that ensued was a means of organising and controlling individuals who, up until such times, had lived a nomadic existence. The creation of the word 'god', it is implied, led to the creation of societies and the amalgamation of individuals. This approach is interesting because it demonstrates the power of language and the subsequent meaning that can be derived from the creation of words. Cupitt (1997, p. 18) writes:

> I have argued that the entire supernatural world of religion is a mythical representation of the creative – and also demonic – powers of language

Cupitt's (1997) work reinforces the point that, before one explores the meaning and relevance of any concept, one must pay attention to the historical events that have shaped the way that a word is presented and most importantly perceived by individuals in a society. The factors outlined by Cupitt (1997) are relevant and appropriate when analysing the concept of spirituality. In the past it would appear that the word spirituality was associated with formal religious practice and a theistic philosophy.

An ontological argument

Bradshaw (1994) and Pattison (2001) are unable to separate the use of the word 'spirituality' from its religious (one assumes Judeo-Christian) heritage, arguing that historically, through religion, the word found meaning, having a discourse and context. Pattison (2001, p. 34) suggests that if the word is removed from this association then it

> is lost in the interests of providing bespoke metaphysical marshmallow that is non-specific, unlocated, thin, uncritical, dull and un-nutritious.

These authors imply that the word has a long history that has shaped and provided the word with expression and meaning. When divorced from this, it is in danger of becoming meaningless. Bradshaw's (1994) philosophical position implies that the word 'spirituality' is intimately interwoven within an ontological argument. In her work she presents an ontological heritage of nursing. Bradshaw suggests that historical context and religious association have shaped the metaphysical and epistemological construction of the word 'spirituality' both within society and, more specifically, within nursing. A problem with this perspective is that it fails to satisfy several schools of thought: for example, the atheistic and the humanistic schools that emerged during the course of the 19th century (Burnard, 1988a; Nelson, 1995) that would argue that spirituality is more than just religion. Therefore, these individuals would not share Bradshaw's position because they are opposed to any notion of the existence of God (Burnard, 1988b; Nelson, 1995).

Individuals such as secular humanists and atheists may also dispute and not place any credence upon philosophical positions that are founded primarily within a Christian tradition, since they will not believe in such teachings. Burnard (1988a), who addressed the spiritual needs of atheists and agnostics, supports these perspectives, suggesting that both atheists and agnostics, while not believing or being uncertain about the existence of God, still possess a spirituality that is based on existential philosophy. That is, they are still able to find meaning, purpose and fulfilment in life. Cobb (2001a) draws attention to an emerging debate surrounding the relationship between spirituality and existentialism. Cobb (2001a) argues that existentialism is something separate to the spiritual dimension. Another limitation of Bradshaw's (1994) and Pattison's (2001) position could be interpreted as being culturally restrictive in that it does not fit the cultural changes within many contemporary and pluralistic societies.

Markham (1998) asserts that individuals from different world faiths may not be able to identify with the descriptors used in health care definitions because they reflect a secular version of a Christian form of spirituality. An opposing opinion to this paternalism might be that some individuals from different world faiths who are active within their local community are generating awareness of the factors that are likely to affect their lives, of which spirituality may be one. Markham (1998) also implies that individuals from other world faiths are passive, neither questioning nor influencing the way that communities and societies change. Irrespective of which view one holds, these arguments imply that individuals from other world faiths can and should be encouraged to contribute to the way that the concept of spirituality is being fashioned within health care and society at large. In short, it may be that the rigid association of the religious and theistic approaches to understanding or defining spirituality are now seen by some western societies as outdated and not in keeping with modernist, multicultural, or indeed secular views of the term.

Modernism and secularisation

Presently there appears to be a marked shift from the religious and theistic beliefs to a more generalist or secular perspective of spirituality. Dawson

(1945, p. 249) in his classic work *Progress and Religion* describes the decline of religion and spirituality within modern society:

> We have come to take it for granted that the unifying force in society is material interest, and that spiritual conviction is a source of strife and division. Modern civilization has pushed religion and the spiritual elements in culture out of the main stream of its developments, so they have lost touch with life and have become sectarianized and impoverished.

The empirical evidence that supports this claim is found in the decline in formal religious practice such as church attendance (Carr, 2001; Matheson and Summerfield, 2001) and the fact that individuals no longer profess belief in God (McSherry, 1997). A recent MORI (2003) poll undertaken for the BBC's *Heaven and Earth Show* revealed that, despite the perceived decline in formal religious practice, 60% of the respondents still believe in God. This result reflects the findings of McSherry's (1997) survey which found that many of the nurses, despite not believing in God, acknowledged a transpersonal belief in forces beyond themselves. Hay and Hunt (2000, p. 10) identified similar views:

> We found that the conversations themselves often took on recognizably spiritual dimensions as people wrestled to articulate their own sense of transcendence.

These findings bring into question the notion that western society has become secularised, because there is still recognition that there is more to existence than purely the secular and the material. Individuals seem to have an awareness of a presence greater than or beyond themselves. This awareness may indeed be heightened after such catastrophic events as those of September 11th 2001, when people's awareness of the fragility of life was brought to the fore (Wright, 2002).

Implications of this attitudinal shift from formal religious practice may account for the moves in nursing to establish a definition of spirituality that is all embracing: a definition that may reflect a modernist or postmodern meaning, or as Carr (2001, p. 21) would say a 'contemporary non-theistic spirituality', that seeks to underline the relevance of the concept to all individuals (Stoll, 1989; Murray and Zentner, 1989; Males and Boswell, 1990; Reed, 1992; Tanyi, 2002). Paradoxically the effects of such attempts to establish universality have created a 'secular form of spirituality' that is extremely subjective and diverse. The resulting subjectivity and diversity does not clarify relevance to nursing practice, but brings further confusion. Furthermore, the philosophical credibility of emerging definitions is questionable, indicating that there is a need to explore in more detail their universal application before a secular version of spirituality is cast in tablets of stone.

Definitions of spirituality

The review of the literature suggests there are numerous definitions of spirituality: some anecdotal, based on case scenarios (McSherry, 1996); others rhetorical and analytical in that they generate more questions than provide answers (Dyson *et al.*, 1997; McSherry and Draper, 1998; Golberg, 1998). By analysing some of the commonly used definitions (Table 2.1) one can gain a sense of the drive in health care to establish an authoritative (Narayanasamy, 2001), almost eclectic definition (Cobb, 2001).

The selection of definitions presented suggests that spirituality can be defined and interpreted differently as many of the definitions have several layers of meaning or defining characteristics. Reed (1992) views spirituality as interconnectedness, within the individual, the environment, and with a transcendent being. Alternatively, Murray and Zentner (1989) adopt a universal view implying that spirituality is to be found in all people both 'good and bad'. Males and Boswell (1990) outline the mysterious, mystical component, emphasising that a functioning intellect is not a prerequisite to spirituality. Tanyi (2002), seeking to offer clarification of spirituality, provides a definition that is existentially based. From this brief analysis it is understandable why the concept is subjective and confusing, because it can mean different things depending upon individual interpretation and preference.

Emerging taxonomy

This review suggests that the word 'spirituality' could be described as a 'cocktail' because it contains a mixture of components of varying strengths and flavours. This is evident in the work of Narayanasamy (1991, p. 3; 2001, p. 3) who provides a litany of possible variables that may be associated with the term. However, in the second edition of Narayanasamy's (2001) work the notion of a God does not feature in the revised list. Even religion is referred to in the negative form 'something not necessarily religious'. This prominent writer on spirituality within nursing seems to be unconsciously removing the theistic and religious components, signalling (and to some degree endorsing and reinforcing) the disassociation from religion to a more secular and plural-

Table 2.1 Definitions of spirituality in health care spanning the last two decades.

Author(s)	Definition
Stoll (1989, p. 6)	'Spirituality is my being; my inner person. It is who I am – unique and alive. It is me expressed through my body, my thinking, my feelings, my judgments, and my creativity. My spirituality motivates me to choose meaningful relationships and pursuits. Through my spirituality I give and receive love; I respond to and appreciate God, other people, a sunset, a symphony, and spring. I am driven forward, sometimes because of pain, sometimes in spite of pain. Spirituality allows me to reflect on myself. I am a person because of my spirituality-motivated and enabled to value, to worship, and to communicate with the holy, the transcendent.'
Murray and Zentner (1989, p. 259)	'A quality that goes beyond religious affiliation, that strives for inspirations, reverence, awe, meaning and purpose, even in those who do not believe in any good. The spiritual dimension tries to be in harmony with the universe, and strives for answers about the infinite, and comes into focus when the person faces emotional stress, physical illness or death.'
Males and Boswell (1990, p. 35)	'It is not easy to define spirituality since it concerns the way in which men and women may understand their existence and the action which comes from an understanding; the knowledge of things both within an individual and of the existence and importance of things beyond him or her. 'It is important to point out this knowledge is not the grasp of intellectual facts but rather a reverence for mysteries of life which no-one can fully understand. It is not, therefore, something which can be regarded as being unattainable for people with learning difficulties.'
Reed (1992, p. 350)	'Specifically spirituality refers to the propensity to make meaning through a sense relatedness to dimensions that transcend the self in such a way that empowers and does not devalue the individual. This relatedness may be experienced intrapersonally (as a connectedness within oneself), interpersonally (in the context of others and the natural environment) and transpersonally (referring to a sense of relatedness to the unseen, God, or power greater than the self and ordinary source).'
Tanyi (2002, p. 506)	'Spirituality is a personal search for meaning and purpose in life, which may or may not be related to religion. It entails connection to self-chosen and or religious beliefs, values and practices that give meaning to life, thereby inspiring and motivating individuals to achieve their optimal being. This connection brings faith, hope, peace, and empowerment. The results are joy, forgiveness of oneself and others, awareness and acceptance of hardship and mortality, a heightened sense of physical and emotional well-being, and the ability to transcend beyond the infirmities of existence.'

istic approach. Therefore, conceptually it appears there are several underlying subjective descriptors, or layers, that can be identified within most definitions of spirituality.

It is argued that the descriptors that can be identified within the definitions range from the religious to the existential and the mystical (Murray and Zentner, 1989; Males and Boswell, 1990; Reed, 1992). The descriptors can be arranged into a '*spiritual taxonomy*' which may account for the diversity and subjectivity surrounding the word. A detailed inspection of the taxonomy suggests that each descriptor could be explained by many of the different branches of philosophy, since the concept embraces numerous philosophical arguments, such as cosmology, philosophy of religion, philosophy of mind and body, philosophy of language and philosophy of science. Before explaining the taxonomy there is a need to briefly examine some of the philosophical positions.

A synopsis of the philosophical positions

This section presents a synopsis of the philosophical positions (empiricist, logical positivist, phenomenological and existential), outlining how these positions may view the existence of such a subjective concept as spirituality.

The empiricist position

Thompson (1995) describes how empiricists argue that all knowledge about the world in which individuals exist is acquired through the senses: sight, hearing, touch, smell and taste. All information about the external world is processed through these complex mechanisms. Conclusions are reached about events or things existing in the external world as a result of the observation and subsequent interpretation of the incoming stimuli being processed. This approach implies that individuals have a functioning neurological and cognitive system so that information in the form of stimuli can be processed as it passes through the senses into the brain as impulses. In the external, physical and material realms, individuals are dealing with absolute tangible objects, which exist independently and not relative to anything else.

If an individual has a condition affecting the function of one or more of the senses, then an object in the material physical world would still exist despite the problem with the senses. An example of this would be a blind man walking along the Humber Estuary towards the Humber Bridge. As the man is blind, the Humber Estuary and the Humber Bridge still exist, but are not interpreted by the man's eyes. It is not that the Humber Estuary and the Humber Bridge cease to exist. This example presents an empiricist and materialist philosophy of being.

This empiricist and materialist philosophy of being has difficulty when applied to the concept of spirituality. Empiricists and materialists may argue that all individuals are material beings and their spirituality is formed through the senses. This approach is congruent with the notion of historical religious influences, where the state through the senses directs individuals in that culture or society. Likewise, a child learns about its external and inner world through the vehicle of the senses, and interpretation is reinforced by parental nurturing and chastisement. An illustration may be that the child is rebuked when trying to touch a hot object or the child is encouraged by its parents to say its night-time prayers because God is listening. In these illustrations the parents are providing the child with 'dos' and 'don'ts' in relation to the material and the spiritual aspects of being through the use of the sense and cognitive functioning.

If an individual's spirituality is solely developed through their senses and dependent upon cognitive functioning, then 'spirituality' as a concept as used within nursing may be meaningless. This reductionist view fails to recognise the importance of other non-physical realities, such as thoughts, emotions and feelings, which do not sit comfortably in a rigid empirical position.

Logical positivists

Logical positivists may argue that the definitions of spirituality being used within nursing are not tautologies – true by definition – nor can these definitions be empirically verified. The logical progression would be a total rejection of the word 'spirituality', since its metaphysical nature means that it is not worthy of investigation or explanation. This view is very restrictive and does not place any value or credence upon an individual's expression of his or her beliefs, values and aspects of living which cannot be verified through a rigid empiricism. Therefore, while acknowledging the logical positivist position, it does not mean that the word 'spirituality' is totally void or beyond the realms of analysis.

Limitations

The logical positivist argument does not acknowledge the use of language and the subsequent communication and interaction that may result in the social construction of such concepts as spirituality. The empiricists' and logical positivists' arguments for the development of spirituality fail to take into account any form of interaction or communication that may occur between individuals. The blind man walking along the Humber Estuary may not be able to see the bridge physically, but may make a mental image or visualisation from the descriptions communicated to him by a friend. The ability and power of language to generate meaning and visualisation in the absence of one of the senses cannot be underestimated. Walker *et al.* (1999) have demonstrated the power of relaxation combined with guided imagery (visualising host defences destroying tumour cells) in enhancing the quality of life and the host's immune response in women suffering from breast cancer, although the clinical significance of this is not yet clear.

This emerging body of evidence is a useful illustration that reinforces the importance of the power of language, communicated between individuals or societies to convey meaning. It also brings into question the suitability of a strict empiricist approach in learning about the world. This is because thoughts, feelings and beliefs may not only be acquired through an individual's senses. The illustration offered demonstrates how the ears can compensate for the eyes, but through interaction with a variety of people and situations individuals live and gain experience of the world in which they live.

Other philosophical positions therefore need to be considered that may better explain the acquisition and formation of the concept of spirituality. If one gives further consideration to the strict empiricist approach, are there issues surrounding the ability of individuals to rationally question and formulate their own knowledge and understanding about a subject or event? Initially a child is rebuked for wanting to touch a hot object. After the experience the child learns or associates the word 'hot' with parental displeasure, and after several rebukes knows not to touch the object in question. As the child develops and experiences more of life, words such as 'hot' take on a new meaning. The child understands that its parents, when using the word 'hot', were protecting it from danger. The child learns to understand the language. This illustration demonstrates that individuals learn about life, deriving subsequent meaning by experiencing events and situations.

The manner in which individuals learn about their world and more specifically 'spirituality' strikes at the very essence of concepts and knowledge, necessitating the need to briefly explore Wittgenstein's (1953) view on the nature of concepts and knowledge. Wittgenstein (1953, p. 4) describes the purpose behind the 'ostensive teaching of words' which is necessary 'to establish an association between the word and the thing'. It would appear that this principle may apply to the area of spirituality. Through education and academic debate, nursing has now been primed to understand the word 'spirituality'. The net effect is that we now have sectors of the population who have dissimilar associations, imaginations and understanding of the word.

Phenomenology and existentialism

The phenomenological and existentialist branches of philosophy might best explain the concept of spirituality. Talbot (1995) outlines how phenomenology owes its origins to the philosopher Husserl (1859–1938) and others. The aim of this approach is to understand the basic structure of phenomena as perceived and experienced by individuals. This can be achieved by analysing verbal interpretations. Phenomenology seeks to establish a definition or meaning of phenomena as lived and experienced by an individual. Current definitions of spirituality embrace this perspective, since they imply that spirituality is unique and individually determined since everyone is exposed to different life experiences. This approach, unlike a rigid empiricism, places credence upon the internal world of beliefs, values and emotions that are deemed relevant to spirituality (Thompson, 1995).

Thompson (1995) describes how existential philosophy (Heidegger (1889–1976) and Sartre (1905–1980)) is concerned with issues surrounding meaning and purpose in life, essentially how individuals relate and interact with their world. Like phenomenology, this branch emphasises that individuals are not inanimate objects detached from the world but actively engaged in it. Existential philosophy is not reductionist (separating the mind and body), but integrational, since it supports the assumption that the body works as a whole. The senses do not act independently of the mind.

Frankl (1987, p. 74), the founder of a school of existential psychotherapy, recalling events in the Second World War concentration camps, reinforces the importance of physical mental and spiritual integration:

> The prisoner who had lost faith in the future – his future – was doomed. With his loss of belief in the future, he also lost his spiritual hold; he let himself decline and become subject to mental and physical decay.

Individuals need to find meaning and purpose, even in the most atrocious of situations. An inability to find meaning can have the direst consequences. An example of the need to find meaning in illness is provided by Simsen (1985), who used an existential approach in her research to establish how patients coped with illness and hospitalisation.

No branch of philosophy is without its sceptics and criticisms. Major limitations of the phenomenological and existentialist branches are that, whilst trying to identify the meaning of a phenomenon for the individual, they may not be able to formulate universals. These branches are concerned with the individual's lived experience and engagement in life. They reinforce and support the argument that abstract concepts such as spirituality may not be universally defined. Phenomenology and existentialist branches are beneficial in identifying individually determined descriptors which might explain a phenomenon such as spirituality.

Theory versus concept

It could be argued that perhaps one of the most effective ways of managing the exploration of any concept is to undertake a concept analysis (Walker and Avant, 1983). This type of approach to conceptual development was firstly decided against as this type of exercise has been undertaken by other authors (Cawley, 1997; Golberg, 1998). Secondly, the area of focus was not so much concerned with constructing or developing insight into the defining characteristics and properties associated with spirituality. Rather, the purpose of this review was to investigate the coherence of a particular area (theory) as presented within nursing literature. Paley (1996, p. 577) writes:

> Theories are word-structures, and the place assigned to any word within the structure is that which gives the word its meaning.

This notion of theories 'first', rather than concepts is important and may assist in the clarification of 'spirituality'. Paley's position is that the meaning of any term is made specific and arguably clearer when it forms part of a theory. This argument can be applied to 'spirituality'. Rather than focusing on concept clarification that is cyclical and to some degree fragmenting, nursing (and indeed health care) needs to recognise that individuals, rather than constructing 'concepts', have already created their own personal theory or theories of spirituality. This shift in emphasis may enable nursing to engage with diversity and difference, signalling a shift away from the desire to create an 'all singing and all dancing' authoritative definition.

The taxonomy explained

Having looked at some of the philosophical arguments that may be associated with the concept of spirituality there is now a need to explain in more detail the emerging taxonomy (Table 2.2).

The descriptors incorporated in the taxonomy are not rigid or fixed. The order in which they appear is dynamic in that they are individually determined and develop across a life span, according to an individual's worldview or reli-

Table 2.2 A taxonomy of spirituality.

Descriptors							
Theistic	**Religious**	**Language**	**Cultural, political, social ideologies**	**Phenomenological**	**Existential**	**Quality of life**	**Mystical**
Belief in a supreme being, cosmological arguments, not necessarily a 'God' but deity	Affiliation – belief in a God, undertaking certain religious practices, customs and rituals	Individuals may use certain language when defining spirituality, such as inner strength, inner peace	An individual may subscribe to a particular political position or social ideology that influences and governs their attitudes and behaviours. dependent upon world faith – religious tenets	One learns about life by living and learning from a variety of situations and experiences both positive and negative	A semantic philosophy of life and being, finding meaning, purpose and fulfilment in all of life's events	Although quality of life is not explicit in definitions, it is implicit	Relationship between the transcendent, interpersonal, transpersonal, life after death

LEFT . . . . RIGHT

Consideration

- The order or sequencing of the descriptors present in the taxonomy is individually determined depending upon one's beliefs, values and life experience or worldview.
- The taxonomy is restrictive in that it implies the ability to intellectualise supporting the position that such definitions are exclusive and restrictive.
- The taxonomy implies that an individual's worldview will determine his or her definition of spirituality.
- The descriptors listed in the taxonomy are not exhaustive because they may well be infinite.
- The taxonomy suggests two forms of spirituality: the 'old' and the 'postmodern'. The old = religious and theist while the 'the postmodern' = Phenomenological and existentially focused.

Reflective questions

- Look at the taxonomy and ask yourself what factors have shaped your understanding of spirituality?
- Where would you locate your spirituality on the taxonomy?

gious belief. Contemporary definitions imply that the descriptors may change as a direct result of illness or emotional stress (Murray and Zentner, 1989). However, problems arise with the universal application of the descriptors because some of the ones being used may not be readily recognised or understood by all people, as previously suggested.

Individually tailored tartan

The taxonomy suggests that there are no constant elements: threads that are common to every individual in how they may perceive or define spirituality. The threads are continually in a state of flux with no consistency in the tapestry or weave that they create. The idea that we all weave our own pattern or fabric is apparent. In the Scottish Highlands an individual could be distinguished or identified as belonging to a particular clan by the tartan worn. This cannot be said of spirituality, since the tartan woven is unique and specific to the individual and to some extent the society in which he or she lives or worldview that he or she shares. This means that spirituality will be uniquely determined by the individual, but there may be some commonalities between individuals or groups. The fact that we all create our own definition of spirituality brings into question 'universality' and the general application and usage of the term.

Consideration surrounding the development of the taxonomy

Although this review of the literature and definitions of spirituality could be considered extensive, it does not include all of the definitions of spirituality identified due to the sheer volume and apparent repetition of themes. The taxonomy presented captures and reflects the major themes surrounding the language of spirituality as presented within nursing and health care definitions (see Table 2.1). With this point in mind deliberation must be given to the representativeness and relevance of the definitions for other disciplines for example theology, religious and pastoral studies. Therefore this taxonomy is perhaps not as comprehensive as other taxonomies that have been used to explore concepts within nursing (for example Morse *et al.*, 1990). However, it is a start to help to resolve some of the persistent debates surrounding the concept and language of spirituality.

Variation in meaning

Using abstract terms

The construction of the taxonomy not only highlights the 'cocktail' nature of spirituality but also reinforces that the word is associated with a variety of meanings. The problem associated with the different meanings of particular words is not just specific to the area of 'spirituality'. Cash (1990, p. 250), for example, outlines potential problems with the use of abstract terms such as 'nursing', when discussing the concept of universals, by drawing on the notion of family resemblance. More recently the notion of 'caring' has come under scrutiny, with individuals having very definite views as to whether we can categorically say what caring is (Paley, 2002a) and whether or not caring can be defined by its component parts (Deary *et al.*, 2002).

The evidence presented suggests that spirituality is another abstract term. There are no universals, since the word 'spirituality', as discussed, represents and means distinct things to *all* individuals depending upon their worldview. This means that there is no single common denominator in the term that can be applied universally. Spirituality is associated with many descriptors, making the formulation of a common or universal 'constant' definition theoretically impossible. The 'common denominator' may vary between individuals, cultures and societies. The result is the fabrication of multiple definitions of spirituality each trying to incorporate the length, breadth and depth of the taxonomic diversity or, as stated earlier, taking an eclectic approach (Cobb, 2001). The preoccupation with devising such inclusive definitions means that there is a loss of philosophical credibility in meaning and language, since it can be seen that there is nothing that is common across all instances of the use of the term spirituality (Cash, 1990).

The 'old' and 'new' forms of spirituality

Focusing upon the classes in the taxonomy indicates that there may be two main forms of spirituality. Firstly, there is the historical or 'old' traditional form, which is based on religious and theocentric descriptors. This form of spirituality is tangible and in a sense justifiable because such indicators as belief in a God or attendance at formal religious activity can provide a constant explanation. It is suggested that nurses can attend more easily to an individual's spiritual need(s) stemming from a religious belief because the intervention required can often be readily recognised and the outcome, to a certain degree, quantifiable. This approach would fit with Bradshaw's (1994) and Pattison's (2001) views because the word derives its meaning from a specific association and context.

The second type of spirituality emerging has been classified as the new 'postmodern form'. This type is very subjective, reflecting society's and the individual's preoccupation with the material, sectarianised aspects of life. This form of spirituality contains an infinite number of descriptors that may be phenomenologically and existentially determined such as meaning and purpose in life, creativity, and relationships. They may also reflect the different values, beliefs and attitudes that guide and shape individuals from some world faiths that are sometimes not acknowledged in the Judeo-Christian approach espoused in health care. Nurses in practice may experience difficulty in attending to patients whose spiritual needs arise out of such a definition because they may be subjective, making them hard to address.

Practice illustrations

A health care worker who is a practising Christian may relate to many of the descriptors in the taxonomy, addressing the theistic and religious, and accommodating their belief in Jesus Christ. However, a patient who does not believe in any God but derives meaning, purpose and fulfilment in life through his or her work and relationships with others may adopt a more existentialist view; for example, a secular humanist (Harrison and Burnard, 1993). These two perspectives illustrate that individuals may identify with one or all of the descriptors within the taxonomy, depending upon their own moral worldview. The illustration suggests that what changes is the sequencing and priority of the descriptors from one individual to the next. Individuals will create and identify with those layers of meaning that suit their interpretation and understanding of spirituality, whether this be religiously focused or existential or even a combination of all descriptors. The taxonomy highlights the subjective and personal nature of spirituality. Relating this back to Markham's (1998) concern for individuals from non-Christian traditions, they might not be able to identify with any of the descriptors presented in this taxonomy reflecting the definitions of spirituality used in nursing, thereby bringing into question the notion of universality.

It may be that the two different forms of spirituality are now in dispute. In relation to the taxonomy the 'old' form is located to the left of the axis whilst the 'new modern' form is located to the extreme right. There is also an argument that many individuals would fall in the middle of the continuum, indicating a third form of spirituality, which is not necessarily fundamental or extreme. The third approach may support McSherry's (1997) findings that, despite nurses not practising or having a formal religious belief, they still believe that spirituality is concerned with the transcendent. Irrespective of which form of spirituality one subscribes to, the diversity or different layers of meaning indicate that it may be hard to establish connotational meaning.

Connotational meaning

When thinking of the connotational meaning of a particular word one is usually alluding to its precise dictionary definition (Vivian, 1968). This point is worth considering, since the word 'spirituality' is usually not defined (Oxford Paperback Dictionary, 1983) but used as an adverb (describing word) for spiritual matters. Therefore the word 'spirituality' does not have its own connotational meaning. This means that one must first look to the words 'spirit' or 'spiritual' for a set of defining characteristics. 'Spiritual' (Oxford Paperback Dictionary, 1983, p. 646) means 'of the human spirit or soul, not physical or worldly, of the church or religion'.

These defining characteristics support the taxonomy that has been presented, reflecting an historical or 'old' form of spirituality. The defining characteristics do not incorporate or reflect the sectarianized contemporary understanding of spirituality. Vivian (1968, p. 9) presents a possible explanation for this:

> Because all things possess a very large, if not infinite, number of features, it is not always easy to decide which of them are defining and which are accompanying (and goes on to say). There are inevitably some characteristics which are not obviously one or the other. Failure to distinguish between them however, can often lead to foolish disagreements.

This quotation highlights the difficulties in establishing a universal definition of spirituality. How does one determine or distinguish between defining characteristics (those essential to a definition) and what are accompanying characteristics, which can apply to a word but are not essential for definition. The taxonomy suggests that there could be a litany of items that could be either defining or accompanying which may vary between an individual's and a society's worldview. The list of both defining and accompanying characteristics could be infinite. It is this inability to define spirituality precisely that has led to disagreement and confusion. The word has become ambiguous in that it could be said not to have any denotational meaning or value.

Denotational meaning

The denotational meaning of a word is the class or group to which it refers. Vivian (1968) using the word 'Unicorn', illustrates how some words used in our language have connotational meaning (they can be described), but possess no denotational meaning because the groups denoted do not or have never existed. Spirituality, like the mystical Unicorn, is another such word. We have multiple descriptors, or layers of meaning, which are individually determined, but no specific group to which they can be applied unless viewed from affiliation to a religious belief. The confusion and misconceptions surrounding spirituality originate because individuals and groups promote and advocate their own meaning of spirituality that has a different set of connotations and denotations – thus supporting Markham's (1998) argument of relevance to individuals of different world faiths. If issues surrounding definition are not sensitively challenged the result may be the formation of negative attitudes or scepticism of the word. This dissatisfaction with the word seems to be emerging within health care.

Emotive powers

There are probably many nurses, when asking patients about their spiritual beliefs, who are told 'I don't go in for any of that religious stuff'. These emotive powers still surround the word 'spirituality'. The move towards a more secular, sectarianised and pluralistic view of spirituality or adoption of the 'new' form means that many of the apprehensions, misconceptions and fears previously associated with the word are being challenged. This is certainly evident within Anglo-American cultures and health care.

Emotive powers can be destructive, inhibiting and disabling for individuals and societies, preventing personal growth and achievement. The emotive powers surrounding spirituality need to be sensitively and culturally challenged and perhaps managed through education and practice (Harrison and Burnard, 1993; Ross, 1996; Bradshaw, 1997; McSherry and Draper, 1998).

Universality

It has been suggested that current definitions of spirituality, while attempting to be all-embracing, are not universal. If one strips away the descriptors, or layers of meaning, then implicit within many contemporary definitions is the notion of a functioning intellect – the ability to reason. For a more detailed account of this debate see McSherry (2001). Close scrutiny of the definitions offered (see Table 2.1) finds a number of descriptors used. Murray and Zentner (1989, p. 259) use the word 'strives', while Reed (1992, p. 350) uses the phrase 'propensity to make meaning'. These authors suggest that the ability to reason, the notion of competence, is an essential ingredient in developing one's spirituality. Intellect within this debate means the ability to use reasoning to appraise critically situations or events in order to gain a deeper insight and understanding. If these assumptions are correct then it would appear that contemporary definitions are not universal because they appear to exclude a large number of individuals who have neurological or cognitive impairment, being deprived of the ability to intellectualise or reason. The logical question that follows is, 'Do such individuals have the capacity to develop or possess spirituality?'

If a purely empiricist argument was applied then the propensity of such individuals to develop their own spirituality would be restricted. Again, this position may best be illustrated by an example from practice. What happens when someone who has developed their own unique spirituality suffers a stroke or develops a degenerative disorder like dementia that alters their ability to reason? Do such individuals no longer possess spirituality?

This illustration highlights the lack of universality within contemporary definitions because they do not apply to all groups of individuals either on the bases of religious belief or functioning intellect. Males and Boswell's (1990) definition of spirituality for individuals with learning difficulties suggests an urgent need for nursing to look beyond the written word to the connotations implicit within contemporary definitions. If there is to be a 'common language' or 'understanding' associated with spirituality in health care then attention must be paid to the literal and, more importantly, the hidden meaning of the word.

Implications for practice and education

The ambiguity and misconceptions that still surround the meaning of spirituality may prevent the application of the concept within practice and education. If there is confusion around the literal and hidden meanings of the word, in that it means different things to individuals from diverse faiths, then this will have implications for nurses in the course of their clinical practice. The taxonomy outlined suggests that there may be 'diverse spiritual taxonomies', all with the potential for conflict between the different descriptors, or layers of meaning. For example, a nurse whose spirituality is defined by association with descriptors on the left of the taxonomy caring for a patient whose spirituality is defined by association with descriptors on the right may come into conflict. The patient may view the nurse as a threat in that they fear the potential for persuasion or proselytising. The same threats may operate in reverse. Another concern stemming from Markham's (1998) argument is if a patient with a strong religious belief (not of the Judeo-Christian tradition) requires health care then they might not be able to identify with the terminology or definitions of spirituality being presented.

Interestingly, there have been two documented cases of nurses being brought before the UKCC (now the Nursing and Midwifery Councils' Professional Conduct Department) associated with this aspect of care (Cobb, 2001b; Castledine, 2005).

The situations described may be prevented or diffused if nurses have sufficient self-awareness surrounding their own spirituality and an insight into the fact that not all individuals will share the same understanding of the word. Having awareness of the potential for diverse spiritual taxonomies will help alert nurses to the need for caution and sensitivity when addressing spiritual or religious matters.

Bradshaw (1997) suggests that spirituality is something that cannot be taught in a formal didactic sense – since spirituality or spiritual awareness is developed through experience and exposure to situations across the life span, whilst McSherry and Draper (1998) believe that the spiritual dimension should be formally integrated within nursing curricula – implying that spirituality and spiritual care should be addressed both theoretically and practically.

The more religiously focused may suggest that the hospital chaplain or different religious leaders should undertake this educative role, while the existentialist or humanist may argue that spirituality is so broad that it comes into all domains of nurse education, and therefore any competent lecturer should be able to address the concept. From the information presented it would appear that we cannot have 'real' action, either clinically or educationally, unless there is a compromise and an understanding (a consensus) that it is acceptable to have different meanings of the word 'spirituality'.

A way forward

A way forward in the 'language of spirituality' debate is not to focus upon restrictive arguments of definition, but through qualitative research, grounded theory, ethnography, and phenomenology examine the reciprocal interactions of individuals, patients, practitioners, and diverse cultures, generating a deeper insight into how people 'perhaps' with differing worldviews understand the word. This may move the debates surrounding spirituality from a 'cognitive' and 'academic' process to one that embraces social practice. By generating such insights the meaning of spirituality may become more focused and embodied in practice, and a language of spirituality may be developed that is relevant at all levels – conceptual, clinical and educational – accommodating and reflecting diversity. At present we need to accept that there are diverse spiritual taxonomies which individuals may identify with and adopt.

Key points

- It would appear that there is no such thing as a universal definition of spirituality and the theoretical probability of creating one is virtually impossible.
- Historically the word derived meaning, connotational and denotational, from its association with religion and theistic beliefs - 'old' form. However, the legacy and emotive powers surrounding the word still remain.
- Presently, there is a conscious move to fashion a definition of spirituality that is modern, reflecting secular, material and sectarianized ideas - 'post modern' form of a Christian version of spirituality (Markham, 1998).
- In society it appears that there is a deliberate shift to remove the restrictive components of spirituality such as the religious and the theistic. However, if attempts to do this were successful some authors (Bradshaw, 1994; Pattison, 2001) would argue 'what are we left with?' The result could be a word void of any real meaning or relevance so broad and universal that it becomes meaningless.
- Individuals fashion and manufacture their own unique definition of spirituality. The taxonomy illustrates that such definitions may embrace the religious or the sectarian descriptors, layers of meaning, contained within contemporary definitions. It may be that the language used means that current attempts to establish a theoretically universal definition within nursing are misguided.

Part II: Theoretical sensitivity: exploring key issues

Introduction

Part I explored some of the conceptual issues associated with the language of spirituality. Part II, rather than focusing upon conceptualisation, explores four primary issues, identifiable within the nursing and health care literature, associated with the emergence of spirituality. In short, these are the notion of Judeo-Christian bias, 'holism', moral relativism and managerialism. These areas were considered significant and pivotal to the arguments in existing literature. Therefore, because of their primary and significant nature they provided a framework or guide for this grounded theory study investigating the meaning of spirituality.

Reflective question

- Why do you think the concept of spirituality become fashionable within health care?

First, the section revisits the argument that attempts at defining the word 'spirituality' as used within nursing reflect a secularised version of 'Christian spirituality', the descriptors of which may not be applicable or understood by all people, especially some of the world faiths. Secondly, it is argued that interest in the spiritual dimension has originated out of unrest and discontent with the scientific reductionist model which seems to prevail within health care. It would seem that this discontentment has witnessed a refocusing upon a holistic approach to individuals. However, this debate warrants closer inspection if the position of spirituality within it is to be understood. Thirdly, some contemporary research alludes to the fact that the provision of spiritual care is morally relative: that is, spiritual care may only be provided if the nurse shares a similar moral position to that of the patient. Fourthly, it is suggested that the rediscovery of the spiritual dimension is an attempt by the nursing profession to challenge the status quo or shed the constraints imposed on them by a paternalistic, managerial system which seems to control all aspect of care delivery.

Purpose of Part II literature review

The purpose of this part of the literature review was to identify and explore some of the contemporary debates and concerns being generated within the health care literature surrounding the concept of spirituality and the provision of spiritual care. The rationale for examining these concerns was to highlight the issues to be investigated, setting the parameters and describing possible relationships that exist. By focusing upon these key issues it would allow several seemingly discrete areas of theoretical and conceptual debate to be pulled together. This activity assisted in raising my awareness so that theoretical sensitisation (a process whereby the researcher develops an 'awareness' for the area to be investigated) could occur.

This part of the literature review offers my perspective and interpretation of how several phenomena may be influencing and shaping the manner in which 'spirituality' is defined and perceived within health care. The literature review does not present a formal substantive theory for testing but a loosely structured set of assumptions and philosophical views that I hold. However, these assumptions and philosophical views have originated from, and been constructed within, the confines of existing literature reinforcing my attempts at becoming 'theoretically sensitised' with contemporary debates and developments surrounding 'spirituality'. The key issues to be explored throughout this thesis are structured around the following set of assumptions or ideas (Table 2.3)

Placing these assumptions within the context of existing literature

It would seem that there is a drive in health care (nursing) to create a definition of spirituality that is universal or all-inclusive (McSherry and Draper, 1998). This is reflected in the generalised and pluralistic language of contemporary definitions (Murray and Zentner, 1989; Males and Boswell, 1990; Reed, 1991). The language used in the construction of these definitions is very general, vague and secular in the sense that it tries to avoid over-emphasising the religious component, highlighting issues of transcendence and existentialism. This activity could be interpreted as a subconscious act to try to divorce – indeed remove – the religious element from spirituality. The impact of this could be far-reaching for chaplains, indeed for all whose spirituality is expressed and shaped through religious belief and affiliation.

Table 2.3 Identifiable issues.

Issue 1
Is there a relationship between the provision of spiritual care and individuals from different world faiths? There is a growing unease with the definitions of spirituality used in health care. The argument is that definitions being formulated reflect a secular version of Judeo-Christian spirituality – not taking into account the variants that exist between individuals from different world faiths. The hidden danger is that such individuals may not be able to identify or understand the form of spirituality being instituted or advocated.
Issue 2
Why has interest in the spiritual dimension gained such popularity within contemporary health care? Possible explanations for this might originate from the notion of holism and dissatisfaction with the scientific-reductionist models of health care.
Issue 3
Is the provision of spiritual care morally relative; that is, dependent upon the nurse's own moral position or understanding of the concept? Emerging research indicates that spiritual care is more likely to be provided by nurses who possess insight into their own spirituality.
Issue 4
Is the rediscovery of the spiritual dimension of nursing a move by nurses to challenge the status quo or shed the constraints imposed on them by a managerial system that seeks to control? It might be that interest in the spiritual dimension is seen as a chance to regain some charge over aspects of care that are mysterious – beyond the realms of audit and measurement – thereby challenging modern day reforms that seek to quantify care.

However, closer analysis of such definitions suggests that these moves towards a universal or authoritative definition may be misguided, inaccurate and importantly contradictory in the sense that instead of being universal they distinguish features that may not be recognised or appropriate for some groups of people (McSherry, 2000). Furthermore, the definitions intimate certain prerequisites that may be necessary for the formation and development of spirituality and spiritual awareness, the need to be introspective, and the need for a 'functioning' intellect.

Issue 1 – Potential danger: a Christian understanding of spirituality

Markham (1998, p. 74) alerts the health care professions to a potential danger, because current definitions of spirituality being constructed may be perceived as a secular form of a 'Christian understanding of spirituality'. This means that some members from the diverse world faiths may not be able to identify with emerging definitions because of inharmonious perceptions and understanding of the word. Markham (1998) goes on to suggest that there are three identifiable components or themes present within nursing and health care definitions of spirituality of Anglo-American origin (Table 2.4).

Markham (1998, p. 74) indicates that these three components might have significant meaning for individuals from Judeo-Christian traditions who are familiar with the descriptions used:

> Christians would view this as a recognisable, albeit a minimal understanding of spirituality. So for a Christian, a person is not simply a body, but a mind (or spirit or soul) as well. Life has meaning because the Christian believes that we live in a universe intended by God. And our reason for existing is to worship the transcendent God who is the source of goodness, love and beauty. Therefore a Christian will recognize the descriptions of 'spirituality' despite the generalized language.

The quotation raises several important considerations when addressing the concept of spirituality within nursing from theoretical, clinical and educational perspectives. Theoretically the implications of fostering and perpetuating what appear to be universal, broad, secular definitions of spirituality might have the effect of alienating individuals from different world faiths who may not be able to identify with the terminology and descriptions used.

Evidence derived from two primary sources reinforces that health care and nursing have unknowingly perpetuated a definition of spirituality that is

Table 2.4 Markham's Descriptors – indicating a secular form of Christian spirituality.

- There is a conscious effort to move away from the reductionist or scientific–medical model, which seeks to fragment or compartmentalise individuals.
- Spirituality is associated with an existential philosophy concerning the need to invest life with meaning, purpose and fulfilment.
- There is an acknowledgement of the transcendent – a general awareness of something greater or beyond the individual.

potentially 'Judeo-Christian' biased. First there is a growing realisation and acknowledgment by researchers in spirituality that their study sample was not representative in that the majority of participants identified with Western religions (Hungelmann *et al.*, 1985; Emblen and Halstead, 1993; Cavendish *et al.*, 2000; Taylor *et al.*, 2003). This means that any insights gained and subsequent theory developed by default must reflect a Judeo-Christian perspective, thereby perpetuating a bias.

Secondly, writers from some of the Eastern religious traditions are now engaging with the debates and drawing attention to the potential bias (Rassool, 2000; Mayet, 2001). Further, there is a growing amount of publication from a broad range of religious, ethnic, cultural traditions being written on the subject (Narayanasamy and Owens, 2001; Chiu, 2001; Shirahama and Inoue, 2001). Generating this cultural and religious dialogue must go some way towards challenging the potential bias that has existed.

Clinically, HCPs may not be aware of the religious and cultural needs of individuals from differing world faiths and that the application of a 'one size fits all' approach to individuals from diverse religious and ethnic groups may be perceived as cultural ignorance and offensive. As Gilliat-Ray (2001, p. 136) recognises, these populations of people are not 'monolithic' because they possess internal diversity in terms of language, ethnicity, race and gender. Therefore the teaching of spirituality will need to take into account this diversity and the impact it may have upon the interpretation of the word spirituality. Perhaps in the past this level of awareness was not so developed. However, before blaming nursing for being bigoted, there is a need to consider the religious traditions that have influenced Western societies and thought. It may be that the manner in which 'spirituality' is being developed and articulated within nursing reflects historical norms, patterns and religious traditions.

Religious traditions

Perhaps one of the most detailed accounts outlining the nature of religious tradition and influences on society is offered by Ninian Smart in *The Religious Experience of Mankind* (1969, p. 11). Smart writes:

> To understand human history and human life it is necessary to understand religion, and in the contemporary world one must understand other nations' ideologies and faith in order to grasp the meaning of life as seen from perspectives often very different from our own.

Smart indicates that consideration needs to be given to the religions present within any culture because their ideologies, doctrines and traditions may have influenced how that particular society has evolved. Therefore, while Markham

(1998) is correct to alert the nursing profession to the limitations within emerging definitions of spirituality, consideration must also be given to religious influences that may have guided and shaped individuals' perceptions of the term. It could be argued that historically the Western world has been primarily influenced by Christian thought and tradition, which has resulted in the construction and perpetuation of secular forms of Christian spirituality within nursing. Widerquist and Davidhizar (1994, p. 647) stress that historically nursing had its roots in the Christian concept of ministry, highlighting that there may not be a conscious attempt to alienate or discriminate against other world faiths but a subconscious reflection of how deeply Christian values, philosophies penetrate Western thought and traditions.

One approach to this question of religious bias may be to explore the antecedents of the National Health Service (NHS). At the time of its inception in 1948, the NHS was created to meet the needs of the 'indigenous population', who, one can assume rightly or wrongly were 'White' and from the Christian tradition. Evidence to support this premise can be found in the work of Olumide (1989) and Beckford and Gillat (1996), whose findings are endorsed by Lie (2001, p. 184) describing how each NHS hospital usually had a chapel, and appointments of clergy were primarily from the Church of England. This apparent display of cultural insensitivity was not intentional, but affirms Smart's (1969) argument that different religious dimensions permeate all echelons of human life and society, including the NHS.

The prevailing religion influencing British society in 1948 was possibly the Church of England and Christian philosophy. This assertion may account for the apparent Judeo-Christian bias in the NHS and the caring professions. Having stated this, the current trend to revise the composition and structure of chaplaincy provision (SEHD, 2002; DOH, 2003b) is a positive step to meet the diverse religious needs of people living within the UK. A summary of the major religions that may need to be represented in the NHS might reflect those identified in the 2001 census (Table 2.5), keeping in mind regional variations.

Contemporary health care – changing trends

Since the Second World War Britain can no longer be viewed as monocultural but multicultural. British society is now composed of individuals and communities from a diverse range of ethnic groups, resulting in a diversity of religious traditions. Evidence to support this cultural shift is found in the 2001 National Census Statistics, which provided a detailed exposition of the composition of the UK population (Office for National Statistics, 2002). The majority ethnic group is 'white' (91.7%) with the minority ethnic groups accounting for (7.9 %) of the total population. There is a slight increase in the percentage

Table 2.5 The UK population: by religion, April 2001.

	England and Wales	Scotland	Northern Ireland	UK	UK %
Christian	**37338486**	**3294545**	**1446386**	**42079417**	**71.6**
Roman Catholic	*	803732	678462	n/a	n/a
Other Christian	*	344562	102221	n/a	n/a
Church of Scotland	*	2146251	*	n/a	n/a
Presbyterian Church in Ireland	*	*	348742	n/a	n/a
Church of Ireland	*	*	257788	n/a	n/a
Methodist Church in Ireland	*	*	59173	n/a	n/a
Buddhist	**144453**	**6830**	**533**	**151816**	**0.3**
Hindu	**552421**	**5564**	**825**	**558810**	**1.0**
Jewish	**259927**	**6448**	**365**	**266740**	**0.5**
Muslim	**1546626**	**42557**	**1943**	**1591126**	**2.7**
Sikh	**329358**	**6572**	**219**	**336149**	**0.6**
Other religion	**150720**	**26974**	**1143**	**178837**	**0.3**
All religions	*40321991*	*3389490*	*1451414*	*45162895*	*76.8*
No religion	7709267	1394460	45909	n/a	15.5
Not stated	4010658	278061	187944	n/a	7.3
All no religion/not stated	*11719925*	*1672521*	*233853*	*13626299*	*23.2*
Base	*52041916*	*5062011*	*1685267*	*58789194*	*100*

Source: Census, April 2001, Office for National Statistics

of minority ethnic groups identified in 1991 census (6.0%). The 2001 census reveals that the three largest minority ethnic groups are Pakistani, Asian and African. These changing social trends must be taken into account when looking at health care provision and nursing. These statistics suggest that all HCPs will be providing services to individuals from minority ethnic groups, but obviously there will be regional variations. Statistics providing a breakdown and distribution of ethnic groups across the different regions in the UK are provided (Table 2.6).

The following commentary from the Office for National Statistics (2001) on the April 2001 Census provides a very useful analysis and demographic profile of the region in which this investigation was conducted:

Table 2.6 Distribution of ethnic groups across regions, April 2001 census.

		North East	North West	Yorkshire and the Humber	East Midlands	West Midlands	East	London	South East	South West	England	Wales	England and Wales	Scotland	Northern Ireland	UK Base = 100%
White	%	4.5	12	8.57	7.2	8.63	9	9.42	14	8.9	82.5	5.3	87.8	9.16	3.09	54153898
Mixed	%	1.8	9.2	6.65	6.37	10.8	9	33.4	13	5.5	95	2.6	97.6	1.89	0.49	677117
Indian	%	1	6.9	4.89	11.6	17	5	41.5	8.5	1.6	97.6	0.8	98.4	1.43	0.15	1053411
Pakistani	%	1.9	16	19.58	3.72	20.7	5	19.1	7.8	0.9	94.6	1.1	95.7	4.25	0.1	747285
Bangladeshi	%	2.2	9.2	4.36	2.45	11.1	7	54.4	5.4	1.7	97.3	1.9	99.2	0.7	0.1	283063
Other Asian	%	1.3	5.9	4.98	4.77	8.45	5	53.7	9.5	2	96	1.4	97.4	2.5	0.1	247664
Black Caribbean	%	0.2	3.6	3.77	4.72	14.5	5	60.7	4.9	2.2	99.2	0.5	99.6	0.31	0.1	565876
Black African	%	0.5	3.3	1.98	1.89	2.47	4	78.1	5.1	1.3	98.1	0.8	98.8	1.05	0.1	485277
Black Other	%	0.4	5.4	3.41	3.72	10	5	61.8	5	2.4	97.7	0.8	98.5	1.16	0.4	97585
Chinese	%	2.4	11	4.99	5.22	6.51	8	32.4	13	5.1	89.2	2.5	91.7	6.59	1.68	247403
Other	%	1.8	5.8	4.11	3.19	6.11	6	49	13	4	93.1	2.2	95.3	4.15	0.56	230615
All minority ethnic groups	%	1.3	8.1	6.98	5.86	12.8	6	44.6	8.5	2.4	96.2	1.3	97.5	2.19	0.27	4635296
All ethnic groups	%	4.3	11	8.45	7.1	8.96	9	12.2	14	8.4	83.6	4.9	88.5	8.61	2.87	58789194

Source: Census, April 2001, Office for National Statistics

> In ... [Name of Region deleted] 91.7 per cent of people identify themselves as being White British compared with 87.0 per cent in England as a whole.
>
> The highest minority ethnic group in the region is Pakistani, which account for 2.9 per cent of people, twice the proportion across England as a whole (1.4 per cent).
>
> Across the region, other ethnic minorities have a smaller percentage of the population. In all except the mixed group it was less than half the average for England as a whole.
>
> The proportion of people who say they are Christian is slightly higher in [Name of Region deleted] (73.1 per cent) than in England (71.7 per cent).
>
> Those who stated their religion was Muslim (3.8 per cent) is slightly higher than the average for England (3.1 per cent).
>
> [Name of Region deleted] has a smaller proportion of Buddhists, Hindus, Jews, Sikhs and other religions than the average for England.
>
> Source: Census, April 2001, Office for National Statistics

World wide travel and immigration

Sampson (1982) indicates that mass travel and immigration may be responsible for the Western world experiencing a change in the religions that are now inherent within many communities. However, this approach is rather simplistic and does not seem to look at some of the more complex sociological and psychological reasons that may lead to emigration, immigration and social migration, or indeed the need to seek asylum. Narayanasamy (1999b, p. 664) uses the phrase ‘push and pull factors’ when exploring reason why individuals may want to leave their country of origin. As a result of some of these factors some large urban cities and towns now contain individuals from diverse religious and cultural backgrounds, living, working and caring together. Sociological, cultural texts talk about ‘ethnic majority’ and ‘ethnic minority’ groups. The 2001 census statistics confirm that ‘White’ is still the majority population within the UK (Office for National Statistics, 2002). The BBC (2003), in what could be interpreted as a form of xenophobia, stresses that there are now two regions within Britain that

> ... have more blacks and Asians than white people for the first time ever. White people made up 39.4% of the population in Newham, east London, and 45.3% in Brent, north west London.

These statistics underline that there are regional variations; importantly, they reinforce the need for cultural sensitivity. This awareness must be extended so that it is reflected in the dialogue surrounding spirituality within health care. Failure to respond to the ethnic diversity will mean the perpetuation of a definition and understanding of spirituality that is homogeneous and not heterogeneous in that it will represent the views and opinions of the ethnic majority.

Sampson (1982, p. 1) states:

> Nowadays, nurses, doctors and patients may be from different cities, regions, countries, religions and cultures. Somehow they must meet the challenge of understanding each other first, before attempting to anticipate the needs of patients who come from different ethnic backgrounds.

Sampson highlights that there will be a need for cultural and religious sensitivity when considering matters of spiritual care. A consideration not mentioned is the need for cultural sensitivity when exploring theory development. Markham (1998) agrees with this approach suggesting that harmonisation of the concept of spirituality may only be achieved if individuals within nursing and health care listen to the disagreement concerning definitions of spirituality that might be raised by other world faiths and if all engage in the emerging debate. A starting point for any debate is for each 'camp' to set out their stall.

Spirituality and differing world faiths

It is not possible within this text to provide a detailed account of all the major world religions. There are numerous publications providing explanations of the beliefs and practices of many of them, for example Neuberger (2004), Carson (1989) and Narayanasamy (1991, 2001). However, what might be useful is to provide a summary as to how these communities perceive spirituality. Markham (1998) provides one such summary, intimating how 'spirituality' is perceived by Islam, Judaism, Hinduism and Buddhism. In Islam, spirituality is understood as an eradication of self – the Muslim becomes lost or lives life according to the will of Allah. In Judaism the normal and ordinary events of life are elevated to higher meaning through belief in a God who is mysterious and transcendent. In Hinduism there is a refocusing not upon a transcendent dimension but inwardly upon oneself. Through a process of introspection individuals can find their true or 'cosmic' self. Finally, in Buddhism spirituality is concerned with a realisation that everything in life is transient and that the correct way of life or 'Nirvana' is reached by following certain guiding principles.

A shared understanding

Another possible explanation for the perpetuation of secular forms of Christian spirituality is that western society assumes that other world faiths and cultures have a shared understanding of the term when this is not necessarily correct. This may originate from the fact that many world faiths have common rituals and practices that have been taken to represent spirituality, such as prayer and meditation, when in reality there are great differences in matters of theology and perceptual understanding (Sampson, 1982; Markham, 1998).

Fragmentation of spirituality

A review of the work undertaken by many authors writing on the subject of spirituality in health care reveals that the prevailing view is that spirituality incorporates three broad elements – transcendence, existentialism and the notion of universality. Conversely, an interesting perspective is being promulgated bringing into question the blanket application of these terms. The consequences of this perspective will have significance to all faiths and denominations, and will be relevant to those without any. Cobb (2001a, p. 3) suggests that the notion of existentialism or the '*existential perspective*' is something separate to and distinct from spirituality, proposing that the difference is found in the inability of existentialism not to look beyond the universe of human subjectivity. While Cobb's (2001a) perspective is welcome and provoking, one must consider the impact of these views upon a much wider audience. In divorcing or removing the existential element from spirituality the question that must be asked is 'What are we left with?'. The response may well be another layer of academic and philosophical wrangling that does not bring clarity to the debates surrounding spirituality, but instead results in an extra layer of division and fragmentation.

The danger with this fragmentation is that it can be applied to all the elements of spirituality, existentialism, transcendence and religious belief. If we argue that all of these are separate from and not relevant to understanding spirituality, then the term is in danger of becoming obsolete and redundant. Further, how does one explain the notion of spirituality when applied to individuals whose spirituality is not predicated on any of the above philosophies? The principle of universality assumes that the term spirituality is relevant to all individuals, regardless of religious faith or creed. Spirituality is present in those who do not profess or believe in any deity or supreme being.

Alternative categories

Harrison and Burnard (1993) suggest that there are three categories of individuals to consider when exploring the universal notion of spirituality. First, there are those whose spirituality originates from a belief in a religious faith. The second category is those who are non-believers. Harrison and Burnard (1993) divide this category into three subgroups: Atheists, Agnostics and Secular Humanists. Atheists are those individuals who categorically deny and denounce the existence of any god. Agnostics, in the absence of any concrete evidence to prove or disprove the existence of a god, tend to remain silent and ambivalent on the matter. An alternative belief is held by secular humanists, who suggest that people are alone and responsible for their own destiny in that there is no god responsible for them – ultimately they are responsible for themselves. Interestingly the third category is classified as the spiritual neutral. For these individuals the belief in a god or the notion of atheism is totally unnecessary to their beliefs or worldview. These categorisations and polarisations are discernable in much of the published literature (Cawley, 1997). They provide some explanation of how individuals' perceptions of spirituality may be catalogued. Yet superficial application and perpetuation of these classifications will not explain how an individual's spirituality is shaped in that they adopt a generalist not an individualised approach.

Developing cultural and spiritual awareness

In an attempt to combat and to rectify the imbalance with regard to the Judeo-Christian bias and the seemingly apparent failure to recognise that ethnic diversity exists within the National Health Service, there has been a growing movement to educate and develop cultural awareness. This attempt to raise awareness across all sectors and levels of care delivery, while a resolute step to eradicate and remove some of the racial tensions that prevail, may be counterproductive in the delivery of individualised care.

Transcultural nursing

There has been a vast amount of literature written on the subject of 'transcultural nursing', pioneered by Madeleine Leininger in the mid-1950s (Leininger, 2001) or now more accurately known as 'Leininger's Culture Care Theory of Nursing' (Cohen 1992, p. 1149). Since its inception, 'transcultural nursing' has been presented under several synonyms, for example culture and diversity, or cultural sensitivity. This interest has witnessed the publication of some extremely useful resources that outline the specific religious beliefs and practices of many of the world religions (Henley and Schott, 1999; Holland and Hogg, 2001). However, the pendulum may have swung too far, in that, rather than informing and alerting HCPs to potential needs, such resources are interpreted literally, which may result in some HCPs adopting a very blinkered and prescriptive approach, for example believing that all Muslims eat 'halal food', or Jews eat a 'kosher diet'.

Cash (2000) and Gilliat-Ray (2001) have expressed the danger of generalisation and the failure of nursing to acknowledge that diversity does exist within many cultures. Gilliat-Ray is correct, alerting HCPs to the danger of over-simplification and generalisation, yet her criticisms seem rather harsh and disproportionate when directed to some nursing writers. What Gilliat-Ray fails to acknowledge is that one of the writers that she vehemently criticises (Aru Narayanasamy) was possibly the first nurse in the UK trying to break down barriers and address some of the inadequacies that existed in this area.

It is not only nurses who are trying to redress this imbalance. Chaplains have also engaged with these issues and, again, there is a vast amount of literature appearing addressing the area of spiritual and pastoral care (Cobb and Robshaw, 1998; Orchard, 2001). Indeed, many of these writers will be referred to throughout this book. However despite the contributions of chaplains and religious, pastoral, and practical theologians (Willows and Swinton, 2000), there still exist some omissions and deficiencies that are impacting on the provision of culturally sensitive religious, pastoral and spiritual care within the NHS.

Reflecting diversity in chaplaincy provision

Orchard (2001), when taking about 'presence' in the meeting of spiritual needs, looks at the reverse, 'absence', using research (Orchard, 2000) undertaken within London hospitals and highlighting which communities are not represented within the health care team. It would appear that some of the minority ethnic and faith groups are not proportionately represented within chaplaincy teams. However, it would be wrong to generalise and say that this applies across the board, because several NHS Trusts are trying to redress this by actively recruiting individuals from some of the minority faith groups into funded posts.

Tide of change

It could be argued that nurses, closely followed by chaplains, are the professional groups that have made the greatest contribution in researching and developing the area of spirituality and spiritual care. The tide is changing as there is a growing realisation within 'medicine' of the need to take seriously this subjective but nevertheless important dimension of people's lives (Astrow *et al.*, 2001; Koenig, 2002; Larimore, 2001). With more and more empirical research being undertaken and published, spanning all spectrums and specialities of health care provision, there is emerging a significant evidence base that alludes to the importance of 'spirituality' in maintaining individuals' sense of health and well-being, and indeed their quality of life (Dossey, 1993; Ross, 1995).

With this point in mind, a trawl of the *British Medical Journal* (BMJ) spanning the last decades, using key words such as 'spirituality' and 'spiritual care' indicates that there is growing interest within medicine in the 'spiritual dimension'. By far the greatest interest has been from psychiatry, with some individuals making a major contribution, challenging colleagues to regain this element of their practice (Culliford, 2002a,b; Cook, 2004). Similarly, more is appearing surrounding 'cultural awareness'. This is evident with a growing number of medics from diverse faith communities writing on the subject (for example Sheikh and Gatrad, 2000). It must be stated that the levels of debate and conceptualisation are still in their infancy, when compared to other professional groups who have grappled with the 'thorny' issue of spirituality (Swinton and Narayanasamy, 2002) for several decades. However, this activity is a positive indicator, signalling medicine's desire to contribute and join the multidisciplinary dialogue.

Key points

- The need for multicultural dialogue in the area of spirituality is essential if an inclusive and representative model (theory) of spirituality that accommodates and reflects the increasing level of diversity within health care settings is to be developed.
- This review of the literature demonstrates that the concept of spirituality can no longer be termed an 'Anglo-American' debate.
- There is a growing body of evidence that 'spirituality' within health care is being researched, debated, and applied in many countries around the world, including the USA (Burkhardt, 1991), Netherlands (Cusveller, 1998), Australia (Fry, 1998; Thomas and Retsas, 1999) and Japan (Chiu 2001; Shirahama, and Inoue, 2001) and within different faith communities, for example Christian (Conco, 1995) and Muslim (Rassool, 2000).

Issue 2 – Holism and health care practice

Introduction

It would appear that the concept of 'holism' has become fashionable within nursing, and more recently this has infiltrated the whole of health care. Further, it has been argued that holism or the provision of holistic care cannot be considered such unless spirituality is an integral part of this process.

> **Activity 2.2 Drawing holism**
>
> Draw on a piece of paper an illustration or diagram that best represents your understanding of the concept of holism.
>
> This exercise will help you understand the debates outlined in the following section.

The word 'holism' originates from the Greek word *holos*, meaning 'whole' (Griffin, 1993; Ham-Ying, 1993). Pearson *et al.* (2005) indicate that the phrase 'holism' was first used by Jan Christian Smuts, a South African philosopher, in 1926. Pearson *et al.* (2005) reinforce that originally the philosophy had nothing to do with health care. However, since its inception, the philosophy of holism has been adopted by the nursing profession, possibly in an attempt to challenge the scientific model that prevails. Perhaps the nursing profession was attracted to this philosophy because the term 'holism' implies that all dimensions of our lives are equally important to our functioning and well-being – 'The whole is greater than the sum of its parts' (Patterson, 1998, p. 287). In contrast, the biological and medical models of care are perceived to be in opposition to the term, since they separate individuals into functional mechanistic units or biological systems at the expense of seeing the whole person and their situation

Several authors (Buckle, 1993; Griffin, 1993; Kolcaba, 1997; Patterson, 1998; Woods, 1998) have explored and discussed the term 'holism', and they conclude that because the word is surrounded by subjectivity, it is hard to give a precise definition of what constitutes holism. Ham-Ying (1993) implies that nurses do not have an adequate understanding or educational preparation into the concept of holism and the result may be that holistic care will not be fully operational within the context of nursing practice. With this point in mind it might be useful to present how the term is defined within nursing.

A nursing definition of holism

Holism is a common feature in many nursing models (Pearson *et al.*, 2005) and it could be argued that it has guided and shaped the direction of nursing care throughout its inception and evolution. The Churchill Livingstone (1996, p. 176) pocket dictionary for nurses does not offer a definition of holism but defines *holistic* as 'In a nursing context, caring for the whole patient – total patient care'. The 18th edition (Brooker, 2002, p. 411) elaborates on this, stating:

> ...relating to the theory of holism. It considers that individuals function as a whole rather than as separate parts or systems. Holistic nursing care takes account of physical, psychological, emotional, social and spiritual aspects → total patient care.

This description reinforces the notion that holistic care concerns the entire person. A possible reason why these terms are open to misinterpretation is that, like spirituality, a great deal of uncertainty still surrounds them. Buckle (1993) argues that the term 'holism' is used inaccurately because it is used interchangeably with the word 'complementary', thus underlining the confusion and misconceptions surrounding the use of the term. From this brief analysis of the term 'holism', it would appear that there is some degree of ambiguity about what the word exactly means. Despite these uncertainties, the relevance and benefits of using these terms in the provision of health and nursing care cannot be dismissed.

In summary, the word 'holism' is used to describe the 'whole' and the adjective 'holistic' is used to describe the application of the term to practice, for instance 'We provide holistic care'. There is recognition that all parts of an individual share equal importance in a balanced manner. If we are providing holistic care then we attend to all dimensions of an individual with the same amount of importance. Orchard (2000, p. 139) suggests 'all right-thinking professionals may want "a part" in providing spiritual care' because of its central position in holistic care.

Explaining holism

Holism can be defined as recognition that all dimensions of the individual – physical, social, psychological and spiritual – are attended to with equal importance (McSherry, 2006). 'The whole is greater than its constituent parts' is one phrase often used to describe holism (Bradshaw, 1994, p. xix). If one subscribes to this view, then 'holism' is about looking at the entire individual, since all dimensions equal the whole person. It is not about fragmenting and reducing individuals into manageable units, but appreciating how all the units of the person may be interconnected, interacting with each other. This 'whole' approach to holism is not often reinforced in health care. Instead, the terms 'holistic care' or its synonym 'total patient care' are often used.

'Holism' is often depicted diagrammatically as a circle or square divided into quarters. This approach to holism is still 'reductionist', because the person is divided into manageable units. For example, the quarters are often labelled *physical*, *social* and *psychological*, with *spiritual* tagged on at the end – an afterthought. Sadly, this approach to holism is still evident in contemporary health care.

A limitation of this segmental or reductionist model is that it does not emphasise how all dimensions of the person are integrated and dependant upon each other in order to maintain a sense of physical, psychological, social and spiritual well-being or a state of harmony. Ross (1997b, pp. 9–10), referring to Brewer's (1979) *Model of Spiritual Well-being*, reinforces the integrating nature of spirituality. She writes:

> However, the point to note is the way in which the spiritual dimension pervades all other dimensions.

While Ross's (1997b) work is not specifically focusing on the question of holism, it does highlight that the spiritual dimension is fundamental to the philosophy.

Scientific versus holistic care

Perhaps one of the main drivers that has resulted in re-emergence of the spiritual dimension of care as a welcome and to some degree attractive addition to nursing and health care is the desire to move away from a purely scientific, biomedical approach. The medical model, based on scientific theory, quantification, and physicalism has dominated and shaped the progress and delivery of health care (Woods, 1998). One of the legacies of this trend for nurses has been the devolution of medical tasks down to the nursing profession. It could be argued that devolution has been detrimental to nursing care. Devolution of tasks and a growing emphasis upon specific treatment modalities combined with a preoccupation with systems and organs has resulted in nurses becoming concerned with the potential for fragmentation and dehumanisation of the person (Thorne, 2001). These developments have led to the institution of specialist nurses, nurse consultants and an array of other practitioners with extended roles, adhering to prescribed protocols and procedures.

The peril for nursing is that, rather than the individual person being the focal point of treatment, the condition or pathology becomes the priority. The concern is that if this trend continues, rather than providing holistic care in an integrated manner, the care becomes reductionist. This means that all the professionals and specialists involved in the delivery of a patient's care contribute their expertise, focusing upon their specific area and adding to the picture, whereas, in the past nursing seemed to emerge from a 'spiritual heritage' that viewed the patient as an integrated 'whole'.

Religious communities recognised that caring for the soul was synonymously linked with attending to the 'whole' person (McSherry, 2006). It could be argued, rightly or wrongly, that this notion of integrated care was lost with the emergence of philosophical reasoning and the enlightenment that occurred around the time of the renaissance (Bradshaw, 1994). The philosopher René Descartes (1569–1650) is considered the founder of 'dualism' – the separation of mind and body now referred to as 'Cartesian Dualism'. Pearson *et al.* (2005) describe how the 'mind' – immaterial – became the province of clerics and the 'body' – material – was given over to physicians because it was prone to malfunction. The notion of a mind and body split implies superiority of one over the other. Paley (2002b) draws attention to some of the misunderstanding and misrepresentations surrounding Descartes' philosophies. He starts his defence by suggesting that Descartes is possibly the most reviled philosopher in history. This is because of the destructive impact that his theories have allegedly had upon the medical and nursing professions in terms of fragmentation and dehumanisation of the person. Despite these misgivings, the positive impact that 'dualism' and 'reductionism' have had upon the medical professions must be acknowledged.

The contribution that science and medicine have made in eradicating disease and pioneering treatments cannot be underestimated. It is not a simple case that holism is superior to reductionism. This moral stance fails to recognise the interplay between both paradigms. In order to understand people there is a need to understand all their parts. Flamming (2001, p. 263) recognises this need for moderation:

> Reductionism and holism should have a symbiotic, nonhostile relationship. They are partners, not adversaries. By definition, wholes need parts, and parts need wholes.

This will necessitate breaking down individuals into their constitute parts so that a greater understanding of how distinct parts impact upon the 'whole' may be gained.

Woods (1998) proposes a resolution to the debate by offering two forms of holism: 'strong' and 'weak'. The 'strong' form is defined by adherence to three canons: reductionism is incompatible with holism, the whole is greater than the sum of its parts, and parts cannot be understood in isolation from the whole. Adherence to these tenets would make nursing impossible. Further, the implications of this approach for the provision of spiritual care would be disastrous. 'Strong' holism is incompatible with the notion of multidisciplinary working, a philosophy and practice that underpins the very essence of spiritual care.

'Weak' holism is characterised by flexibility, making it more practical for nursing. This type of holism recognises the importance of the relationship between the parts and the whole. Yet what is important is recognition of the context in which the whole is defined. Woods (1998) suggests that the significant whole for many nurses will be the individual patient. The nurse may revise his or her view of the individual to include other wholes, such as family or environment. The notion of flexibility and being individually focused provides a potential framework for explaining the relationship between holism and spirituality.

Holism and spirituality

The unseen and inherent danger for health care is the perpetuation of a 'strong' version of holism that, if promulgated, may 'fragment' or detach spirituality from the heart of holistic care. Elsdon (1995) highlights the integrating and unifying force of spirituality within the context of people's lives, asserting that as an individual's physical health recedes greater emphasis and importance may be placed upon the spiritual dimension.

Bradshaw's (1994) concern is that if 'spirituality' is isolated and viewed out of context, in that it is set aside and viewed in isolation as an area for attention or study, then it may become disengaged. Rather than providing 'integrated care', individuals are fragmented and the spiritual dimension becomes another category or box to be completed, another aspect of care to be attended to. The net effect may be that there is a dislocation of the spiritual, a loss of integrity in that the individual is no longer viewed as a 'whole' but as a discrete set of manageable mechanistic units.

Key points

- This analysis of 'holism' reveals that spirituality and how it operates and resides within peoples' lives is very mysterious and subjective. The precise nature of this relationship will possibly be the source of many debates for years to come.
- Health care cannot be delivered in a holistic manner if spirituality is removed from the notion of holism. This removal may occur at two levels. Firstly, spirituality is omitted or does not feature in the philosophy of holism or, secondly, spirituality is fragmented out and seen purely as a separate entity to be addressed.
- In essence, spirituality could be described as the thread: the force that penetrates, integrates and harmonises all dimensions of a person in an equal, unique, hidden and mysterious manner.

Issue 3 – Moral relativism

The notion of moral relativism and the provision of spiritual care has been alluded to within several research studies and papers (for example Neuberger, 2004; Waugh, 1992; Schoenbeck, 1994; Clark, 1997; Cavendish *et al.*, 2000). Waugh (1992) identifies that nurses who possessed spiritual awareness are more likely to recognise and respond to patients presenting with a spiritual need. However, what is not explicit within research investigating spirituality and the provision of spiritual care is whether there are limitations or boundaries which nurses will not cross in the delivery of spiritual care. Devlin (1996) suggests that our own moral and personal beliefs may act as 'baggage', preventing the delivery of nursing care to individuals with divergent views to our own.

Activity 2.3 Does spirituality apply to all?

Some of the nurse participants were given the following scenario:

> Current definitions of spirituality seem to operate around principles that are good and acceptable to society. How would you feel if a patient admitted into your care identified as their religion witchcraft, occult or voodoo?

How would you have responded?

Devlin (1996, pp. 58–9) writes:

> Through the personal baggage questionnaire, we are able to see that we each of us as carers carry our baggage. This baggage comes from our family background, the newspapers we read, the views of our friends, the influences of our teachers, our culture and so on. It is imperative that career carers are aware of their own personal baggage and how it may influence care provision.

Closer inspection of Devlin's quotation suggests that the degree to which a health care professional or a 'career carer' may become involved in the provision of spiritual care may be morally relative to his or her own personal view or position concerning the subject. Such views may be developed and determined by cultural values, beliefs and experiences during the processes of socialisation.

Murray's and Zentner's (1989, p. 259) definition of spirituality is interesting in terms of the moral relativism debate because it states 'even in those who do not believe in any good'. This phrase implies that spirituality as a concept is equally relevant to individuals who could be perceived or judged by societies as intrinsically (morally) bad or evil – for example in past times Adolf Hitler and, in more recent times Osama Bin Laden and Saddam Hussein.

The notion of good and bad in relation to spirituality requires consideration of some important ethical issues, raising the spectre of 'moral relativism'. Empirical research and conceptual debates imply that the delivery of spiritual care and the effectiveness of subsequent interventions may be predicated on two factors: firstly, that an individual possesses awareness of the importance of this dimension within him- or herself, and secondly, that the degree to which an individual will engage with spiritual matters may be influenced by his or her own preconceptions and moral baggage surrounding the concept.

The idea of moral relativism needs careful and sensitive management, because what might be perceived as being morally, socially and, therefore, ideologically acceptable by the standards of one group or society may be judged as perhaps unethical, illegal and totally unacceptable when contrasted against the standards and ideologies of a different group. Fry (1998) affirms that nurses are not passive onlookers in their interaction and dealings with patients. On the contrary, she stresses that the worldview held by a nurse will ultimately determine the type of care provided.

Resolution of this potential dilemma may be 'self-awareness', meaning tolerance and the suspension of making rash judgments (Fry, 1998). The idea of being totally non-judgmental is probably unrealistic, in that the mere fact of being human means that we all make judgments. It could be argued that this is intrinsic to human nature. Rather, individuals may need awareness of what judgment is potentially being made, ensuring this is suspended and preventing it from being expressed. Cusveller (1998, p. 272) corroborates this: 'The nurse's spirituality has to fit the spiritual dimension of nursing. She has to be "cut from the right wood"'.

Harrison and Burnard (1993, p. 98) offer several reasons for nurses confronting their own spirituality and becoming 'spiritually aware', stressing the benefits gained by having heightened awareness of one's own beliefs in this area. They suggest that by 'confronting their own spirituality' nurses will have an increased awareness that will enrich all interventions and interactions with the patient. The implications of this debate are far-reaching in terms of how individuals manage and relate to diversity and whether an individual's moral relativism can be shaped through educational processes.

Key points

- Serious consideration needs to be given to the educational preparedness of HCPs in meeting their patients' spiritual needs.
- There is a pressing call for exploration of some of the ethical implications of undertaking such activity. Firstly, is it right that health care programmes should be asking individuals to consider a dimension of care that they may have never considered previously? Secondly, should educational programmes raise such awareness and actively seek to broaden people's understanding in this area? Basically, should people's understandings of spirituality be challenged and potentially changed? These ethical questions seem to have been overlooked in the health care literature.
- Conversely, there is an abundance of publications that could be described as dogmatic and prescriptive and which call for the education of all HCPs in spiritual matters through the development of self-awareness. If the concept of moral relativism does have an important role to play in the provision of spiritual care, then these issues warrant further research and investigation by all the health care professions.

Issue 4 – Managerialism[2]: introduction

The provision of spiritual care is firmly fixed on the health care agenda. If one looks at both political and professional legislation, one cannot fail to acknowledge that 'spiritual care' is gaining prominence. There is a clear emphasis being directed towards practitioners to attend to this dimension of people's lives. The growing number of government guidelines (NAHAT, 1996; SEHD, 2002; DOH, 2003a) is reassuring in that they draw attention toward the importance of spirituality emphasising that meeting the spiritual needs of service users is a fundamental part of health care. However, what is not clear within these guidelines is what evidence has been used to formulate them. The danger is that these guidelines make assumptions surrounding people's needs in terms of receiving spiritual care. The literature review reveals that little research has been undertaken within the UK searching for the opinions of the general public with regard to their understanding of spirituality and what their expectations might be in terms of receiving spiritual care. This type of insight is required because it could be used to inform government guidelines, thus preventing assumptions being made.

Political context

There has been a drive to establish spirituality as an important and integral part of health care provision, both politically and professionally. Reference to spirituality can be found in government publications (DOH, 2001) and is implied in codes of professional practice (NMC, 2002). The first major 'political' attempt to locate responsibility for the delivery of spiritual care by NHS staff was the Patient's Charter (DOH, 1991) supported by the DOH Circular HSG (92) 2 *Meeting the Spiritual Needs of Patients and Staff* (1992). The Patient's Charter (1991, p. 12), and more recently *Your Guide to the NHS* (DOH, 2001, p. 29) state:

> NHS staff will respect your privacy and dignity. They will be sensitive to, and respect, your religious, spiritual and cultural needs at all times.

The DOH Circular HSG (92) 2 provides guidance on how to meet the standard, highlighting spirituality as an important dimension of people's lives.

---

2 Aspects of this section are reprinted from McSherry, W., Cash, K. and Ross, L. (2004) Meaning of spirituality: implications for nursing practice. *Journal of Clinical Nursing*, **13**, 934–41. Copyright 2004 with permission from Blackwell.

These documents affirm the place of spirituality within the context of health care, supporting the desire to provide holistic care. Orchard (2000) suggests that these initiatives have led to confusion and false expectation with regard to patients' rights. It could be argued that these initiatives highlight a political agenda that has been created for the provision of spiritual care without giving any real consideration to the implications of this for staff or patients. It is not clear whether any form of consultation was undertaken with patients, key stakeholders or NHS staff prior to the development of these initiatives.

In response to some of the confusion and difficulties that local NHS were experiencing in translating and implementing the Patient's Charter (1991), the National Association of Health Authorities and Trusts (NAHAT) (1996) published the document *Spiritual Care in the NHS: A Guide for Purchasers and Providers*. The primary aim of this publication was to assist providers of health care to implement the charter standards associated with spiritual care. The political and professional developments outlined in this document seem to imply that patients and NHS staff have a clear, shared understanding of the concepts of spirituality and spiritual care.

The Department of Health (DOH) has recently undertaken a listening exercise, canvassing views and thoughts on its document *NHS Chaplaincy Guidance: Meeting the Spiritual and Religious Needs of Patients and Staff* (DOH, 2003b). This exercise is now closed, but it signals a positive attempt by the DOH to consider and, hopefully, act upon people's opinions and concerns with regards to the future direction of spiritual care.

Reflective question

- Do guidelines aid health care professionals in the delivery of spiritual care?

Statutory bodies

The United Kingdom Central Council (UKCC) and (one can assume) the newly formed Nursing and Midwifery Council (NMC), in its publication *Requirements for Pre-registration Nursing Programmes* (NMC , 2002, p. 14), declare that the following competency should be achieved for entry on to the professional register:

> Undertake and document a comprehensive, systematic and accurate nursing assessment of the physical, psychological, social and spiritual needs of patients, clients and communities

While this competency statement was evident in Rule 18 A (UKCC, 1986), it has been revised to include the assessment of communities, thus extending and raising the profile of spiritual assessment. Furthermore, this competency seems to firmly locate responsibility for spiritual assessment in nursing without giving any consideration to any practical implications (McSherry and Ross, 2002).

Reflective questions

- What is meant by competency in spiritual care?
- How might competency in spiritual care be evaluated?

Looking at the above policy documents and the NMC competency statements, it seems that two assumptions have been made by policy makers, and more recently by professional regulatory bodies:

- Patients and nurses are aware of their own spirituality and understand the concept as presented in health care terms.
- Patients and users of health care facilities expect to have their spiritual needs addressed.

These two assumptions signal a desire to establish and raise awareness of the importance of spirituality within the context of people's lives. However, one must question the motives and origins of these acclamations. If this is an attempt by the government to genuinely meet the essential human needs and rights of all people, then it should be embraced. Alternatively, if the development of institutional polices and procedures that prescribe 'spiritual and culturally sensitive care' is a managerial and bureaucratic attempt to control and prevent the ever-growing threat of public litigation, then this must be questioned. By being prescriptive and asking nurses and HCPs to assess and attend to the spiritual needs of patients, the NHS is fulfilling its obligation. However, if practitioners then fail to attend to these needs, they may be brought to account or task for any omissions.

This managerial 'top down approach' will not motivate or empower those who are directly involved in the provision of spiritual care. Rather, it will infuriate and subject them to another level of bureaucracy and form filling. This concern is expressed by Govier (2000, p. 34–5) when discussing the need for spiritual care to be provided within a systematic process:

> Otherwise the information remains of little use, fulfils the purpose of 'form-filling' and contributes to an increasing volume of perfunctory paperwork.

This quotation highlights that there is already a realisation within nursing that managerialism is 'rampant', seemingly driven by the ever-looming threat of litigation (Simmons, 2002). However, it is naïve to think that increasing paperwork will dissipate or remove the threat of litigation. In response to this threat, the government has reacted with the institution of 'Clinical Governance' in striving for clinical excellence (NHS Executive, 1996). Greater emphasis is being placed on the need for transparency and accountability of Trusts and health care practitioners to achieve standards, benchmarks of care. Spirituality is subsumed under the standard Maintaining Privacy and Dignity in the Essence of Care' (DOH, 2003a).

Evidence of managerialism

In an attempt to meet the above policy, many sections of health care are developing local strategies and formulating standards to demonstrate their efforts at implementing such or similar recommendation. This is evident in the growing number of publications that address areas such as spiritual assessment (Catterall *et al.*, 1998; Johnson, 2001), spiritual care (Cressey and Winbolt-Lewis, 2000) and spiritual audit (Hunt *et al.*, 2003). The driver for all this activity is undoubtedly political. For example, in Annex 2 (DOH, 2003b, p. 32) is a letter from the Chief Officer of Hospital Chaplaincies Council, sent to executives of NHS Trusts and chaplaincy networks. One paragraph reinforces the consequences of failing to address spiritual matters with patients:

> If Trusts fail to set up an adequate system for allowing patients to be asked about their spiritual care whilst in hospital and to register their consent for this information to be passed on, they could themselves be liable under The Human Rights Act 1998, should a patient claim that s/he was denied the right enshrined in Article 9 of the ECHR to manifest his or her religion, in worship, teaching, practice and observance.

This paragraph sends a very clear message to all involved in the provision of health care. It highlights that the fundamental right of all individuals is to express, and be supported in, their religious and spiritual needs. Interestingly, the DOH (2003a) guidelines, while seemingly prescriptive in terms of what HCPs should be undertaking in relation to the provision of spiritual care, fall short of offering any real guidance, firstly, in relation to what constitutes spiritual care, and secondly, in how spiritual care needs might be assessed and addressed. The assumption made, as previously stated, is that staff will be aware, feel comfortable and have the skills to provide spiritual care. Further, there is no real reference or acknowledgement given to the potential emotional cost upon staff. Neither is there any real indication of the resources that will be made available to support them in their endeavours. After all, people working in the NHS also possess spiritual needs. The guidelines do not really appreciate the collaborative nature of spiritual care, in that very little reference is made to the involvement of other professionals other than chaplaincy.

The DOH (2003a) guidelines are a useful illustration of the perils of imposing managerialism and bureaucracy in relation to spiritual care. One cannot deny that individuals' human rights are of paramount importance and should be upheld. However, in relation to spiritual care, perhaps there is an urgent need to establish with diverse patient groups what these needs might be. Further, there is a need to consult with all health care professionals to see what is realistic in terms of the support that they can provide and what they feel they may require in terms of educational preparedness to engage with spiritual issues.

Resolution of managerialism

As previously indicated, the Scottish Executive Health Department (SEHD) (2002) published their *Guidelines on Chaplaincy and Spiritual Care in the NHS in Scotland (NHS, HDL (2002) 76)*. It must be stressed that these guidelines do appear more comprehensive, acknowledging the need for consultation with all parties involved in the provision of spiritual care and what such involvement may cost in terms of resources. One criticism of the guidelines is that they present a very hierarchical structure. This structure utilises a 'top down approach' apportioning responsibility to key people within the organisation. This type of framework is in opposition to the voice of practitioners. Oldnall (1996) asserts that the spiritual agenda should be driven by practice, not by a managerial and bureaucratic system.

A counter argument is that if the governing bodies do not take responsibility for the promotion and monitoring of spiritual care, such services may become very disparate and may, indeed, be totally ineffective. By instigating some managerial and bureaucratic control, spiritual care will be accessible by all and delivered in a fair and equitable manner. However, politicians and civil servants must not forget to listen to the voice and concerns of HCPs that will surely be expressed when such guidelines are 'enforced' and evaluated. At present, it is not totally clear what the concerns of HCPs and patients are with regard to 'spirituality and spiritual care' since very little research, or indeed clinical audit, has been conducted in this area.

Key points

- This section has presented and analysed four key issues within the contemporary nursing and health care literature that may be influencing interest and theory development in spiritual care.
- The discussion outlines that the questions and concerns that are associated with the meaning of spirituality and the provision of spiritual care are multi-faceted, complex and often interrelated.
- It is suggested that nursing and health care need to slow down and consolidate theory development to avoid constructing a definition of spirituality that is theoretically insensitive, contradictory and restrictive.
- There is a pressing need for nursing and health care to evaluate its progress and achievements to date (and there are many) in this area so that a new route and course can be steered, if pitfalls and conceptual and practical 'minefields' are to be avoided.

Part III: Selected overview of empirical research

Introduction

In this part of the literature review the findings of a review and a critique of the nursing research that investigate spirituality and spiritual care are presented. Rather than conducting a critique of each individual quantitative and qualitative study, they have been grouped together and are discussed collectively. Two central themes arising from the review are described and the implications of these for this investigation are outlined. The concluding section provides an outline of the international and UK studies utilising 'grounded theory' inquiry spanning 1985–2000.

Reflective questions

- Is it realistic to think that an individual's perceptions of spirituality and spiritual care can be measured?
- How might measurement of spirituality or spiritual care practices enhance the delivery of spiritual care?

Purpose of and scope of review

Having undertaken earlier reviews of the conceptual and theoretical sources, this review concentrated on locating empirical literature. The databases again searched were CINHAL and MEDLINE, spanning the period 1991–2003. The rationale for just focusing on the above timeframe was that I had previously undertaken an extensive search and critique of the empirical literature as part of my previous research and publications (McSherry, 1997, 2000, 2006) and still had all these resources.

Key words such as 'spirituality', 'spiritual', and 'spiritual' care were used in combination with the word 'research', including the terms 'quantitative', 'qualitative' and 'grounded theory'. The terms 'nurse', 'nursing' and 'patient' were also used. The search was restricted by ensuring that the identified source contained an abstract and was written in English, and the research method was clearly stated. In addition to the electronic searches, manual searching was undertaken to look at reference lists in published works. A total of 40 resources were identified. These included original research papers, dissertations and theses (totalling 36; see Table 2.7). Papers that were derived from dissertations/theses (totalling 4) are identified as such within the summary. Perhaps more studies would have been identified if the words 'religious' and 'beliefs' had been used. I am aware of some studies that may have fallen into this category (King *et al.*, 1995; Dein and Stygall, 1997; Hay and Hunt, 2000).

Reflective question

Why do qualitative research methods seem to be the preferred way of investigating the spiritual dimension?

Table 2.7 Findings of the literature search.

	Year	Country of origin	Authors	Type	Sample size	Sample	Area of focus
1	1991, (1994)*	USA	Burkhart	Qualitative	12	Appalachia women	Describing spirituality
2	1991	USA	Reed	Quantitative	300	100 hospitalised adults with incurable cancer 100 hospitalised adults with no serious illness and 100 well non-hospitalised adults	Determine terminally ill and non-terminally ill patients preferences for spirituality related interventions
3	1992	USA	Highfield	Quantitative	50	27 nurses 23 patients with primary lung cancer	Spiritual health of oncology patients and how well nurses assess spiritual health
4	1992	UK	Waugh	Multiple methods	793	Qualified nurses	Perceptions of spirituality
5	1993	UK	Harrison and Burnard	Qualitative	10	Qualified nurses	Understanding spirituality
6	1993	UK	Narayanasamy	Quantitative	33	Registered nurses	Educational preparedness to meet patients' spiritual needs
7	1993	USA	Emblen and Halstead	Qualitative	38	7 chaplains 19 surgical patients 12 nurses	Defining spiritual needs and interventions
8	1994	UK	Kearney	Qualitative	11	Patients with MS	Spiritual coping
9	1994 and 1995	USA	Taylor *et al.*	Quantitative	181	Cancer nurse clinicians	Attitudes, beliefs and definitions of spiritual care
10	1995	Australia	Harrington	Qualitative	10	Registered nurses	Perceptions of spirituality
11	1995	USA	Clark and Heidenreich	Qualitative	63	Critical care patients	Nursing interventions
12	1995	USA	Conco	Qualitative	10	Christian volunteers	Christian patients' views of spiritual care
13	1997a	UK	Ross	Qualitative	10	Elderly patients	Understanding spirituality

Table 2.7 *(continued)*

	Year	Country of origin	Authors	Type	Sample size	Sample	Area of focus
14	1997, (2002)*	UK	McSherry	Quantitative	559	Qualified and unqualified nurses	Perceptions of spirituality
15	1997, (1999)*	USA	Walton	Qualitative	13	Myocardial patients	What spirituality means
16	1999	Australia	Thomas and Retsas	Qualitative	19	Terminal cancer	Spiritual meanings people with terminal cancer give to life experiences
17	2000	USA	Cavendish *et al*.	Qualitative	12	Well adults	Spiritual factors/growth
18	2000	USA	Walton and St Clair	Qualitative	11	Received a cardiac transplant	What spirituality means to heart transplant patients
19	2001	UK	Carroll	Qualitative	15	Hospice nurses	Exploration of the nature of spirituality and spiritual care
20	2001	USA	Chiu	Qualitative	15	Chinese immigrants with breast cancer	Spiritual resources
21	2001	UK	Wright	Quantitative	151 hospices 194 Trusts	Senior chaplains	Features of spiritual care
22	2001	USA	Hermann	Qualitative	19	Hospice patients	Identify dying patients' definitions of spirituality and their spiritual needs
23	2001	Finland	Kuuppelomaki	Quantitative	328	Nurses working in-patient wards	Spiritual support for terminally ill patients
24	2001	UK	Narayanasmay and Owens	Qualitative	115	Post-registration nurses	Response to spiritual needs of patients
25	2001	USA	Daalemann et al	Qualitative	35	17 women diabetic patients Type 2 18 women with no self-identified illness	Patient-reported, health-related spirituality
26	2001	USA	Stranahan	Quantitative	102	Nurse practitioners	Spiritual perceptions and attitudes about spiritual care/practices
27	2001	Sweden	Strang and Strang	Qualitative	20 patients 16 next of kin	Brain tumour patients	Spiritual thoughts and coping

Table 2.7 *(continued)*

	Year	Country of origin	Authors	Type	Sample size	Sample	Area of focus
28	2001	Japan	Shirahama and Inoue	Qualitative	10	People living in a farming community	Explore the concept of spirituality
29	2001	USA	Tuck *et al.*	Quantitative	52	Males living with human immunodeficiency virus (HIV)	Relationship between spirituality and psychosocial factors2002
30	2002	USA	*Arnold et al.*	Multiple methods	47	Opioid-dependent patients	Determine how spirituality is defined
31	2002	UK	Wright	Qualitative	16 not stated	Key stakeholders in palliative care	Spiritual essence of palliative care
32	2002, (2003)*	UK	Baldacchino	Multiple methods	70	Myocardial infarction patients	Spiritual coping strategies
33	2002	UK	O'Driscoll	Quantitative	463	Nurses	Perceptions of spirituality
34	2002	UK	Narayanasamy et al	Qualitative	10 nurses	Learning disability nurses	Meeting spiritual needs of clients
35	2002	UK	Narayanasmay	Qualitative	15 patients	Chronically ill patients	Spiritual coping mechanisms
36	2003	USA	Taylor	Qualitative	28	Patients with cancer and primary family carer givers	Determine what patients, primary family caregivers expect from nurses regarding the meeting of spiritual needs

*Refers to a paper published from the original dissertation/thesis

The review identified 23 international studies that utilised qualitative methodologies (for example phenomenology, ethnography and grounded theory), with eight originating from within the UK. In terms of quantitative studies, only 10 international studies (13 if including the three studies that had used multiple methods) were identified. Perhaps one explanation for this disparity in research methods might stem from the deeply subjective and personal nature of spirituality, which means that some form of rapport needs to be established between the researcher and the participant. This can be hard to achieve in several forms of quantitative research: for example, survey methods that employ questionnaires.

Ross (2006) provides an overview of the research papers published on spiritual care between 1983 and October 2005. Her paper provides suggestions and recommendations for future direction of research in this emerging field.

Central themes identifiable in the empirical literature

Identifiable within the empirical literature are two central themes. The first theme is linked with perceptions of spirituality and spiritual care, while the second theme surrounds the enhancement of spiritual care practices, primarily for patients.

Perceptions of spirituality and spiritual care

The quantitative and qualitative studies reviewed appear to focus predominantly upon specific groups' perceptions of spirituality. The word 'perception' is used as an umbrella covering words such as beliefs, attitudes and understandings of spirituality. For example, within the UK Waugh (1992), Harrison and Burnard (1993), McSherry (1997) and more recently O'Driscoll (2002) have examined nurses' perceptions of spirituality and spiritual care, working predominantly within the National Health Service. The findings of these investigations validate that spirituality is perceived as a universal, multifaceted phenomenon. The findings also reveal that nurses are prepared to be involved in the provision of spiritual care. However, not all nurses felt that they were able to meet their patients' spiritual needs satisfactorily. Other researchers have concentrated on the perceptions of service users. For example Hermann (2001) interviewed dying patients about their understanding of spirituality, while Kearney (1994) and latterly Strang and Strang (2001) discussed issues of spirituality with patients living with neurological disorders such as multiple sclerosis or brain tumours. These investigations demonstrate that some patients may have difficulty in articulating what constitutes spirituality. However, the studies reveal that patients were prepared to talk about their spiritual beliefs, identifying spirituality as an important factor in helping them cope with their illness or impending death.

Another positive benefit of the research investigating perceptions of spirituality and spiritual care is that some of the studies have led to the development of several scales that assist researchers to measure aspects of the spiritual dimension, for example the Spiritual Well Being Scale (SWB) (Paloutzian and Ellison, 1979), the Spirituality and Spiritual Care Rating Scale (SSCRS) (McSherry, 1997; McSherry *et al.*, 2002), Spiritual Assessment Inventory (SAI) (Hall and Edwards, 2002) and the Spiritual Coping Strategies Scale (SCS) (Baldacchino, 2002; Baldacchino and Buhagiar, 2003). These instruments have been used successfully in a variety of situations with diverse groups of individuals, and provide valuable insights into how individuals perceive spirituality and how spirituality can be a powerful force in coping with illness and disease.

Additionally, research that targets the spiritual care practices of specialist practitioners has been undertaken. For example, Taylor *et al.* (1994) used a questionnaire to determine what spiritual care practices oncology nurses used in their dealings with patients. Frequent practices identified in this investigation were praying with patients, referring to chaplains, and the use of presence as well as listening and talking to patients. Taylor *et al.* (1994) were concerned with the findings because a question mark was raised about the nurses' commitment to, or confidence in, providing spiritual care, suggesting that this was not as strong as it could be.

Stranahan (2001) examined the spiritual perceptions and practices among nurse practitioners working in a range of clinical situations; interestingly, the term 'nurse practitioner' was not defined. This is important because the term 'practitioner' can have many meanings, given the proliferation in specialist roles. Like Taylor *et al.*'s (1994) study, this investigation also established that practitioners felt uncomfortable in performing spiritual care. Stranahan (2001, p. 100) writes 'More than half (57%) of respondents rarely or never provided spiritual care...'

The findings of all these investigations, if taken literally, imply that despite all the attention and presumed advancement in this area, HCPs are still struggling to recognise and engage with the concepts. However, these findings may be explained by the fact that many of the practitioners may have been providing spiritual care but not labelling it as such. The danger with elucidating and defining spiritual care is that this area of practice is fragmented and viewed as something separate from the everyday practices that HCPs perform (Carroll, 2001).

In summing up, the empirical literature corroborates and substantiates the conceptual, theoretical and anecdotal evidence surrounding spirituality. It affirms that spirituality is personal and uniquely defined by individuals, and that it depends upon one's own personal philosophy or worldview. The studies demonstrate that spirituality may have relevance to all people: believers and non-believers. Yet the principle of universality is precarious in the sense that the language and discourses associated with meaning are not always recognisable. For example, many patient groups linked spirituality with religious beliefs. The studies also provide valuable insight into why a group may view spirituality in a particular manner and the forces that shape their understanding. For example, Burkhardt (1991) identified and described how women in Appalachia viewed their spirituality and the societal forces that shaped this understanding, while Cavendish *et al.* (2000) used grounded theory to clarify the opportunities in life that support or enhance spirituality in well adults living in a region within the USA. More recently, Shirahama and Inoue (2001) conducted an ethnographical study to explore the concept of spirituality and its expressions among persons living in Japanese farming community. These investigations demonstrate that perceptions and understandings of spirituality may be shaped by a variety of social, cultural or regional factors such as religious beliefs, ideologies and historical associations.

While the empirical studies provide a valuable insight into how spirituality may be perceived and defined by specific populations, there was a noticeable lack of comparative studies. Comparative in this instance means simultaneously contrasting the perceptions of two or more groups of participants (for example nurses, patients, chaplains or physicians) or studies that have compared the perceptions of the same professional group (for example nurses working in a variety of specialities such as critical care, palliative care, mental health or learning disabilities). It seems that many of the studies undertaken have targeted a specific group. For example, Narayanasamy *et al.* (2002) obtained critical incidents from learning disability nurses in an attempt to understand how they meet the spiritual needs of the people for whom they care. This type of research is valuable in that it provides insights into the perceptions and practices of a specific professional group. However, the results cannot be generalised to a wider audience (Carroll, 2001).

The empirical literature highlights that a large proportion of the research undertaken focused upon the role of the nurse. In addition, much of the research has been conducted by nurses. However, several studies were identified within the UK that had been conducted by chaplains (Wright, 2001, 2002; O'Driscoll, 2002). Only four comparative studies were identified that sought the perceptions of more than one group.

Reed (1991) used a questionnaire to explore preferences for spirituality related to nursing interventions with terminally ill and non-terminally ill hospitalised adults, contrasting their views with those of well adults. The findings of this investigation emphasised the need for nurses to be sensitive to the spiritual needs of all patients, not just those with a religious belief. Highfield

(1992) investigated the spiritual health of oncology patients by contrasting nurses' and patients' perspectives. The study revealed that gender difference may be influential in undertaking an assessment of a patient's spiritual health, because males were less inclined to talk about spiritual issues. Emblen and Halstead (1993) used a descriptive qualitative design to collect interview data to establish how patients, nurses and chaplains defined spiritual needs and interventions. The findings demonstrate a need for nurses and chaplains to work collaboratively in meeting patients' spiritual needs.

Most of the comparative studies described have been conducted in the USA and employed quantitative methodologies or a combination of multiple methods, with the exception of Emblen and Halstead (1993), who used grounded theory. Comparative investigations are important because they shed light on the disparities and commonalities in understanding between participant groups. In addition, they provide researchers with an opportunity to explore possible reasons, explanations and potential solutions. The literature search indicates that no additional comparative studies have been undertaken in the USA. The literature search reveals also that none were identified that originated within the UK. This is interesting because Ross (1997a, p. 714), who identified a need for such research (having undertaken a pilot study of elderly patients' perceptions of their spiritual needs and care) writes:

> A study comparing both nurses' and patients' interpretations of spiritual needs and care would help clarify what spiritual needs and spiritual care are and would highlight the type of help that patients might welcome with their spiritual needs.

It appears that there is an urgent need for comparative studies to investigate the discrepancies that exist between HCPs' and patient groups' perceptions of spirituality and spiritual care. The results of such investigations could be used to inform future policy initiatives and guidelines that surround spiritual care.

The empirical literature verifies that an exclusive language of spirituality may have been created within health care. Several authors stress the need for HCPs to avoid using and generalising unfamiliar terminology in their dealings with patients (Taylor *et al.*, 1995; Hermann, 2001). This argument could be extended also to diverse cultural groups. A major limitation of many of the studies reviewed is the lack of cultural and religious diversity. Many of the studies were comprised of very small samples and, because of the homogeneous nature of the subjects in terms of religious belief, professional group and area of residency, these limit the generalisability of the findings.

There is a growing expectation in the empirical literature that the composition of study samples should reflect the ethnic and religious diversity that exists within a pluralistic society. With regard to investigating the spiritual dimension there is a growing realisation by researchers that the insights previously developed may not have meaning for individuals from many of the Eastern religious traditions, who, it seems, have been under-represented in earlier research. My interpretation of this situation is that there has not been a conscious attempt to exclude such groups. On the contrary, one plausible explanation may be that the samples used have reflected the majority population working or residing in those areas at the time of conducting the investigation.

Beside, there may well have been difficulties in identifying and recruiting individuals from diverse ethnic groups due to language barriers. Other sociological factors may also have been operational: for example, perceptions of authority, how the information will be used and confidentiality if researchers are from the same ethnic group. Having stated this, there is now a pressing need to ensure that future investigations into spirituality and spiritual care do reflect the ethnic and religious diversity that exists within those regions. By including the perceptions of the minority ethnic and religious groups a richer insight into the concept of spirituality will be gained.

Enhancement of spiritual care practices

One of the central themes identifiable within the empirical literature is linked to the enhancement of spiritual care practices. As indicated, several of the investigations have focused primarily upon the spiritual care interventions of HCPs who were primarily nurses. The empirical literature appears judgmental of HCPs who do not demonstrate a familiarity and fluency with the language of spirituality and the practice of spiritual care (Taylor *et al.*, 1995). Enhancement of spiritual care practices can be explained by two subcategories. Firstly, there are those investigations that make recommendations to enhance patient care by making inferences, for example by developing the technical skills and competence of HCPs, which will lead to improvements in spiritual care. Technical skills means nurturing the HCPs' own personal awareness of spirituality in conjunction with education to develop skills to address patients' spiritual needs. Secondly, there are those studies that attempt to enhance spiritual care practices by offering insight into the experiential world of patients.

Several of the studies reviewed that explored HCPs' perceptions of spirituality and spiritual care assume that deficits in relation to the provision of spiritual care may be remedied through education (Harrington, 1995; Taylor *et al.*, 1994, 1995; Kuuppelomaki, 2001). It is assumed that education will remove the discomfort and unease that some HCPs feel when addressing spiritual needs. However, what is not explored in the educational debates is whether it is ethical to change HCPs' perceptions of spirituality. Neither is there any real exploration of the economic or emotional cost of providing spiritual care

(Walter, 2002). Furthermore, an assumption seems to be made that all HCPs want to, and should be, attending to the spiritual needs of service users.

The empirical literature revealed a growing number of investigations that examined the spiritual well-being of specific patient groups. These studies focus upon individuals living with acute or chronic illness or diseased systems, such as endocrine, neurological and cardiac systems. This form of specialisation is in keeping with the medical and reductionist models that prevail within health care. Clark and Heidenreich (1995) interviewed 63 patients in a critical care unit, identifying nursing interventions that may enhance patients' spiritual well-being. Walton (1997) explored the relationship of spirituality in patients recovering from acute myocardial infarction and patients undergoing heart transplantation (Walton and St Clair, 2000). Daalemann *et al.* (2001) used focus group interviews to elicit the understandings of spirituality of female patients with type 2 diabetes and how they viewed its impact upon their health and well-being, while Arnold *et al.* (2002) used focus groups to establish patients' attitudes concerning the inclusion of spirituality into addiction treatment. More recently, Baldacchino (2002) (using combined methods) conducted a longitudinal study into the spiritual coping strategies of Maltese patients who had suffered their first acute myocardial infarction. She concluded that maintaining an individual's spiritual well-being may be a precursor to the relief of anxiety and depression. All these studies demonstrate that spirituality can be a powerful force that enables the patient to endure illness and hospitalisation. In addition, these studies may highlight aspects of spiritual care that are unique to these individual groups. However, the fundamental message communicated within these investigations is the central role that HCPs play in maintaining patients' spiritual well-being.

A major limitation of the quantitative studies reviewed that, while they offered valuable insight into a broad range of issues pertaining to spirituality and spiritual care, this insight was often superficial in that they were unable to convey the full extent of a participant's beliefs or feelings. The quantitative studies were not capable of exploring the complexity of the area or of portraying and conveying the meaning, feeling and emotion that an individual or group had regarding the issue(s) under investigation. It would appear that, because of the sensitive and personal nature of spirituality, qualitative research is more suitable for exploring this dimension.

Limitations and omissions within existing empirical studies

1. Investigations have been initiated principally by nurse researchers and directed mainly upon nurses' perceptions of spirituality and spiritual care practices.

2. Very few comparative studies were located that contrasted simultaneously the views of two or more groups.
3. The study samples have been homogeneous, reflecting the views of specific cultural, professional or client groups.
4. The quantitative studies were not really capable of exploring the complexity of spirituality.

Outline of studies using grounded theory methodology

The literature search revealed that internationally eight grounded theory investigations had been conducted exploring diverse aspects of spirituality: two in the UK and six abroad. The literature review established that grounded theory has been the most frequently used qualitative methodology in the exploration of the spiritual dimension. The reason for this is that grounded theory allows the researcher to discover attitudes, meanings and characteristics. In addition, this method allows the researcher to explore a phenomenon that is not readily visible and that may mean different things to different people. Grounded theory enables the researcher to construct and test out existing theory.

The availability of these published studies was certainly one of the deciding factors in choosing this methodology over the other qualitative approaches. These studies were a valuable resource in describing and orientating oneself with the methodological processes involved in this form of inquiry. On a cautionary note, Stern (1994) suggests that grounded theory has been eroded because of a 'do-it-yourself' approach to the method. That is, researchers learn by reading a book or a chapter in book. Stern argues that as a consequence there has been 'generational erosion' through inadequate mentorship. With this point in mind it was reassuring that I had an experienced grounded theorist on my supervision team.

The six international studies identified, in chronological order, are Hungelmann *et al.* (1985); Burkhardt (1991); Thomas and Retsas (1999); Walton (1997); Cavendish *et al.* (2000); and Walton and St Clair (2000). The two UK studies were Harrison and Burnard (1993) and Kearney (1994). The significant properties of each of the studies are summarised in Table 2.8. The studies also fall into the two central themes outlined in the introduction to this section.

Chronologically the studies ranged from 1984–2002. It must be stressed that this list is not exhaustive and there may well be more undergraduate and postgraduate research available within nursing and other disciplines. One recommendation arising from this book is that there is a pressing need for some form of collaboration to establish a central database in which this type of information can be collated and made accessible to all researchers interested in this dimension of care within the UK and wider international community.

Summary points

- Part III of the literature review outlined two central themes identifiable within the empirical literature associated with perceptions of spirituality and spiritual care.
- The review demonstrates that both quantitative and qualitative methods have made a significant contribution in elucidating the concept of spirituality.
- The section describes how quantitative studies have been significant in terms of developing insight into perceptions of spirituality and spiritual care. A limitation with some of the quantitative investigations is that they have been unable to offer a deep insight into the personal and socially constructed world of individual experience.
- In addition, the review suggests that few qualitative studies have been undertaken comparing and contrasting simultaneously the views of diverse groups.

Conclusion

The three parts of the literature review provide the reader with an overview of the conceptual and theoretical issues surrounding spirituality and spiritual care. Part I provided a conceptual analysis of spirituality highlighting how language and meaning are deeply subjective. Part II presented a framework sensitising the reader to some of the constructs and arguments that are shaping the emergence of spirituality within contemporary health care. Finally, Part III offered a review of the empirical evidence, highlighting how there is a need for further qualitative research to gain deeper insight into the personal meanings and significance of spirituality.

Table 2.8 Summary of grounded theory investigation.

Authors	Year	Purpose	No. participants	Theory developed
Hunglemann *et al.*	1985	Determine defining characteristics of spiritual well-being	$n = 31$ no breakdown by gender provided	Basic social process of harmonious interconnectedness was discovered with two major themes that applied to all categories harmony and connection.
Burkhardt	1991, 1994	Identify and describe how women in Appalachia view their spirituality and to describe characteristics of spirituality as understood by these women	$n = 12$ females	Common understanding of spirituality that was identified – a unifying force that shapes and gives meaning to the pattern of one's self becoming and connecting.
Harrison and Burnard	1993	Explore trained nurses' perceptions of spirituality both personally and professionally in order to highlight their knowledge and understanding	$n = 10$ no breakdown by gender provided	Three higher order headings: the concept of spirituality; spirituality and nursing practice, and the spirituality of nurses. General categories identified were definitions of spirituality; relevance and importance to the nurses role; manifestations of patients' spiritual needs; nurses' beliefs relating to the 'why' of suffering; nurses' beliefs relating to mortality; and nurses' sources of hope and strength.
Kierney	1994	Investigate the role of spirituality as a coping mechanism in multiple sclerosis viewed from the patients' perspective	$n = 11$ 6 female 5 male	Spirituality was viewed as an effective strategy helping patients cope with chronic illness, discover meaning in illness and suffering, combat loneliness and isolation, satisfy the human desire to give and receive love, redress the balance between lack of locus of control due to chronic illness, and encourage hope and a positive outlook.

Table 2.8 *(continued)*

Authors	Year	Purpose	No. participants	Theory developed
Walton	1997, 1999	Discover what spirituality means for patients with an acute myocardial infarction and to identify patients' perceptions of how spirituality influences their recovery	$n = 13$ 4 female 9 male	Core category 'receiving presence' had three subcategories: divine presence, presence of friends, family, or community; and presence of health care providers. 'Receiving presence' also permeated three subcategories: developing faith, discovering meaning and purpose, and giving the gift of self.
Thomas and Retsas	1999	Construct a grounded theory explaining how the spirituality of people with terminal cancer develops	$n = 19$ 12 female 7 male	Identification of one single unifying core category labelled 'transacting self preservation'. This process is dependent upon three behaviours: 'talking it all in', 'getting on with things', and 'putting it all together'.
Cavendish *et al.*	2000	Explicate the opportunities that occur in life that either support or enhance spirituality in adult	$n = 12$ 8 female 4 men	Two overall domains emerged as significant to participants: physical domain and metaphysical domain. Seven themes emerged from domains – connectedness, beliefs, inner motivating factors, divine providence, understanding the mystery, walking through and life events.
Walton and St Clair	2000	Identify what spirituality means to heart transplant patients and to identify perceptions of how spirituality influences illness and recovery	$n = 11$ 4 female 7 male	Two core categories were identified: enduring illness and sustaining hope.

References

Arnold, R. M., Avants, S. K., Margolin, A. and Marcotte, D. (2002) Patients' attitudes concerning the inclusion of spirituality into addiction treatment. *Journal of Substance Abuse Treatment*, **23**, 319–26.

Astrow, A. B., Pulchalski, C. M. and Sulmasy, D. P. (2001) Religion, spirituality, and health care: social, ethical and practical considerations. *The American Journal of Medicine*, **110**, 283–7.

Baldacchino, D. (2002) Spiritual coping of Maltese patients with first acute myocardial infarction: a longitudinal study. *Unpublished PhD Thesis*, University of Hull, England.

Baldacchino, D. R. and Buhagiar, A. (2003) Psychometric evaluation of the Spiritual Coping Strategies scale in English, Maltese, back-translation and bilingual versions. *Journal of Advanced Nursing*, **42**(6), 558–70.

British Broadcasting Company (2003) *At a Glance Census Results* Available from http://news.bbc.co.uk/1/hi/uk/2756993.stm. Accessed April 2004.

Beckford, J. and Gillat, S. (1996) *The Church of England and Other Faiths in a Multifaith Society*. Department of Sociology, University of Warwick, Coventry.

Bradshaw, A. (1994) *Lighting the Lamp: The spiritual Dimension of Nursing Care*. Scutaria Press, London.

Bradshaw, A. (1996) The legacy of Nightingale. *Nursing Times*, **92**(6), 42–3.

Bradshaw A. (1997) Teaching spiritual care to nurses: an alternative approach. *International Journal of Palliative Nursing*, **3**(1), 51–7.

Brewer, D. C. (1979) Life stages and spiritual well-being. In: *Spiritual Well-being: Sociological Perspectives* (ed. D. O. Moberg). University Press of America, Washington.

Brooker, C. (ed.) (2002) *Churchill Livingstone's Dictionary of Nursing*, 18th edn. Churchill Livingstone, Edinburgh.

Buckle, J. (1993) When holism is not complementary. *British Journal of Nursing*, **2**(15), 744–5.

Burkhardt, M. A. (1991) Exploring understandings of spirituality among women in Appalachia. *Doctoral Dissertation*, University of Miami, Florida.

Burkhardt, M. A. (1994) Becoming and connecting: elements of spirituality for women. *Holistic Nursing Practice*, **8**(4), 12–21.

Burnard, P. (1988a) Searching for meaning. *Nursing Times*, **84**(37), 34–6.

Burnard, P. (1988b) The spiritual needs of atheists and agnostics. *Professional Nurse*, December, 130–2.

Carr, W. (2001) Spirituality and religion: chaplaincy in context. In: *Spirituality in Health Care Contexts* (ed. H. Orchard), Chapter 1. Jessica Kingsley, London.

Carroll, B. (2001) A phenomenological exploration of the nature of spirituality and spiritual care. *Morality*, **6**(1), 81–98.

Carson, V. B. (1989) *Spiritual Dimensions of Nursing Practice*. W. B. Saunders, Philadelphia.

Cash, K. (1990) Nursing models and the idea of nursing. *International Journal of Nursing Studies*, **27**(3), 249–56.

Cash, K. (2000) Foreword. In: *Making Sense of Spirituality in Nursing Practice: An Interactive Approach* (W. McSherry). Harcourt Brace, Edinburgh.

Castledine, G. (2005) Senior nurse who demeaned the spiritual beliefs of patients and staff. *British Journal of Nursing*, **14**(14), 745.

Catterall, R. A., Cox, M., Greet, B., Sankey, J. and Griffiths, G. (1998) The assessment and audit of spiritual care. *International Journal of Palliative Nursing*, **4**(4), 162–8.

Cawley, N. (1997) Towards defining spirituality. An exploration of the concept of spirituality. *International Journal of Palliative Nursing*, **3**(1), 31–6.

Cavendish, R., Luise, B. K., Horne, K., Bauer, M., Medefindt, J., Gallo, M. A., Calvino, C. and Kutza, T. (2000) Opportunities for enhanced spirituality relevant to well adults. *Nursing Diagnosis*, **11**(4), 151–63.

Chiu, L. (2001) Spiritual resources of Chinese immigrants with breast cancer in the USA. *International Journal of Nursing Studies*, **38**, 175–84.

Churchill Livingstone (1996) *Churchill Livingstone's Dictionary of Nursing*, 17th edn. Churchill Livingstone, Edinburgh.

Clark, C. and Heidenreich, T. (1995) Spiritual care for the critically ill. *American Journal of Critical Care*, **4**(1), 77–81.

Clark, C. C. (1997) Recognizing spiritual needs of orthopaedic patients. *Orthopaedic Nursing*, **16**(6), 27–32.

Cobb, M. (2001a) *The Dying Soul: Spiritual Care at the End of Life*. Open University Press Buckingham.

Cobb (2001b) Walking on water? The moral foundations of chaplaincy. In: *Spirituality in Health Care Contexts* (ed. H. Orchard), Chapter 5. Jessica Kingsley, London.

Cobb, M. and Robshaw, V. (1998) *The Spiritual Challenge of Health Care*. Churchill Livingstone, Edinburgh.

Cohen, J. A. (1992) Janforum: Leininger's culture care theory of nursing. *Journal of Advanced Nursing*, **17**, 1149.

Conco, D. (1995) Christian patients' views of spiritual care. *Western Journal of Nursing Research*, **17**(3), 266–76.

Cook, C. C. H. (2004) Addiction and spirituality. *Addiction*, **99**, 539–51.

Cressey, R. W. and Winbolt-Lewis, M. (2000) The forgotten heart of care: a model of spiritual care in the National Health Service. *Accident and Emergency Nursing*, **8**, 170–7.

Culliford, L. (2002a) Spiritual care and psychiatric treatment – an introduction. *Advanced Psychiatric Treatment*, **8**, 249–60.

Culliford, L. (2002b) Spirituality and clinical care. *British Medical Journal*, **325**, 1434–5.

Cupitt, D. (1997) *After God: The Future of Religion*. Weidenfeld & Nicolson, London.

Cusveller, B. (1998) Cut from the right wood: spiritual and ethical pluralism in professional nursing practice. *Journal of Advanced Nursing*, **28**(2), 266–73.

Daalemann, T. P., Cobb, A. K. and Frey, B. B. (2001) Spirituality and well-being: a exploratory study of the patient perspective. *Social Science and Medicine*, **53**, 1503–11.

Dawson, C. (1945) *Progress and Religion: An Historical Enquiry*. Sheed and Ward, London.

Deary, V., Dearly, I. J., McKenna, H. P., McCance, T. V., Watson, R. and Hoogbriun, A. C. (2002) Elisions in the field of caring. *Journal of Advanced Nursing*, **39**(1), 96.

Dein, S. and Stygall, J. (1997) Does being religious help or hinder coping with chronic illness? A critical literature review. *Palliative Medicine*, **11**, 291–8.

Devlin, A. B. (1996) Ethics and the spirituality of caring. In: *Exploring The Spiritual Dimension of Care* (ed. E. Farmer), Chapter 4. Quay Books, Wiltshire.

Department of Health (1991) *Patient's Charter*. HMSO, London.

Department of Health (1992) HSG (92)2: *Meeting the Spiritual Needs of Patients and Staff*. HMSO, London.

Department of Health (2001) *Your Guide to the NHS*. Department of Health, London.

Department of Health (2003a) *Essence of Care: Patient-focused Benchmarking for Clinical Governance*. Department of Health, London.

Department of Health (2003a) *NHS Chaplaincy: Meeting the Religious and Spiritual Needs of Patients and Staff*. Department of Health, London.

Dossey, L. (1993) *Healing Words: The Power of Prayer and the Practice of Medicine*. Harper, San Francisco.

Dyson, J., Cobb, M. and Forman, D. (1997) The meaning of spirituality: a literature review. *Journal of Advanced Nursing*, **26**, 1183–8.

Elsdon, R. (1995) Spiritual pain in dying people: the nurse's role. *Professional Nurse*, **10**, 641–3.

Emblen, J. D. and Halstead, L. (1993) Spiritual needs and interventions: comparing the views of patients, nurses and chaplains. *Clinical Nurse Specialist*, **7**(4), 175–82.

Emdon, T. (1997) Cry freedom. *Nursing Times*, **93**(40), 35–8.

Flamming, D. (2001) Duelling dualisms: a response to Thorne's 'People and their parts: deconstructing the debates in theorizing nursing's clients'. *Nursing Philosophy*, **2**, 263–5.

Frankl, V. E. (1987) *Man's Search for Meaning: an Introduction to Logotherapy*. Hodder and Stoughton, London.

Fry, A. (1998) Spirituality, communication and mental health nursing: the tacit interdiction. *Australian and New Zealand Journal of Mental Health Nursing*, **7**, 25–32.

Fowler, J. (1981) *Stages of Faith*. Harper & Row, San Francisco.

Gerrish, K. (1997) Preparation of nurses to meet the needs of an ethnically diverse society: educational implications. *Nurse Education Today*, **17**, 359–65.

Gilliat-Ray, S. (2001) Sociological perspectives on the pastoral care of minority faiths in hospital. In *Spirituality in Health Care Contexts* (ed. H. Orchard), Chapter 10. Jessica Kingsley, London.

Golberg, B. (1998) Connection: an exploration of spirituality in nursing care. *Journal of Advanced Nursing*, **27**, 836–42.

Govier, I. (2000) Spiritual care in nursing: a systematic approach. *Nursing Standard*, **14**(17), 32–6.

Greenstreet, W. (1999) Teaching spirituality in nursing: a literature review. *Nurse Education Today*, **19**, 649–58.

Griffin, A. (1993) Holism in nursing: its meaning and value. *British Journal of Nursing*, **2**(6), 310–12.

Hall, J. (1997) The search inside. *Nursing Times*, **93**(40), 36–7.

Ham-Ying, S. (1993) Analysis of the concept of holism within the context of nursing. *British Journal of Nursing*, **2**(15), 771–5.

Harrington, A. (1995) Spiritual care: what does it mean to RNs? *Australian Journal of Advanced Nursing*, **12**(4), 5–14.

Harrison, J. and Burnard, P. (1993) *Spirituality and Nursing Practice*. Avebury, Aldershot.

Hay, D. and Hunt, K. (2000) *Understanding the Spirituality of People Who Don't go to Church*. A report on the findings of the Adults' Spirituality project at the University of Nottingham.

Henley, A. and Schott J. (1999) *Culture, Religion and Patient Care in a Multi-Ethnic Society*. Age Concern, London.

Hermann, C. P. (2001) Spiritual needs of dying patients: a qualitative study. *Oncology Nursing Forum*, **28**(1), 67–72.

Highfield, M. F. (1992) Spiritual health of oncology patients: nurse and patient perspectives. *Cancer Nursing*, **15**(1), 1–8.

Holland, K. and Hogg, C. (2001) *Cultural Awareness in Nursing and Health Care*. Arnold, London.

Hungelmann, J., Rossi, E. K., Klassen, L. and Stollenwerk, R. M. (1985) Spiritual well-being in older adults: harmonious interconnectedness. *Journal of Religion and Health*, **24**(2), 147–53.

Hunt, K., Cobb, M., Vaughan, L. K. and Ahmedzai, S. H. (2003) The quality of spiritual care – developing a standard. *International Journal of Palliative Nursing*, **9**(5), 208–15.

Johnson, C. P. (2001) Assessment tools: are they an effective approach to implementing spiritual health care within the NHS? *Accident and Emergency Nursing*, **9**, 177–86.

Kearney, S. (1994) Spirituality as a coping mechanism in multiple sclerosis: the patient's perspective. *Unpublished dissertation*, Institute of Nursing Studies, University of Hull, England.

King, P., Speck, P. and Thomas, A. (1995) The Royal Free interview for religious and spiritual beliefs: development and standardisation. *Psychosocial Medicine*, **25**, 1125–34.

Koenig, H. G. (2002) *Spirituality in Patient Care: Why, How, When and What?* Templeton Foundation Press, Radnor, Pennsylvania.

Kolcaba, R. (1997) The primary holisms in nursing. *Journal of Advanced Nursing*, **25**, 290–6.

Kuuppelmaki, M. (2001) Spiritual support for terminally ill patients: nursing staff assessments. *Journal of Clinical Nursing*, **10**, 660–70.

Larimore, W. L. (2001) Providing basic spiritual care for patients: should it be the exclusive domain of pastoral professionals? *American Family Physician*, **63**(1), 36–40.

Lie, A. S. J. (2001) No level playing field. In *Spirituality in Health Care Contexts* (ed. H. Orchard), Chapter 14. Jessica Kingsley, London.

Leininger, M. M. (2001) *Culture Care Diversity and Universality: A Theory of Nursing*. Jones and Bartlett, Boston.

Macquarrie, J. (1972) *Paths in Spirituality*. SCM Press, London.

Macrae, J. (1995) Nightingale's spiritual philosophy and its significance for modern nursing. *Image: Journal of Nursing Scholarship*, **27**(1), 8–10.

Males, J. and Boswell, C. (1990) Spiritual needs of people with a mental handicap. *Nursing Standard*, **4**(48), 35–7.

Markham, I. (1998) Spirituality and the world faiths. In: *The Spiritual Challenge of Health Care* (eds. M. Cobb and V. Robshaw), Chapter 6. Churchill Livingstone, Edinburgh.

Matheson, J. and Summerfield, C. (2001) (eds.) *Social Trends No. 31*, p. 235. Stationery Office, London.

Mayet, F. (2001) Diversity in care the Islamic approach. In: *Spirituality in Health Care Contexts* (ed. H. Orchard), Chapter 13. Jessica Kingsley, London.

McSherry, W. (1996) Raising the spirits. *Nursing Times*, **92**(3), 48–9.

McSherry, W. (1997) A descriptive survey of nurses' perceptions of spirituality and spiritual care *Unpublished MPhil Thesis*, University of Hull, England.

McSherry, W. (2000) *Making Sense of Spirituality in Nursing Practice*. Churchill Livingstone, Edinburgh.

McSherry, W. (2006) *Making Sense of Spirituality in Nursing and Health Care Practice*, 2nd edn. Jessica Kingsley, London.

McSherry, W. (2001) Spirituality and learning disabilities: are they compatible? *Learning Disability Practice*, **3**(5), 35–8.

McSherry, W. and Draper, P. (1998) The debates emerging from the literature surrounding the concept of spirituality as applied to nursing. *Journal of Advanced Nursing*, **27**, 683–91.

McSherry, W. and Ross, L. (2002) Dilemmas of spiritual assessment: considerations for nursing practice. *Journal of Advanced Nursing*, **38**(5), 479–88.

McSherry, W., Draper, P. and Kendrick, D. (2002) The construct validity of a rating scale designed to assess spirituality and spiritual care. *International Journal of Nursing Studies*, **39**(7), 723–34.

MORI (2003) *Three In Five 'Believe In God'*. `http://www.mori.com/polls/2003/bbc-heavenandearth.shtml` Accessed April 2004.

Morse, J. M., Solberg, S. M., Neander, W. L., Bottoroff, J. L. and Johnson, J. L. (1990) Concepts of caring and caring as a concept. *Advances in Nursing Sciences*, **13**(1), 1–14.

Murray, R. B. and Zentner, J. B. (1989) *Nursing Concepts for Health Promotion*. Prentice Hall, London.

Narayanasamy, A. (1991) *Spiritual Care: a Practical Guide for Nurses*. Quay, Lancaster.

Narayanasamy, A. (1993) Nurses' awareness and educational preparation in meeting their patients' spiritual needs. *Nurse Education Today*, **13**(3), 196–201.

Narayanasamy, A. (1999a) Learning spiritual dimensions of care from a historical perspective. *Nurse Education Today*, **19**, 386–95.

Narayanasamy, A. (1999b) Transcultural mental health nursing 1: benefits and limitations. *British Journal of Nursing*, **8**(10), 664–8.

Narayanasamy, A. (2001) *Spiritual Care: a Practical Guide for Nurses and Health Care Practitioners*, 2nd edn. Quay, Wiltshire.

Narayanasamy, A. (2002) Spiritual coping mechanisms in chronically ill patients. *British Journal of Nursing*, **11**(21), 1461–70.

Narayanasamy, A. and Andrews, A. (2000) Cultural impact of Islam on the future directions of nurse education. *Nurse Education Today*, **20**(1), 57–64.

Narayanasamy, A. and Owens, J. (2001) A critical incident study of nurses' responses to the spiritual needs of their patients. *Journal of Advanced Nursing*, **33**(4), 446–55.

Narayanasamy, A., Gates, B. and Swinton, J. (2002) Spirituality and learning disabilities: a qualitative study. *British Journal of Nursing*, **11**(14), 948–57.

National Association of Health Authorities and Trusts (1996) *Spiritual Care in the NHS: A Guide for Purchasers and Providers*. National Association of Health Authorities and Trusts, Birmingham.

National Health Service Executive (1996) *Promoting Clinical Effectiveness: a framework for Action in and Through the NHS*. HMSO, London.

Nelson, S. (1995) Humanism in nursing: the emergence of the light. *Nursing Inquiry*, **2**, 36–43.

Neuberger, J. (2004) *Caring for Dying People of Different Faiths*, 3rd edn. Radcliffe Medical, Abingdon.

Nursing and Midwifery Council (2002) *Requirements for Pre-registration Nursing Programmes*. NMC, London.

Nursing and Midwifery Council (2004) *NMC Code of Professional Conduct: Standards for Conduct, Performance and Ethics*. NMC, London.

O'Driscoll, P. J. (2002) A study of the perceptions and understanding of spirituality and spiritual care of the nurses of the Basildon & Thurrock General Hospitals Trust. *Unpublished MA Dissertation*, University of Leeds, England.

Office for National Statistics (2002) *Census 2001*. HMSO, London. `http://www.statistics.gov.uk/census2001/census2001.asp`

Oldnall, A. (1996) A critical analysis of nursing: meeting the spiritual needs of patients. *Journal of Advanced Nursing*, **23**, 138–44.

Olumide, O. (1989) Towards a non-racist fulfilment of the 1948 Health Act's recommendations about spiritual care for all patients and staff in NHS hospitals in the UK. *Unpublished dissertation*, University of Bradford, England.

Orchard, H. (2000) *Hospital Chaplaincy: Modern, Dependable?* Sheffield Academic Press, Sheffield.

Orchard, H. (ed) (2001) *Spirituality in Health Care Contexts*. Jessica Kingsley, London.

Oxford Paperback Dictionary (1983) 2nd edn. Oxford University Press, Oxford.

Paley, J. (1996) How not to clarify concepts in nursing. *Journal of Advanced Nursing*, **24**, 572–8.

Paley, J. (2002a) An archaeology of caring knowledge. *Journal of Advanced Nursing*, **36**(2), 188–98.

Paley, J. (2002b) The Cartesian melodrama in nursing. *Nursing Philosophy*, **3**(3), 189–92.

Patterson, E. F. (1998) The philosophy and physics of holistic health care: spiritual healing as a workable interpretation. *Journal of Advanced Nursing*, **27**(2), 287–93.

Pattison, S. (2001) Dumbing down the spirit. In *Spirituality in Health Care Contexts* (ed. H. Orchard), Chapter 2. Jessica Kingsley, London.

Paloutzian, R. F. and Ellison, C. W. (1979) Developing a measure of spiritual well-being. In *Spiritual Well-being, Loneliness and Perceived Quality of Life* (chair R. F. Paloutzian). Symposium presented at the annual meeting of the American Psychological Association, New York.

Pearson, A., Vaughan, B. and Fitzgerald, M. (2005) *Nursing Models for Practice*, 3rd edn, Chapters 5 and 6. Butterworth-Heinemann, Oxford.

Quality Assurance Agency for Higher Education (2001) *Nursing Benchmark Statements: Health Care Programmes*. Quality Assurance Agency for Higher Education, Gloucester.

Rassool, H. G. (2000) The crescent of Islam: healing, nursing and the spiritual dimension. Some considerations towards an understanding of the Islamic perspectives on caring. *Journal of Advanced Nursing*, **32**(6), 1476–84.

Reed, P. (1991) Preferences for spirituality related nursing interventions among terminally ill and non terminally ill hospitalised adults and well adults. *Applied Nursing Research*, **4**(3), 122–8.

Reed, P. (1992) An emerging paradigm for the investigation of spirituality in nursing. *Research in Nursing and Health*, **15**, 349–57.

Ross, L. (1996) Teaching spiritual care to nurses. *Nurse Education Today*, **16**, 38–43.

Ross, L. (1997a) Elderly patients' perceptions of their spiritual care: a pilot study. *Journal of Advanced Nursing*, **26**, 710–15.

Ross, L. (1997b) *Nurses' Perceptions of Spiritual Care*. Avebury, Aldershot.

Ross, L. (2006) Spiritual care in nursing: an overview of the research to date. *Journal of Clinical Nursing*, **15**(7), 852–62.

Schoenbeck, S. L. (1994) Called to care: addressing the spiritual needs of patients. *The Journal of Practical Nursing*, September, 19–23.

Scottish Executive Health Department (2002) *Guidelines on Chaplaincy and Spiritual Care in the NHS Scotland (NHS HDL (2002) 76)*. Scottish Executive, Edinburgh.

Sheikh, A. and Gatrad, A. R. (2000) *Caring for Muslim Patients*. Radcliffe Medical Press, Oxford.

Shirahama, K. and Inoue, E. M. (2001) Spirituality in nursing from a Japanese perspective. *Holistic Nursing Practice*, **15**(3), 63–72.

Simsen, B. (1985) Spiritual needs and resources in illness and hospitalisation. *Unpublished Masters Thesis*, University of Manchester, England.

Smart, N. (1969) *The Religious Experience of Mankind*. Collins, London.

Stern, P. N. (1994) Eroding grounded theory. In: *Critical Issues in Qualitative Research Methods* (ed. J. M. Morse). Sage, Thousand Oaks.

Stranahan, S. (2001) Spiritual perceptions, attitudes about spiritual care, and spiritual care practices among nurse practitioners. *Western Journal of Nursing Research*, **23**(1), 90–104.

Strang, S. and Strang, P. (2001) Spiritual thoughts, coping and 'sense of coherence' in brain tumour patients and their spouses. *Palliative Medicine*, **15**, 127–34.

Stoll, R. I. (1989) The essence of spirituality. In: *Spiritual Dimensions of Nursing Practice* (ed. V. B. Carson), Chapter 1. W. B. Saunders, Philadelphia.

Strauss, A. and Corbin, J. (1998) *Basics of Qualitative Research*, 2nd edn. Sage, Thousand Oaks.

Swinton, J. and Narayanasamy, A. (2002) Response to: A critical view of spirituality and spiritual assessment by P. Draper and W. McSherry (2002) *Journal of Advanced Nursing*, **39**, 1–2. *Journal of Advanced Nursing*, **40**(2), 158–60.

Talbot, L. A. (1995) *Principles and Practice of Nursing Research*. Mosby, London.

Tanyi, R. A. (2002) Towards clarification of the meaning of spirituality. *Journal of Advanced Nursing*, **39**(5), 500–9.

Taylor, E. J., Highfield, M. and Amenta, M. (1994) Attitudes and beliefs regarding spiritual care: a survey of cancer nurses. *Cancer Nursing*, **17**(6), 479–87.

Taylor, E. J., Amenta, M. and Highfield, M. (1995) Spiritual care practices of oncology nurses. *Oncology Nurses Forum*, **22**(1), 31–9.

Taylor, E. J. (2003) Nurses caring for the spirit: patients with cancer and family caregiver expectations. *Oncology Nursing Forum*, **30**(4), 585–90.

Thomas, J. and Retsas, A. (1999) Transacting self-preservation: a grounded theory of the spiritual dimension of people with terminal cancer. *International Journal of Nursing Studies*, **36**(3), 191–201.

Thompson, M. (1995) *Philosophy*. Hodder & Stoughton, London

Thorne, S. E. (2001) People and their parts: deconstructing the debates in theorizing nursing's clients. *Nursing Philosophy*, **2**, 259–62.

Tuck, I., McCain, N. L. and Elswick, R. K. (2001) Spirituality and psychosocial factors in persons living with HIV. *Journal of Advanced Nursing*, **33**(6), 776–83.

Turner, P. (1996) Caring more, doing less. *Nursing Times*, **92**(34), 59–60.

United Kingdom Central Council for Nursing, Midwifery and Health Visiting (1986) *Project 2000 – A new preparation for practice*. UKCC, London.

Vivian, F. (1968) *Thinking Philosophically: An Introduction For Students*. Chatto & Windus, London.

Walker, L. G., Walker, M. B., Ogston, K., Heys, S. D., Ah-See, A. K., Miller, I. D., Hutheon, A. W., Sarkar, T. K. and Eremin, O. (1999) Psychological, clinical and pathological effects of relaxation training and guided imagery during primary chemotherapy. *British Journal of Cancer*, **80**(1/2), 262–8.

Walter, T. (1997) the ideology and organization of spiritual care: three approaches. *Palliative Medicine*, **11**, 21–30.

Walter, T. (2002) Spirituality in palliative care: opportunity or burden? *Palliative Medicine*, **16**, 133–9.

Walton, J. (1997) Spirituality of patients recovering from an acute myocardial infarction: a grounded theory study. *Unpublished doctoral dissertation*, University of Missouri, Kansas City.

Walton, J. (1999) Spirituality of patients recovering from an acute myocardial infarction: a grounded theory study. *Journal of Holistic Nursing*, **17**(1), 34–53.

Walton, J. and St Clair, K. (2000) 'A beacon of light': spirituality in the heart transplant patient. *Critical Care Nursing Clinics of North America*, **12**(1), 87–101.

Waugh, L. A. (1992) Spiritual aspects of nursing: a descriptive study of nurses' perceptions. *Unpublished PhD Thesis*, Queen Margaret College, Edinburgh.

Widerquist, J. and Davidhizar, R. (1994) The ministry of nursing. *Journal of Advanced Nursing*, **19**, 647–52.

Willows, D. and Swinton, J. (2000) *Spiritual Dimensions of Pastoral Care: Practical Theology in a Multidisciplinary Context*. Jessica Kingsley, London.

Wittgenstein, L. (1953) *Philosophical Investigations*. Basil Blackwell, Oxford.

Woods, S. (1998) Holism in nursing. In: *Philosophical Issues in Nursing* (ed. S. Edwards), Chapter 4. Macmillan, London.

Wright, M. C. (2001) Chaplaincy in hospice and hospital: findings from a survey in England and Wales. *Palliative Medicine*, **15**, 229–42.

Wright, M. C. (2002) The essence of spiritual care: a phenomenological enquiry. *Palliative Medicine*, **16**, 125–32.

Wright, S. (1997) Free the spirit. *Nursing Times*, **93**(17), 31–2.

Wright, S. (2002) Out of the ashes. *Nursing Standard*, **16**(24), 24.

CHAPTER 3

Identifying the issues: the research question

Introduction

This brief chapter presents the study aim and objectives. These have been formulated to meet the discrepancies and omissions discussed (Chapter 1). The rationale for having one broad study aim and objectives is provided. It is argued that the aim and objectives provided a flexible framework that directed the investigation.

Activity 3.1 Study aim

Read the 'Study Aim' presented below. Answer the following questions:

- Is the aim of the investigation clear?
- Do you think the aim to be realistic and achievable?
- Why is it important to have a broad aim?

Study aim

> The purpose of this investigation is to explore the subjective nature of spirituality and spiritual care by using existing theory to reflect upon the way in which health care professionals, patients and the public perceive the concept from within diverse care settings and with differing religious/worldviews.

Strauss and Corbin (1998, p. 41), when discussing the formulation of research questions, suggest that the question should be open and broad so that areas can be addressed comprehensively and not so specific that it 'excludes discovery'. They also suggest that the research question sets the parameters of the study. Initially these may well be broad, becoming 'more specific or focused during the research process as concepts and their relationships are discovered'.

In an attempt to be more focused and to provide the study with more direction, the broad question was set against three objectives. Porter and Carter (2000, p. 18) deem this to be an acceptable approach when structuring a research study. They describe how a study may consist of a 'research question' which is 'a general statement of the purpose of the study', which may then be broken down into specific objectives to be achieved.

By identifying a broad question with specific objectives the flexibility of the study was maintained while providing specific goals/targets, thus providing a possible framework around which the study could operate and the data analysis be managed.

The research objectives

■ Objective I

To examine the assumption that spirituality is a universally recognised and understood concept within the context of nursing and health care.

■ Objective II

To develop insight into HCPs', patients' and the public's understanding of spirituality and spiritual care within diverse care settings, for example palliative and acute care including areas such as medical, surgical and intensive care.

■ Objective III

To produce a model of spirituality in order to generate a deeper understanding of the concept for use within nursing and the wider health care community in order to shape future practice and education.

References

Porter, S. and Carter, D. E. (2000) Common terms and concepts in research. In: *The Research Process in Nursing*, 4th edn (ed. D. F. S. Cormack), Chapter 2. Blackwell Scientific, Oxford.

Strauss, A. and Corbin, J. (1998) *Basics of Qualitative Research*, 2nd edn. Sage, Thousand Oaks.

CHAPTER 4

Investigating spirituality and spiritual care: methods

Overview

This chapter presents and discusses the research design, explaining why grounded theory was selected as the preferred method for investigating the area of spirituality. This chapter also describes other methodological issues that were involved in the research process, such as selection of the sample, research setting, data collection, data analysis and a review of the ethical issues that impacted on the study.

Grounded theory as the chosen method

The rationale is given for selecting a qualitative research design over a quantitative one and for choosing grounded theory as the preferred qualitative method to address the study aim. Following this debate, the grounded theory method will be explored, addressing some of the pros and cons associated with this approach. Finally, an outline will be presented as to how grounded theory best suited the aim and objectives of the study.

Activity 4.1 Quantitative and qualitative research

Before proceeding any further with this section can you write down your understanding of the terms 'quantitative' and 'qualitative'?

The distinctions between these approaches to research will be explained in the following section.

Rationale for qualitative over quantitative research

The 'selected review' of the studies in Chapter 2 revealed that spirituality has been investigated using the full spectrum of research methods incorporating both quantitative and qualitative designs and some comparative studies employing multiple methods in order to triangulate and to provide meaning to the phenomenon. The studies that were reviewed reveal that the subjective and abstract nature of 'spirituality' presents major obstacles in researching this area from a purely quantitative perspective. Spirituality seems to be beyond the realms of scientific inquiry and purely quantitative methods. A logical extension of this argument would be to assume that such a subjective dimension would best suit qualitative research designs.

The quantitative versus qualitative research debate has rumbled on for several decades, especially within nursing and health care, and does not seem to have abated. This is evident in a recent editorial in a leading international nursing journal (Watson, 2002; Draper and Draper, 2003) and the response it engendered. Interestingly, the spiritual dimension has not been exempt from the quantitative/qualitative debate. As indicated, there is a preference for qualitative over quantitative methodologies when investigating matters pertaining to spirituality.

Perhaps this preference for qualitative methods is best explained by comparing and contrasting the characteristics of quantitative and qualitative methodologies. Burns and Grove (1997, p. 28) provide a useful insight into the different characteristics of quantitative and qualitative methodologies. This is adapted below (Table 4.1) with an additional column that highlights the relevance and appropriateness of each qualitative characteristic for the investigation of spirituality.

The quantitative characteristics underline that the primary tenet of quantitative research is that it operates around the ability to measure rigorously, objectively and systematically, generating data for statistical analysis (Carter, 2000). The focal point in quantitative research is on control, seeking to establish relationships between variables under investigation. Burns and Grove (1997, p. 791) define quantitative research as:

> A formal, objective systematic process to describe, test relationships, and examine cause and effect interactions among variables

The emphasis upon control, rigour and measurement do not seem to suit the spiritual dimension, which is deeply personal, individual, subjective and mysterious, and seemingly beyond any manipulation because such properties do not lend themselves to scientific measurement.

Conversely, qualitative research is concerned with processes and meanings that are not 'rigorously' measured. Denzin and Lincoln (1998) assert that

Table 4.1 Characteristics of qualitative and quantitative methodologies.

Quantitative research	Qualitative research	Relevance of qualitative characteristics to this investigation
Hard science	Soft science	Dealing with abstract terms and processes
Focus: usually concise	Focus: usually broad	Focus of the study is very broad
Reductionistic	Holistic	Spirituality is an integral part of the 'whole person'. Holistic approaches emphasised within nursing
Objective	Subjective	Investigation is dealing with a subjective dimension
Reasoning; logistic, deductive	Reasoning: dialectic, inductive	Theory development is inductive
Basis of knowing: cause-and-effect relationship	Basis of knowing: meaning, discovery	Aim of the investigation is to establish meaning and discover new insights into the spiritual dimension and practices of individuals
Test theory	Develop theory	Test existing theory and offer new insights
Control	Shared interpretation	No variables to control, all participants' interpretations were valid
Instruments	Communication and observation	Interviews, observations and field notes were used as a means of obtaining data
Basic element of analysis: numbers	Basic element of analysis: words	Micro- and macro-analysis of interview transcripts
Statistical analysis	Individual interpretation	Theory developed reflective of my interpretation of data
Generalisation	Uniqueness	Emphasis is not upon generalising findings but upon reflecting the reality and uniqueness of individual participants

qualitative researchers are interested in the socially constructed nature of reality and the dynamic processes that exist, such as the relationship between the researcher and what is being studied. Denzin and Lincoln (1998) propose that qualitative researchers are more concerned with understanding an individual's perceptions of the world and seeking insight and illumination of people's interpretations of facts rather than generating numerical data for statistical analysis (Porter, 2000). These characteristics of qualitative research seem to suit the spiritual dimension because they accommodate the uniqueness of individuals, highlighting that the concern is not about absolutes, but about diversity and difference. This brief analysis of the principal characteristics of quantitative and qualitative methodologies reveals that both can make a valuable contribution in explaining phenomena, for example spirituality.

Despite the realisation that both methodologies have an important part to play in explaining phenomena, the current trend in the health care professions, especially nursing, is still a strong preference for quantitative research over qualitative methods. Fondness for systematic reviews and randomised control trials over other forms of qualitative evidence demonstrate this favouritism. McSherry *et al.* (2002a, p. 11) talk about 'strengths of evidence', in which they refer to Muir Gray's (1997) classification and ranking of evidence. Their evaluation of this classification affirms preference for quantitative methods:

> However, a limitation of this hierarchy is that it places scientific or quantitative research studies with higher status than qualitative studies.

The reasons why quantitative studies are perceived as superior to qualitative investigations is because of the credence placed on objectivity, control, causal relationships and statistical analysis. In light of this discussion, the ideal of ever achieving evidenced-based spiritual care is perhaps an anathema. This is in part due to the nature of spirituality, which does not satisfy the characteristics of hard science. The principal characteristics of quantitative research do not suit the investigation of broad exploration of spirituality. Hard science attempts to make generalisations, while spirituality is more about capturing unique interpretations, meaning that the entire area is deeply skewed and open to much speculation.

Within quantitative research emphasis is placed upon validity (that is, the investigation measures what it is designed to measure) and reliability (that the same results will be obtained if the study were to be replicated under the same conditions). Because of the nature of spirituality the concepts of validity and reliability are a little more precarious. It would be very hard to control all the miscellaneous variables that influence and shape an individual's spirituality. Therefore, in qualitative studies the emphasis is not so much upon validity and reliability but on the truthfulness and integrity of the research findings.

It has been shown that quantitative and qualitative research are two very distinct and unique methods used for the investigation of phenomena. Although both approaches have fundamental differences and specific characteristics, they can be developed, combined and integrated within some research designs. Both these approaches have played a crucial role in the exploration and clarification of spirituality and spiritual care, a concept that I would say is largely qualitative by nature but which does have elements that can be quantified and analysed statistically (McSherry, 1997).

The aim of this section is not to perpetuate the debate that qualitative methods are superior to quantitative analysis when investigating spirituality. On the contrary, it is more about selecting a methodology that best answers the research aim in an attempt to provide deeper insight into the issue under investigation. To dismiss and exclude quantitative research in the investigation of spirituality would be naïve. This is because such studies do shed light upon this important dimension for humankind (Baldacchino, 2002). The exploration of some of the quantitative characteristics affirms that using solely this approach to investigate the spiritual dimension may be problematic because it may fail to capture the essence of and meanings associated with the language of spirituality, thus supporting the need for qualitative inquiry. The following paragraphs present the reasons and arguments for selecting grounded theory as the preferred research method.

Rationale for grounded theory approach over other qualitative methods

When undertaking any research there is a fundamental need to assess and evaluate the approach and methods being used to question their suitability for a specific investigation. After spending considerable time in reading and developing my understanding of qualitative methods, and especially 'ethnomethodology', as this was the preliminary method considered, I began to feel a growing unease.

Garfinkel (1967 p. 11) writes:

> I use the term 'ethnomethodology' to refer to the investigation of the rational properties of indexical expressions and other practical actions as contingent ongoing accomplishments of organized artful practices of everyday life.

My interpretation of the literature suggested that the ethnomethodological approach seemed to focus predominantly upon the language that individuals use to describe their world. Yet the literature review revealed that there may be more to understanding spirituality than the language and descriptors used to define it. It seemed that there are many more variables to consider in relation to how individuals arrive at an understanding of spirituality; for example, cultural, religious and socio-political factors and the impact of illness and disease.

Another consideration was the need to understand why interest in spirituality had emerged within nursing and health care, again exploring possible reasons for this (for example discontentment with the scientific reductionist approach to individuals requiring health care and the subsequent emergence of the holistic movement). A purely ethnomethodological approach seemed too restrictive, and previous research using this method had been predominantly undertaken within social institutions such as prisons or schools. I also felt uncomfortable with the approach because there were some difficulties in trying to relate the main principles of ethnomethodology to the concept of spirituality – in reality it felt as if I were trying to put a square peg into a round hole. After discussing these concerns with my supervision team, I re-examined other forms of qualitative methods, identifying and deciding upon grounded theory, partially because this method had been employed successfully when investigating 'spirituality' and because I felt comfortable with the methodology in relation to its ability to meet the aims and objectives of the investigation.

Overview of grounded theory

Grounded theory was developed by Glaser and Strauss (1965, 1967, 1968) during work they carried out on death and dying, and, in particular, into how hospital staff interacted with dying patients. This influential research led to the publication of two classic books: *Awareness of Dying* (1965) and *Time for Dying* (1968).

Activity 4.2 The term 'grounded theory'

Spend a couple of minutes focusing upon on the term 'grounded theory'. Ask yourself:

What does this phrase or each of the words suggest to you about this research method?

Grounded theory is an approach to qualitative research in which the researcher develops a theoretical framework to allow understanding of a concept, via a cyclical process of reflection on, and analysis of, the ways in which that concept is used. This process is outlined in the book *The Discovery of Grounded Theory*, in which Glaser and Strauss (1967, p. 7) describe it as an attempt

> ... to strengthen the mandate for generating theory, to help provide a defense against doctrinaire approaches to verification, and to reawaken

and broaden the picture of what sociologists can do with their time and effort.

Grounded theory was a stimulus for new approaches to sociological research. Its development was a counterattack by sociologists upon the scientific community, demonstrating and defending the usefulness of qualitative approaches to research. In reality it was an attack upon the 'great man' theories that had dominated and shaped sociological research and thinking at that time. In addition, it was developed in response to claims by the scientific community that qualitative research was not systematic and lacked rigour (Corbin, 1997). McCann and Clark (2003a) provide a useful overview, tracing its development.

Grounded theory receives its name from the fact that any theory generated is derived from and grounded in data (Glaser and Strauss, 1967; Strauss and Corbin, 1998). It is a theoretical framework for generating theory through the ongoing interaction and interplay between data analysis and data collection. Chenitz and Swanson (1986, p. 3) affirm this when they write:

> Grounded theory is a highly systematic research approach for the collection and analysis of qualitative data for the purpose of generating theory that furthers understanding of social and psychological phenomena.

It could be argued that grounded theory seeks to incorporate many elements associated with scientific methods and is therefore positivistic in approach. Wells (1995) argues that, since the initial inception of grounded theory in the mid-1960s the approach has been refined and extended by its originators and their students.

Philosophical and theoretical underpinnings

Holloway and Wheller (1996) suggest that grounded theory is derived from the insights of Symbolic Interactionism. Mead (1934), who is considered to be the founder of this sociological position, recognised that the concepts of self, mind and society are not separate entities but are all interconnected and influence each other. Chenitz and Swanson (1986, p. 4) indicate that 'Symbolic interaction focuses upon the meaning of events for people in natural or everyday settings'. According to this view, individuals are not passive beings but have the power to shape and manipulate their own world. Bulmer (1971) points out that symbolic interactionism involves interpretations of the way in which an individual's actions are shaped by interaction with others, suggesting that the psychological and sociological contexts in which individuals live are important when considering their behaviour.

Kendall (1999) suggests that symbolic interactionism was developed as an alternative to the grand functionalist theories that had dominated sociological theory during the 19th and early 20th centuries. Functionalist theory operated around the premise that parts of a system have meaning only in relation to the whole. 'System' in a sociological sense refers to society, while subsystems could be family, politics, religion or culture. The role of an individual within society was to maintain the greater system or society. This perspective reduced the individual to a set of functions and processes with no real indication of the interplay and interaction that took place between individuals and the subsystems and how meanings can be perpetuated and transmitted throughout society and to subsequent generations. This limitation of functionalist theory led to the development of symbolic interactionism.

Central characteristics and processes of grounded theory

During the last 30 years grounded theory has not only become fashionable within the field of sociological research but has also been used within other disciplines, for example anthropology, psychology and more recently nursing (Holloway and Wheller, 1996; Wells, 1995). The features or characteristics that must be evident if qualitative research is to be classified as 'grounded theory' will be explored.

In nursing and the wider health care literature there are many articles that provide a descriptive overview of the characteristics and processes involved in grounded theory (Burns and Grove, 1997; Field and Morse, 1985; Holloway and Wheller, 1996; McCann and Clarke, 2003a,b,c, Morse and Field, 1996; Polit and Hungler, 1999). There also exist several scholarly texts (Denzin and Lincoln, 1998; Glaser, 1978; Strauss and Corbin, 1998) which describe in great detail the development and applications of grounded theory as a qualitative methodology. In describing the central characteristics and processes of grounded theory I will draw primarily on nursing and health-related literature.

Primary operations

Grounded theory has seven central characteristics, and the three primary operations commonly referred to are:

- theoretical sensitivity
- theoretical sampling
- constant comparative analysis

Table 4.2 McCann and Clark's (2003, p. 10) seven key characteristics of grounded theory.

- Theoretical sensitivity
- Theoretical sampling
- Constant comparative analysis
- Coding and categorising the data
- Theoretical memos and diagrams
- Literature as a source of data
- Integration of theory

McCann and Clark (2003a) suggest that there are indeed seven key characteristics (Table 4.2). However, closer analysis of these characteristics suggests that they may be accommodated or subsumed under the three primary operations. In addition, by highlighting the individual characteristics this can imply that grounded theory is a staged activity involving a number of unrelated activities, when in reality all these activities may be occurring simultaneously in a cyclical manner.

A brief outline of the three primary operations will now follow the remaining characteristics are discussed under the respective sections within the chapter.

- **Theoretical sensitivity** is about entering the field with an awareness of the key issues so that the researcher is able to give meaning to the data and separate the relevant from the irrelevant. Theoretical sensitivity is about researchers sensitising themselves to the key issues; this can be done through a preliminary review of the literature and by reflecting upon previous personal or professional experience. The emphasis of theoretical sensitivity is about sensitisation (being informed) and not about the researcher imposing an existing framework upon the data.
- **Theoretical sampling** is about the researcher collecting new data to compare emerging categories and properties. Categories are concepts that represent a phenomenon; for example, how people define spirituality. Properties are the characteristics of a category in the above example the properties could be synonymous with religion, supernatural forces/ghosts and ghouls. The properties help to explain and define the category. Theoretical sampling involves the researcher constantly making comparisons (Strauss and Corbin, 1998, p. 201), and as a result they may need to recruit different participants or visits different places in order to develop or test out emerging categories and their properties in order to identifying variations or similarities. This comparative exercise ensures that theoretical saturation

is reached. Strauss and Corbin (1998, p. 143) state that saturation 'is the point in category development at which no new properties, dimensions, or relationships emerge during analysis'. Theoretical sampling is cumulative because each participant adds to previous data collection and analysis thus contributing to theory construction and testing.

- **Constant comparative analysis** is the main approach to data collection, analysis and theory generation. It involves the researcher unearthing the categories and their related properties. The constant comparative method helps the researcher to make comparisons across categories and participant groups (for example, how people from different world religions define spirituality), asking whether there are any marked differences or similarities. The constant comparative method enables a theory to be generated through integrating categories and their properties. In reality, the constant comparative method is a tool which assists the researcher in the creation and writing of the final theory.

This section has provided an overview of the emergence of the grounded theory method, discussing what grounded theory is and what are considered to be the primary operations or key characteristics of grounded theory. A brief explanation of the three primary operations (theoretical sensitivity, theoretical sampling and constant comparative analysis) was presented.

Description of grounded theory, with pros and cons

This section provides a further exploration of what constitutes grounded theory, examining some of the pros and cons of this qualitative method. Grounded theory is again defined, the primary operations are explored in more detail and the relationship and relevance to this investigation are outlined. In addition, the different schools of grounded theory are detailed and some of the methodological concerns associated with this method are discussed.

Definitions of grounded theory

All the definitions offered (Table 4.3) indicate that grounded theory involves a series of systematic, deliberate stages and conscious actions or manipulations on behalf of the grounded theorist. It would appear that such actions are necessary if the research process is to be managed effectively and for the emerging theory to be complete and accurate. These definitions reveal that grounded theory consists of a series of systematic processes and interactions between

Table 4.3 Definitions of grounded theory.

Glaser (1978, p. 2)	'Grounded theory is based on the systematic generating of theory from data, that itself is systematically obtained from social research. Thus the grounded theory method offers a rigorous, orderly guide to theory development that at each stage is closely integrated with a methodology of social research'
Strauss and Corbin (1998, p. 12)	'They mean theory derived from data, systematically gathered and analyzed throughout the research process.'
Strauss and Corbin (1998, p. 158–9)	'Grounded theory is a general methodology for developing theory that is grounded in data systematically gathered and analyzed', arguing that 'A central feature of this analytic approach is "a general method [constant] comparative analysis" (Glaser and Strauss, 1967, p. vii)'

the researcher, data and emerging theory. Thus grounded theory involves the grounded theorist interacting with the social context in which the data is collected.

Analysis of the definitions reveals why it has particular relevance when investigating the area of spirituality. Firstly, the methodology may be useful in testing or refining established theory around spirituality. Secondly, grounded theory is successful in generating new theory or interpreting theory derived from the natural world of individuals and participants. This point is particularly important when trying to establish how spirituality may be understood by diverse groups.

The emphasis placed on the sequential and structured nature implies that the method could be perceived as being very inflexible, causing one to focus more on process rather than creativity. However, this position seems to be in opposition to and contradicts the 'guiding principles' advocated by Glaser and Strauss (1967) who present grounded theory not as a rigid, inflexible method or a method with a specific series of dots that need to be joined. Rather, the pioneers present grounded theory as a qualitative method still very much in its infancy, a form of inquiry that offers a flexible analytical framework for the generation of theory grounded in the data.

In grounded theory the researcher is continuously involved (active), familiar and immersed in every stage of the research process. However, particular emphasis and attention seem to be placed on three primary 'operations': data collection, sampling and theory development.

Primary operations

The 'primary operations' are more commonly known as theoretical sensitivity, theoretical sampling and the constant comparative method of data analysis. The 'operations' are interconnected, occurring simultaneously throughout the research process. They provide a theoretical and procedural framework around which data can be obtained and theory developed. Each of the *'operations'* will be discussed in more detail because they are fundamental to the conducting of a grounded theory inquiry and they are central to and instrumental in developing this thesis. The first operation, 'theoretical sensitivity', was discussed (Chapter 2, Part II). Theoretical sampling and the constant comparative method of data analysis will be explored later in this chapter.

A theme running through the primary operations, and possibly one that is pivotal to all theory development, is the notion of 'reflexivity' (outlined in this chapter). In grounded theory terms, this is an expectation, not an optional extra. This activity permeates the entire research process in the form of procedural, theoretical memo writing; for example, reflecting upon emerging themes and asking questions in order to open up a line of inquiry or to direct theoretical sampling (Strauss and Corbin, 1998).

Reflexivity is the expectation that the grounded theorist needs to suspend previous assumptions and involvement in a specific area. This means that the emerging theory is free from preconceptions and bias. This was particularly important because, as previously indicated, I had undertaken extensive writing and research into this area. Therefore it was imperative that, whilst being theoretically sensitive to some of the debates surrounding spirituality within health care, I did not let this 'prior experience' cloud my judgements or make me formulate preconceived judgements and speculations about what theory was emerging.

Grounded theory, as a methodology, alerted me to this potential pitfall while at the same time accommodating the fact that I am a social being (spiritual being) who creates and recreates social processes. Therefore, previous experience can be included as data and not totally dismissed (Baker *et al.*, 1992). This method of qualitative research, whilst accepting my previous experiences, ensured that I guarded constantly against personal bias by using reflection and introspection.

Schools of grounded theory

In relation to grounded theory inquiry it has been contended that there are now two distinct schools of grounded theory, namely the 'Glaserian' and 'Straussian' or the 'Columbian' or 'Chicago' schools of inquiry. Therefore, one school is based upon its founder (Glaser) while the other is based predominantly upon the work of Strauss. Stern (1994) suggests that the difference in thought centres on the way that the two sociologists view data management and analysis. The Glaserian schools advocate that the grounded theorist must stay true to the data and allow the emergent data to guide theory development. The Straussian school appears to be more conceptually driven or focused with regard to data analysis and interpretation. It adds a further stage, termed 'axial coding', which allows the grounded theorists to make speculations and projections surrounding emerging categories which may then be represented by a paradigm model.

The two contrasting approaches to undertaking grounded theory can confuse the novice grounded theorist and present a dilemma as to which school one should follow. However, closer inspection of the differences in the schools reveals that both may be appropriate. If one solely followed the Glaserian school then a consequence could be a loss of creativity and reflexivity when applied to data analysis, which may lead to premature saturation of categories. However, the notion of adhering to the principles and ideals of the methodology cannot be dismissed. It may be that Glaser is not advocating a form of 'purist' research but is alerting the research community to potential dangers to the initial discovery and underlying methodology principles if one 'strays too far from the path'. Alternatively, strict adherence to the 'Straussian' school may mean that the grounded theorist could be overwhelmed by data, or even misrepresent what the data is revealing, through forcing the data to fit a preconceived 'paradigm model'. The dangers of adhering too rigidly to this approach are described by Kendall (1999) in her study investigating families living with a child who suffers from attention deficit hyperactivity disorder.

The net result of this 'academic argument' is that individuals who consider utilising this method are now unsure as to exactly what is meant by grounded theory. This academic rivalry and uncertainty may have resulted in the methodology being diluted or inappropriately undertaken. Rather than being accused of 'inaccuracy' individual researchers will report that they have used a 'modified' methodology (Smith and Bailey, 1997, p. 26).

The subsequent dilemma for grounded theorists as to which school to follow at the outset of the study, be it Glaserian or Straussian, may have ramifications later in the research study. This is evident in the writings of Norton (1999, p. 35):

> Initially, I felt clear about my aims in terms of data analysis and theory generation. I had researched the process of grounded theory generation thoroughly, and to avoid 'muddling' methods had decided to follow the Glaserian School of grounded theory. However, as I began the process of open and theoretical coding I realised that I was not actually interpreting the data but considering it in a descriptive sense. As the penny

> dropped as to what I should have been doing, I began coding and categorising again, but with a more analytic eye. On reflection, my initial limited analysis was related to a concern that I should be interpreting, categorising and theorising in the right way.

Johnson *et al.* (2001, p. 247), in their paper exploring 'Arguments for "British Pluralism" in qualitative health research', conclude their discussion surrounding grounded theory with the statement: 'but the key point is that there is no "final" version, no one approach which we "must" follow to achieve rigour'. If this recommendation were to be taken literally it would appear that there is no authoritative version of grounded theory. However, to avoid being too descriptive when undertaking data analysis and to guard against 'method slurring', (Baker *et al.*, 1992), I felt the need to be aware of the controversy and criticisms that surrounded both schools of grounded theory. By developing this awareness I was able to suspend making rash and arbitrary decisions. Instead, I was guided by the research question and data analysis, which seems to be the recommended approach to handling this position (Kendall, 1999).

Methodological concerns

As previously stated, with the growing popularity of grounded theory as a form of qualitative inquiry concerns are now emerging that the method is becoming diluted and, seemingly, less rigorous. This loss of rigour arises when individuals who profess to use this method do so only in half measures, not completing all the systematic stages, with the result that no theory is developed (Strauss and Corbin, 1998).

Authors have commented also on the difficulties that some researchers may experience when applying, or adhering to, some of the theoretical constructs of the grounded theory method. Wells (1995) identifies two critical issues concerning the implementation and subsequent evaluation of grounded theory. She suggests that researchers may focus predominantly upon psychological explanations for theory development and not social theory, which was the intended purpose of the method. With respect to evaluation, this may be problematic in the sense that many researchers fail to complete the method due to an inability to identify a core concept that explains all the variability in the generated theory.

Further areas of debate that the novice grounded theorist needs to be aware of are associated with the nature and pragmatics of the method. Cutcliffe (2000) discusses several methodological issues that surround the nature and process of grounded theory, including sampling, creativity and reflexivity, the use of literature and precision. He encourages those proposing to use this method to familiarise themselves with the conflicting opinions that surround these areas.

Coyne (1997, p. 629) analyses the three main forms of sampling that are commonly used in qualitative research: selective, purposeful and theoretical sampling. She concludes that all qualitative sampling methods can be described as purposeful in that the sample is always chosen 'according to the needs of the study'. However, Coyne is always careful in distinguishing theoretical sampling from selective and purposeful sampling methods and suggests it to be more complex and always 'dictated by the data and the emerging theory'. The confusion that surrounds the different forms of sampling and the interchangeability with which such terms are used can be very misleading when embarking on any form of qualitative research.

How grounded theory best addresses the study aim and objectives

Despite some of the above philosophical and methodological considerations, grounded theory was selected because of the following primary features and their potential to achieve the studies aim and objectives.

Firstly, because of the importance placed upon 'theoretical sensitivity' and 'theoretical sampling' these concepts provided opportunities that enabled me to experience the discourse, story and situation as perceived by each participant, taking into account their different social contexts.

Secondly, because of the emphasis upon the constant comparative method, grounded theory has the potential to provide rich data that may provide deeper insight into the phenomena of spirituality as understood by diverse groups. As the literature review revealed, there is a pressing need for existing theory associated with the conceptual and theoretical nature of spirituality and spiritual care to be challenged and refined. The benefit of using this method to test out existing theory is outlined by Glaser and Strauss (1967, p. 4) when they say:

> Grounded Theory can help forestall the opportunistic use of theories that have dubious fit and working capacity

Thirdly, the entire philosophical and theoretical framework of grounded theory, with its links to symbolic interactionism, felt right and suited the investigation of spirituality. The rationale for this is that symbolic interactionism acknowledges the interconnectedness of the individual with many different dimensions. This approach is reflected in some of the theories and models addressing spirituality (Reed, 1992; Stoll, 1989).

Table 4.4 Appealing characteristics of grounded theory.

- Philosophical bases of grounded theory, derived from symbolic interactionism
- Ability to test existing theoretical positions
- **Flexible methodology**
- **Appropriate to practice**
- **Systematic processes and 'similarity to the nursing process'**
- **Constant comparative method of theory development**

Discussion of appealing characteristics of grounded theory

In addition to the three primary features of grounded theory there are four other appealing characteristics of the methodology that had significance for this investigation (Table 4.4). Items highlighted in bold will be discussed in a little more detail within the following section.

Flexible methodology

Glaser and Strauss (1967, p. 31) suggest that using grounded theory as a research method need not necessarily be restrictive or purist in approach. This is evident in the following quotation from their classic book *The Discovery of Grounded Theory: Strategies for Qualitative Research*:

> Grounded theory, it should be mentioned, may take different forms. And although we consider the *process* of generating theory as related to its subsequent use and effectiveness, the *form* in which the theory is presented can be dependent of the process by which it was generated. Grounded theory can be presented either as a well-codified set of propositions or in a running theoretical discussion, using conceptual categories and their properties

This quotation from the pioneers of grounded theory suggests that the researcher or 'grounded theorist' is not bound by a methodological straitjacket. Therefore studies employing this method may not be identical and variation will be evident. This is evident in the growing number of research studies within nursing that have used this method (Wainwright, 1993; Burkhardt, 1994; Walton, 1997). However, the quote does highlight two key words, 'processes' and 'form', which imply that the grounded theorist must give due consideration to primary operations described earlier. Flexibility was important because it enabled me to be creative and open-minded in terms of meeting the primary operations of grounded theory.

Appropriate to clinical practice

One major reason for selecting grounded theory was that this approach has the potential to generate a theory of spirituality which is derived from the reality of nursing and health care practice. The potential for grounded theory inquiry in enhancing patient care and in advancing the nursing profession has been documented (Benton, 2000). Sheldon (1999, p. 47) proposes grounded theory to have the potential to highlight discrepancies in the theory–practice gap, while the construction of theories at a social level 'will advance practice and enhance patient care'. It would appear that current understandings of spirituality are derived from academic study or theoretical propositions that have been unsubstantiated in practice. Oldnall (1995, p. 418) supports this claim when he writes:

> Perhaps one reason why nursing models and theories do not appear to work in clinical practice is because they have evolved in the echelons of academia and have been devolved down to the practitioners to operationalize at a clinical level. This may explain, to some degree, why the concept of spirituality has been omitted totally, or at least not developed sufficiently, in existing theories and models.

Oldnall implies that there is a need for a theory or a model of spirituality to be developed from within the realms of practice. Oldnall (1995, 1996) suggests that there needs to be a paradigm shift in the way that theory is developed. McSherry reinforces this (2006, p. 79), writing:

> Models should not be solely developed in the 'ivory towers of academia' then be expected to work in practice. This top down approach to theory development may overlook and fail to incorporate many issues that are being faced by nurses working on the front line. This approach may have led to the spiritual dimension from being incorporated within contemporary nursing theories and models.

It appears that the contemporary issues surrounding the practical implications and applications arising from some of the conceptual and theoretical bases of spirituality that have been developed need to be tested, substantiated and refined. This process of testing and refining will assist nurses and the allied health professions to understand more fully the conceptual and theoretical base of spirituality at two levels, individually and collectively, when applied to practice.

Systematic processes and 'similarity to the nursing process'

Grounded theory has been described as a series of systematic processes for the generation and testing out of data. As stated earlier, perhaps one attraction of this approach to many professional disciplines is that this form of qualitative inquiry now has a number of texts available that discuss, and almost guide the novice researcher through, every stage of the process. The availability of such texts, combined with the systematic structure, offers a form of security in that reference can always be made to the 'manuals' should a problem arise or a dilemma be encountered. However, this may be a false sense of security in that the instructions available may be contradictory, misleading or imprecise, depending on the sources used. These concerns have been expressed in several publications regarding the grounded theory approach (Anderson, 1991; Backman and Kyngas, 1999). Stern (1994) warns that 'book learners' may fall victim to generational erosion: that is, their reports suffer from incompleteness. They urge all would-be grounded theorists to obtain a suitable mentor in the method.

Perhaps a further reason why this qualitative method has become popular within nursing is because of the similarity that the systematic structure has to using a problem-solving approach or systematic approach to care, commonly referred to as the 'nursing process'. Reflecting on my own reasons for using this method, these two factors did influence my decision. Firstly, I felt that there were sufficient guidelines available and other published studies for reference and clarification. Secondly, I felt comfortable and at ease working with parameters and guidelines to shape and focus the direction of the study alongside data analysis.

Constant comparative methods

Benton (2000) argues that the constant comparative method is at the heart of grounded theory and that the principal method of data analysis is used in theory development. The constant comparative method involves the theorist making comparison of an incident with another incident as data is collected. These comparisons enable the development of categories and their related properties. This type of investigation was felt necessary to test out existing theory and to establish new perspectives or theories into how 'spirituality' is perceived by individuals from diverse groups that hold perhaps quite disparate worldviews. This need has been recognised within the nursing and health care literature (Walter, 1997, 2002; Draper and McSherry, 2002; Swinton and Narayanasamy, 2002; Henery, 2003). With a focus upon the constant comparative analysis method the nature of grounded theory inquiry would allow existing conceptual and theoretical positions to be compared in an integrated manner as the research progressed.

Summary points

- This overview of grounded theory highlights that this form of qualitative inquiry is far from simple and 'perfect'. Indeed, it may be more complex and rigorous than other forms of qualitative methods, with the emphasis upon theoretical sampling, theoretical sensitivity and the constant comparative method.
- The discussion has also indicated potential 'pitfalls' that the neophyte grounded theorist must consider when utilising this form of qualitative inquiry.
- It has been demonstrated that grounded theory inquiry will assist in testing existing theory while generating new knowledge and insights into the concepts of 'spirituality' and 'spiritual care'. Given the nature of grounded theory inquiry, these insights will be derived from, and based upon, the individual participant's own worldview. Consequently, the theory constructed will be based in, and derived from, the real world of the participants.
- The findings of the data analysis will form the basis for new dialogue and debate, generating questions and possible hypotheses for further research.

Selection of the sample

Introduction

This section will present a rationale for the selection of the sample. Firstly, a discussion surrounding theoretical sampling, covering such areas as types of theoretical sampling and the use of comparison groups within grounded theory research, will be outlined. Next, the procedures, such as inclusion and exclusion criteria, setting and sample size relating specifically to the actual sample, will be summarised. Finally, consideration will be given to obtaining the actual sample, discussing questionnaire design and accessing the research population.

Activity 4.3 Selecting a study sample

To ensure that the findings of a research study are representative, what points might you consider when selecting your sample? Jot down your responses so that these can be revisited as you read the reminder of this section.

Theoretical sampling

There are several important features of theoretical sampling that were pertinent to this research study. Firstly, theoretical sampling, rather than being viewed as a method of sampling, is presented as a philosophical underpinning which influences the entire research process. Secondly, the different levels and variations of this method will be explored and the positive gains of using theoretical sampling will be discussed. Thirdly, some of the limitations experienced while using theoretical sampling will be explored.

Initial considerations when undertaking theoretical sampling

Strauss and Corbin (1998, p. 204) provide an overview of 'initial considerations' that the researcher may contemplate in relation to theoretical sampling. These are site and group of study, type of data to be collected, and how long an area should be studied; finally, they provide a summary:

> Initially, decisions regarding the number of sites and observations and/or interviews depends on access, available resources, research goals, and the researcher's time schedule and energy.

This quotation demonstrates that theoretical sampling involves the researcher using his or her own discretion to reflect upon the intrinsic forces (arising from within the researcher/study) and extrinsic forces (arising from within the institution/group) that could impact either positively or negatively upon the sampling procedure. It implies that theoretical sampling is not predetermined at the outset of the study, but that it is constantly evolving and progressing to ensure that the aim of the research is achieved and emerging theory is saturated (Glaser, 1978).

Theoretical sampling as a philosophical underpinning

Rather than focusing upon theoretical sampling as an isolated component within the research process, only concerning issues associated with sample selection, it is more helpful and beneficial to the grounded theorist to see theoretical sampling as a 'philosophical underpinning' which guides and infiltrates all aspects of the research study. If one adopts the first position then the entire research process is viewed, and to some degree managed, in discrete units, or sequential stages, adopting a 'reductionist' approach. A 'reductionist' mentality seems to oppose the original intention of theoretical sampling.

One influential definition is that offered by Glaser and Strauss (1967, p. 45):

> ... the process of data collection for generating theory whereby the analyst jointly collects, codes and analyses his data decides what data to collect next and where to find them, in order to develop his theory as it emerges.

Glaser and Strauss do not view theoretical sampling in a 'reductionist' sense but suggest that theoretical sampling is integrated, permeating every aspect of the research process. The quotation provided supports the position that theoretical sampling, rather than being seen as an isolated or discrete activity, provides a philosophical underpinning for every stage of the grounded theorist's activity. Therefore, theoretical sampling is concerned with the nature of the research and guides and governs all methodological decisions and processes. If theoretical sampling is used as intended, it will ultimately determine the depth and level of the theory developed.

Theoretical sampling was used in this study to maximise and address evolving theory. The sample was selected to clarify concepts that had arisen from the data analysis and which mirrored the evolving theory (Coyne, 1997). As a result of using theoretical sampling, a number of groups with differing worldviews and with diverse religious affiliations participated in the study. Theoretical sampling, as discussed earlier, provided the study with flexibility throughout data collection and ongoing analysis (Glaser and Strauss, 1967). This flexibility was important because it provided scope to discover ideas and connections in the emerging data whilst ensuring that all aspects of the developing categories and theories were covered within and across all groups.

Levels and variations of theoretical sampling

Strauss and Corbin (1998) imply that theoretical sampling operates on the following principle. Initially the researcher will sample broadly to maximise data collection, ensuring that all potential areas are included in the analysis. This type of sampling is referred to as 'open sampling'. Strauss and Corbin (1998) provide four variations of open sampling (Table 4.5).

Three of the four variations of open sampling were utilised throughout the different phases involved in this study. Initially, a small number of nurses and patients were interviewed and the tapes were transcribed and analysed. Each interview added to the emerging categories and themes. This in turn led to the recruitment of more participants into the study, resulting in Phase II and Phase III and the need to utilise the other forms of theoretical sampling: *relational*, *variational* and, finally, *discriminate sampling*.

Relational and variational sampling

As the research progressed and I became more experienced, immersed and 'theoretically sensitive' to the emerging categories and themes, the theoretical sampling became more focused and purposeful. This focusing, which Strauss and Corbin (1998) define as '*relational*' and '*variational*' sampling, ensured that the relationships between emerging codes, categories and themes were explored. This form of sampling ensured potential saturation of themes. The

Table 4.5 Variations of open sampling offered by Strauss and Corbin (1998).

- The researcher may look for particular people, sites or events, where he or she can purposefully gather data related to categories and their properties and dimensions.
- The researcher may systematically identify individuals from a list, going from one person to the next. Or open sampling may be random and based on chance; that is, whoever walks through the door or agrees to participate in the project.
- The researcher, while out in the field, stumbles upon an event, person or situation that may be theoretically significant to the emergent data.
- The researcher returns to the data, reorganising them to identify theoretically relevant concepts.

latter was achieved by recruiting into the sample specific individuals who might assist in maximising differences or similarities within the categories, thus allowing the emerging theory to be shaped and developed. This form of sampling was used predominantly throughout Phase II of the study, when individuals were invited into the study in order to address questions or issues that had come to light either while interviewing or during the analysis of transcripts. This point can be illustrated by the following example. The sampling profiles indicated that, following analysis, there was a need to talk to nurses and patients with a religious belief and those with no religious belief.

Discriminate sampling

As data analysis progressed, sampling became more focused to maximise opportunities for constant comparative analysis. Strauss and Corbin (1998, p. 211) suggest that, at this point, sampling becomes deliberate. This may mean:

> returning to old sites, persons or going to new ones to gather data necessary to saturate categories and complete the study.

This quotation suggests a need to revisit certain sites or groups of people in order to validate incoming data and interpretations. This form of discriminate sampling occurred throughout Phase III of the study. An example of this was the need to revisit Area I in order to maximise saturation of categories and themes.

Summary points

- The three different types and levels of theoretical sampling – initial, selective and discriminate – enabled me to refine and develop the theory.
- Having awareness about the different types of sampling and their purpose enabled me to evaluate constantly the direction of the study to ensure that maximum saturation of categories and themes was achieved.
- The three levels of theoretical sampling allowed me to plan and manage the coding procedures: initial, axial and selective.
- The three phases of the study were guided by the sampling procedures. This focus upon the data meant that the theory generated reflected more accurately what was happening in the field, rather than reflecting my own preconceptions of what I thought should be emerging (Glaser, 1978, p. 38).

Limitations of using theoretical sampling

Whilst undertaking theoretical sampling within this study two difficulties were experienced. Firstly, there is the argument that the researcher is unable to provide a clear profile of individuals participating within the study. Secondly, the researcher is unsure about which groups to recruit in order to develop theory.

The first issue may prove to be a major stumbling block for researchers that propose to utilise this method. Strauss and Corbin (1998), when discussing predetermining the number of participants, accept that the researcher does not have 'prior' knowledge about the number of individuals to be recruited into the study because this cannot be determined before data collection commences. However, many research and ethics committees will not accept proposals for research without some indication of the potential numbers to be involved in the research. The predetermined number of participants that was requested by the two local research committees is presented (Table 4.6). However, the figures that are highlighted bear no resemblance to the final groups recruited into this grounded theory investigation to address the emerging theory. Suffice to say,

Table 4.6 Proposed number of participants.

Nurses	No.
Qualified nurses (acute areas medical)	5
Qualified chronic	5
Qualified Hospice	5
Qualified nurses with no religious belief	5
Qualified nurses with a religious belief	5
?Nurse educators (With a religious and non-religious belief)	5
TOTAL	30
Patients	
Acute areas (medical surgical)	5
Chronic conditions	5
Hospice	5
Non-religious belief	5
Religious belief (differing religions)	5
TOTAL	25

these figures presented were used as a means of satisfying committees, demonstrating that the predetermining of groups does not fit the grounded theory inquiry.

In discussing the second difficulty encountered, theoretical sampling suggests that participants should be selected according to the emerging theory. Theoretical sampling seems to make two assumptions. Firstly, individuals who are asked to participate in the study will possess the required characteristics to advance the emerging theory. Secondly, the researcher has some 'prior knowledge' about where to find such individuals or groups that may lead him or her to believe that they are the correct person(s) to further develop the emerging theory. The question that seems to be arising is which groups or individuals should participate so that detailed comparisons can be made.

Using comparison groups

Glaser and Strauss (1967, p. 48), when discussing the selection of comparison groups in theoretical sampling, provide a possible solution when considering which groups to include. Rather than thinking in terms of 'comparability' of groups they introduce the term 'theoretical purpose and relevance', which can be defined as the extent to which particular group(s) will further develop properties and categories. They argue that these criteria help to maintain a systematic but flexible control over data collection and analysis unlike other forms of 'comparative group' research where controlled comparison of groups and individuals seems paramount and where the control of participants entering the study with similar characteristics is fundamental. By adopting these two criteria, the uncertainties around where to identify and locate the next group were addressed and the focus was placed on theory development rather than trying to compare and match groups. However, this comparison of participants did take place initially, but it was not seen as important or crucial to theory development as the study progressed.

Reflections surrounding theoretical sampling

Reflecting upon the three forms or levels of theoretical sampling used in this investigation suggests that there is some overlap because there is no real demarcation distinguishing each type from the other. The form of theoretical sampling used is determined by the questions to be addressed, the stage of the study and ultimately the quality of the theory to be produced. Closer inspection of theoretical sampling suggests that the researcher purposefully and deliberately recruits individuals into the study to meet the needs of the developing theory. Like Coyne (1997), it could be argued that this approach resembles other forms of sampling procedures used in qualitative research.

On a positive note, theoretical sampling afforded me with flexibility allowing creativity during data analysis. It provided a framework around which the study could be conducted, accommodating economical and other constraints experienced during the course of data collection; for example, access, recruitment of individuals from different world religions and logistical problems associated with travel to sites. Therefore, it would appear that the 'ideal form of theoretical sampling may be difficult to carry out' (Strauss and Corbin, 1998, p. 210). For that reason, many of the decisions made during the sampling procedure were determined by what was available and at my disposal. Strauss and Corbin (1998, p. 210) acknowledge the difficulties in achieving the ideal form of theoretical sampling and offer reassurance: 'Realistically, the researcher might have to sample on the basis of what is available'. There were several points during the course of this study where this principle was applied.

Actual sampling inclusion/exclusion criteria

The following section provides a detailed overview of the individuals recruited and interviewed during the course of the study. In the following paragraphs I will explore the reasons and purposes for using specific groups in this grounded theory inquiry. Key questions will be addressed – 'who' was recruited, 'why' they were recruited and 'where' they were recruited. This section will also explore the inclusion and exclusion criteria that were applied to the groups.

This research involved three distinct populations or groups, these being HCPs, patients, and the public. It must be stressed that initially only nurses and patients were going to be recruited. However, after the ongoing literature review and during data collection, especially during Phase III, this decision was revised so that the emerging theory could be validated and refined on a number of subgroups. This meant that a number of HCPs who were perceived by participants as being central to the provision of spiritual care were recruited into the investigation. Representatives from the major world religions were recruited during Phase I and Phase III. The primary reason for selecting these three target populations was to enable constant comparative analysis to be undertaken. Having a broad range of participants is supported by Morse and Field (1996, p. 129), who suggest: 'There must be an adequate range of participants to provide a full range of variations in the phenomenon so that definitions and meanings are grounded in the data'.

By having a broad range of participants would ensure that the concept of spirituality is explored in depth, accommodating a broad range of social groups and contexts and accommodating diverse understandings.

Participant groups

Nurses

Qualified nurses working in hospice and acute care settings were recruited. The rationale for selecting these two key specialities of nursing was to establish whether there were any similarities or differences in the way nurses working in either area viewed 'spirituality' and provided spiritual care. The nursing sample could also be broken down further by grade. Comparisons could also be made within and across the different specialities: for example, nurses working on medical wards, surgical wards or intensive care units. The reason for only interviewing qualified nurses was that, in essence, it is the qualified nurses who are responsible and accountable for assessing, planning and evaluating nursing care, which one would assume involves a holistic approach. Further, economic constraints meant that restrictions had to be made, indicating a need to focus the study by concentrating only upon qualified nurses. However, I am very much aware that unqualified nursing and ancillary staff do have an important contribution to make in the delivery of all nursing care, including spiritual care (McSherry, 1997; Narayanasamy, 2001). This point was validated during the course of the investigation.

To ensure that the nursing sample was initially representative and similar across all three geographical areas, I tried to identify and match the profiles in all areas in terms of age, gender, grade and working hours (Appendix 1, Tables A1.1–A1.3). Appendix 1 provides demographic information taken from the recruitment questionnaire completed by some of the participants who agreed to partake in the investigation. The rationales for constructing and using the questionnaire are outlined later in the section *'Obtaining the sample'*.

Patients

Patients were recruited from the same geographical locations and specialities from which the nursing samples were drawn (Appendix 1, Table A1.4). One important reason for this was to establish if there were any discrepancies or similarities between the way that nursing staff and patients understood the term 'spirituality' and 'spiritual care'. The patients who participated in this study presented with a range of diverse health problems: acute, ranging from routine orthopaedic surgery to investigations for anaemia; chronic illnesses, including diabetes, respiratory disease, Parkinson's disease; and terminal illnesses. Several patients were diagnosed as suffering from a range of terminal cancers, for example lung, prostate and breast.

World religions

The aim of this investigation was to establish whether the concept of spirituality was universal in the sense that, as a concept, it may be recognisable and have relevance to individuals from diverse religious groups. Recruitment of nurses and patients was homogeneous in the sense that the dominant religion was 'Christianity', with wide denominational variation. Active steps were taken to ensure that the views of all of the major religions to be found in Area II were represented in the investigation. This resulted in individuals being recruited from the following world religions: Islam (2), Hinduism (1), Sikhism (1), Judaism (1) and Buddhism (1). For demographic information pertaining to some participants in this group, see Appendix 1, Table A1.5.

Health care professionals

Most of the allied health professions were recruited into the investigation during Phase III, with the exception of medicine. The professions represented were social work (1), physiotherapy (2), occupational therapy (1) and chaplaincy (7). Again, because of economic constraints, individuals were recruited from the two locations (Area I and Area II) within easy travel distance. The allied health professionals were asked to complete the recruitment questionnaire. For demographic information pertaining to participants in this group see Appendix 1, Table A1.6. The decision not to include representation from the different specialities within medicine warrants some attention. There is a growing realisation within the medical profession of the importance of spirituality to an individual's health, sense of well-being and ultimately quality of life. This omission means that the perceptions of one of the largest professional groups in relation to understanding spirituality and their role in the provision of spiritual care are not represented within this study. Therefore the findings cannot be applied to all professional groups.

General public

'Public' is used as a general term that refers to any participants who were neither patients nor members of any of the allied health professions. This meant that several of the representatives from the major world religions could be classified as 'public' because they were undertaking valuable volunteer roles. Similarly, three individuals who were recruited into the 'world religion' group were carrying out professional roles and vice versa.

> **Reflective question**
>
> What type of inclusion and exclusion criteria might you need to develop when investigating the area of spirituality?

Inclusion and exclusion criteria

Several inclusion and exclusion criteria were established at the outset of the study and these were applied consistently throughout the investigation (Table 4.7). These criteria were felt to be necessary to manage the research process, giving consideration to the economic constraints and logistical problems associated with potential identification and recruitment of some of the participant groups. Care and attention were given when constructing these criteria to ensure that they did not impact upon the potential quality of the data to be collected and the overall credibility and transferability of the findings. The criteria were established to maximise participation while setting parameters that were realistic and fair. These criteria enhanced the quality of the investigation by providing a framework for assessing the suitability of participants to be involved in the investigation.

Table 4.7 Summary of inclusion and exclusion criteria.

Inclusion criteria	Exclusion criteria
Participants aged over 18	Patients aged less than 18
English-speaking	Individuals who could not speak fluent English
Patients hospitalised for more than 48 hours	Patients who had not been in hospital for over 48 hours
Patients admitted to areas/wards participating in the research	Emergency and some acute medical/surgical departments
No acute or chronic mental health conditions	Individuals with acute/chronic mental health conditions
Permission and approval given by consultant providing care for their patients to participate for Area II	Nurses who were not ward-based or working in the inpatient facilities at the hospice
In relation to Area I, patients attending the outpatient/day centre facilities	Student nurses and health care assistants

Patients aged less than 18 years were excluded to avoid issues surrounding parental or guardian consent. However, it was considered that a younger population might present a different perception of spirituality if one considers spiritual development across a lifespan (Carson, 1989). Patients who are not able to speak 'fluent' English were also excluded from the study. The rationale for this criterion was purely economic, in that the cost of identifying, coordinating and indeed employing translators was beyond the finances available.

Patients who were invited to participate must have been in hospital for at least 48 hours or attending the hospice on a regular basis, and therefore having had the opportunity to reflect upon their admission and possible reasons for hospitalisation, and having experience of the type of care that HCPs provided. In light of these variables, consideration needed to be given to the speciality or location from which patients and nurses were to be recruited. It was felt that patients attending emergency and some acute medical/surgical services would not be eligible for inclusion. Given the nature of the interviews and subject matter to be discussed, patients with any form of mental health problem or organic degenerative disease (for example dementia or individuals experiencing any form of acute psychotic episode) were also excluded from the study.

Setting

The research study was carried out within three different institutions located in two different geographical regions in the north of England (Table 4.8). One hospice (Area I) and one large Acute National Health Service Trust (Area III) were in the same region. Area II, also an Acute National Health Service Trust, was selected because of the potential for patients and nurses to be recruited from diverse ethnic groups. To maintain the anonymity of these areas, more specific detail concerning location, for example city, cannot be provided, as this would allow the areas to be easily recognised.

The rationale for selecting a hospice was because of the historical association of spirituality with the hospice movement and because the literature addressing spirituality seemed to suggest that such issues may emerge when individuals are facing death (Rumbold, 2002; Cobb, 2001; Murray and Zent-

Table 4.8 Overview of areas.

Area I	Hospice
Area II	Acute National Health Service Trust – two hospitals used Two specialities: medical (2 wards), intensive care units (1 unit)
Area III	Acute National Health Service Trust – one hospital used Three specialities: medical (1 ward), surgical (3 wards), intensive care units (2 units)

ner, 1989). Caution must be exercised here because I am aware that the hospice does not only meet the needs of the patient living with life-limiting illness, but also offers specialist palliative care, for example pain management and symptom control, to individuals with a range of life-threatening illnesses. Therefore patients recruited into the study through the hospice might well have experience of care provision within both hospice and acute care settings. This was especially evident in one patient's transcript (P14 (Patient, I)):

> You get care in the hospice because you are important to them and there are fewer numbers. In a hospital you are getting medical treatment plus a bit of food.

Reflective question

When conducting a qualitative study do you think it is important to have a large sample size?

Sample size

The question of sample size was guided by the theory underpinning 'theoretical sampling'. That is, there can be no predetermined figure of the number of individuals to be recruited. Holloway and Wheller (1996, p. 78) suggest that a large sample size is not necessary in qualitative research. They indicate that experienced researchers and students usually have to present predetermined and large samples 'to appease' research committees who may know very little about qualitative research. This situation did arise in this investigation and was the main reason for the production of Table 4.6.

Instead, theory development and analysis determined 'when' and 'where' to recruit further participants into the study. This approach is in keeping with that recommended by Strauss and Corbin (1998, p. 292) when they write:

> For most theory-building researchers, data collection continues 'until theoretical saturation takes place.' This simply means (within the limits of available time and money) that the researcher finds that no new data are being unearthed. Any new data would only add, in a minor way, to the many variations of major patterns.

The notion of sample size seems to be a measure of the credibility of a research study, especially within the scientific paradigm where statistical analysis determines the level of confidence in a particular result or research finding. However, it would appear that sample size is an area of debate and uncertainty in both quantitative and qualitative research. Quantitative research is governed by scientific probability-sampling methods, while qualitative studies are guided by non-probability sampling. The net effect of this uncertainty and ambiguity is that most research texts describe in great detail issues associated with what constitutes an adequate sample with respect to quantitative research, but fail to adequately address what would be deemed an adequate sample in qualitative research. Haber (1994, p. 302) attempts to offer some resolution to the debates surrounding sample size suggesting that 'a general rule of thumb' is to always use the largest sample possible.

With respect to qualitative research using a grounded theory design I came across no authority as to what would be classed as an acceptable figure. The grounded theory studies reviewed (Burkhardt, 1991; Harrison and Burnard, 1993; Kearney, 1994; Wainwright 1993; Walton 1997) indicated that final sample size had been determined by two factors: firstly, the point at which theoretical saturation occurred; and secondly, when the grounded theorist felt that availability of resources meant that they had to prematurely suspend data collection. These findings back up previous discussion that sample size in a grounded theory investigation is determined by theoretical saturation and, ultimately, the grounded theorists. Haber (1994) suggests that having too large a sample in qualitative research can be just as disadvantageous because the study might lack the depth and richness of a smaller study. This principle may be pertinent to grounded theory because, instead of focusing on in-depth analysis, the researcher becomes preoccupied with generating more data, moving onto interviews before detailed analysis and the identification of categories and themes are completed.

Obtaining the sample

The groups that were participating in this investigation were recruited from a range of clinical settings. Therefore obtaining these samples involved many stages of negotiation and facilitation. This section will provide a brief overview of how the study sample's participant groups were obtained. Issues of access to each of the areas involved in the investigation will be outlined later in this section.

Nurses

Nurses working in all of the areas involved in the research were accessed through their service manager. They were informed of the research and once their permission and authorisation had been gained I was allowed to approach the respective ward managers. Ward managers were asked to distribute the 'recruitment questionnaire' to all their qualified staff. Acting upon the advice of one of the LRECs, a recruitment questionnaire (see Appendix 4) was developed. This process is covered in greater detail in the section '*Rationale for constructing a recruitment questionnaire*'. Once the nurse questionnaires had been returned, I collated the information and drew up a list of nurses who had agreed to participate further in the investigation by indicating that they would be willing to participate in an interview. These individuals were then contacted by telephone and a mutually convenient date and time to conduct the interview was agreed.

Patients

Initially it was hoped that nurses working within the wards would identify and select patients that they felt would be suitable to participate in the study. A recruitment questionnaire similar in design to that of the nurses was forwarded either in person or by post to the ward managers. They distributed this to all patients in their area and established that they satisfied the inclusion and exclusion criteria. The questionnaires were processed as detailed above. Rather than telephoning, prospective participants were contacted by a letter that contained an information sheet detailing that I would contact them at a later date to establish whether they still wanted to participate in the investigation.

World religions

Representatives from the major world religions were accessed through one of the Trusts' (Area II) chaplaincy department. With the assistance of one of the chaplains, names and contact details of individuals who were willing to act as representative(s) for their particular religions were forwarded to me. The individuals were then approached by me via telephone when their offer of support was verified and a mutually convenient date and time to conduct the interview was agreed. Prior to conducting the interview, consent was gained and the recruitment questionnaire used for nurses completed.

Health care professionals

The processes to obtain allied health professionals to participate in the investigation were very similar to those of the other groups. Individuals were contacted after their line manager or head of department had informed me that they had expressed an interest in being involved in the investigation. Upon receipt of a name and contact details I approached the individuals concerned via telephone and interviews were arranged. Again, prior to conducting the interview consent was gained, and the recruitment questionnaire used for nurses was completed.

General public

With the exception of one individual, all the participants were recruited within the context of a particular group. One individual, an acquaintance, was approached to participate because he had expressed an interest and he fell outside all the other groups. An interview was arranged informally, ensuring that the same procedures pertaining to information and consent were met.

Rationale for constructing a recruitment questionnaire (Appendix 4)

One LREC (Area III) questioned the appropriateness of using nurses to identify patients who would be willing to participate in the investigation. They suggested this was not a valid and rigorous form of recruitment. The following is a paragraph from the letter of correspondence.

> One final concern was raised in the course of our conversation regarding the scientific validity of the study, the Committee had some concerns about the selection of patients in that only those who felt that a spiritual dimension might be approached, thus providing a huge bias. This could easily be remedied by passing a questionnaire to each patient on the ward where subjects were identified, asking whether they would be willing to be interviewed as part of the study, this would least let you know the proportion of your population which had made response.

This recommendation seemed to go against the notion of recruiting and purposefully selecting or, more fundamentally, theoretically sampling using a grounded theory inquiry. It may be that the LREC did not fully appreciate the nature of qualitative research. Initially, it seemed that the committee was trying to fit this qualitative method into a more scientific model. Nevertheless, some major benefits did emerge from adhering to this advice.

With the above recommendation in mind it was decided that a small questionnaire should be constructed and distributed in all areas. This was felt to be necessary because after commencing data collection it soon emerged that the proposed method of recruiting patients and, indeed nurses, to the study was problematic. Allowing nurses to identify and approach patients did not seem to work. There were several reasons for this, including charge nurses being too busy and patients hearing the word 'spirituality' and assuming that it was to do purely with religion, resulting in them not wanting to be involved due to apprehensions and insecurities, seeing this as an opportunity for someone to convert them.

Recruitment questionnaire (design)

Copies of the questionnaires that were designed are provided (Appendix 4). Two separate questionnaires were developed: one for use with patients and the other for use with nurses. The format of both questionnaires was similar, with slight variation in the questions asked. The questionnaire comprised six questions (Table 4.9). Question 3 was different in the nurse and patient questionnaires. In the patient questionnaires, the wording was modified to provide insight into the duration of stay, reflecting differing locations, whether this was the hospice or hospital. Representatives from different world religions and the 'general public' were instructed to omit Question 3 when completing the questionnaire.

Question 4 concerned the respondents' understanding of spirituality. Three of the four statements used in this question are based upon my earlier work using factor analysis to investigating nurses' perceptions of spirituality (McSherry, 1997; McSherry *et al.*, 2002b). The factors were called 'Existential Search', 'Universality' and 'Individuality'. Therefore the statements presented in the recruitment questionnaire addressed these key areas of spirituality with the addition of a fourth statement providing a choice for those individuals who did not have any belief, or specific understanding of spirituality.

Table 4.9 Summary of the six questions.

Q1	Gender
Q2	Age
Q3a,b,c	Length qualified, type of work, grade (health care professionals only)
Q3	Length of stay in hospital or hospice (patient)
Q4	Statement about spirituality
Q5	Religion
Q6	Practising religion
Final section	Willingness to participate in an interview and contact details.

By addressing these areas it was felt that these would provide me with important information about the overall study sample, for example the types of individuals from all the groups who were willing to participate in an interview and those who were not. By analysing questionnaires I was able to build up a substantial profile for each of the areas, highlighting the types of individuals who were willing to be interviewed and those who were not.

The notion of self-selection was therefore problematic, as individuals who expressed an interest in participating may not possess the same perceptions and understanding as those who declined to interview. To differentiate between nurse and patient questionnaires these were printed in two distinct colours – pastel blue for nurses and pastel green for patients. This made identification and sorting much easier.

Problems faced with the distribution of questionnaires

Distribution of the questionnaires was undertaken at different intervals. However, the main determinant of this was access. Once formal approval had been gained then the process of distribution commenced. Therefore initial distribution was in Area I followed by Area II and Area III.

The use of a questionnaire did not overcome the fears and insecurities felt by patients and, to a lesser extent, nurses when they read the word 'spirituality'. I asked Charge Nurses in all the areas to keep an informal log, recording the reasons why patients refused to volunteer for an interview. In almost all the cases patients who refused viewed the word 'spirituality' as being synonymous with religion and did not want to be involved. This reason may account for the low number of patients in Areas II and III (Acute National Health Service Trust) who volunteered for interview, in contrast to Area I (hospice), where there was a large number of volunteers. This finding in itself was significant and perhaps indicated that patients receiving specialist palliative care have a more 'universal' understanding of spirituality, not viewing it synonymously with religion, or perhaps that patients living with a life-limiting illness are more aware of the spiritual dimension.

It emerged soon that the study population was an extremely homogeneous group in that it was predominantly individuals from the Judeo-Christian religion who were represented. I feel that it is important to declare this significant finding because it may have implications upon the overall findings of the study. Morse and Field (1996, p. 129) suggest that such transparency is essential in grounded theory inquiry: 'If the participants are restricted to an homogenous group, this fact must be made clear'. This restriction was not intentional, as earlier discussion suggests, but was enforced, the reason being that individuals from most of the main world religions were not present in the nursing workforce or these groups were not featuring in the questionnaires that were returned by both nurses and patients.

This issue of the sample being homogeneous and possibly not representative in that it was not inclusive of all major world religions presented a major problem. Measures were taken to try to identify how many qualified (ward-based) nursing staff from different ethnic groups were currently employed within Area II. This area was important because this geographical area was known to be more ethnically diverse than the other two. Consideration was given to the major assumption and stereotypical approach that was being made, namely of 'ethnicity' being synonymous with religious affiliation. I was very much aware that 'ethnicity' might not truly reflect or determine whether an individual belonged to a specific world religion. This connection is made by other writers. Narayanasamy (2004, p. 464) writes '... because religion plays a significant role among minority ethnic communities of Muslim, Sikhs and Hindus'. After discussing this assumption with my supervision team it was decided that this could be a valid determinant of an individual's religious affiliation. Therefore this type of data might provide a clearer indication of the potential number of qualified nurses from diverse ethnic groups (and through association major world religions) who were available to be recruited into the study from within a single Trust.

These figures were obtained through the Trust's (Area II) 'Work Force Planning Department' and are presented in Table 4.10. Close analysis of the data suggested that only a minority of the workforce were from diverse ethnic groups and the majority of the workforce classified themselves as White. The data revealed that the areas identified for recruiting potential nurses only employed a small number of individuals from diverse ethnic groups. The table was concerning in that it highlighted that only a small percentage of qualified nurses were from diverse ethnic groups. This presented a further dilemma about how to recruit individuals from diverse groups into the study. The problem of recruiting members of different ethnic groups into health care research is well documented. Burns and Grove (1997, p. 312) suggest potential reasons for this:

> Recruiting minority subjects for a study can be particularly problematic. Minority individuals may be difficult to locate and are often reluctant to participate in studies because of feelings of being used while receiving no personal benefit from their involvement.

Reflection on recruitment of individuals from diverse ethnic groups

A major aim of this study was to identify how individuals from a wide range of ethnic, religious and cultural groups perceived the concept of spirituality.

Table 4.10 Table detailing qualified nursing staff by ethnicity and service area working within Area II.

Service area	Ethnic origin										
	Bangladeshi	**Black – African**	**Black – Caribbean**	**Black – other**	**Chinese**	**Indian**	**Not known**	**Other**	**Pakistani**	**White**	**Grand total**
Acute day services		1	3				1	3	1	67	76
ENT/eye			3	1		1	3	2		70	80
General medicine	**1**	**1**	**1**	**1**			**11**	**19**		**72**	**106**
General Surgery			**2**	**1**			**10**	**3**	**2**	**98**	**116**
ICU		**2**	**2**	**1**		**2**	**5**	**30**	**3**	**142**	**187**
Infection control										2	**2**
Obstetrics and gynaecology		1	8	1	5	2	20	8	3	188	236
Orthopaedics		2	1	2			7	11	1	127	151
Paediatrics			2		1	1	3		3	148	158
Radiography							1			9	10
Renal and elderly		1	4	2		1	2	9	1	70	90
Temporary nurse register		1	2	1	1		43	2		69	118
Theatres		2	4	1			6	25		75	113
Grand total	**1**	**11**	**32**	**11**	**7**	**7**	**112**	**112**	**14**	**1137**	**1444**

Areas highlighted in bold were accessed to recruit participants, nurses and patients.

As discussed, identification and recruitment of individuals from some of the 'minority ethnic groups' proved problematic. The majority group was 'White', accounting for 46 of the 53 participants, with only three of the 'minority ethnic groups' represented accounting for seven participants. Classification was based on the 2001 census categorisations, these being 1 Black African, 1 Black African British, 2 Asian British, 1 Asian and 2 Pakistani. The under-representation of minority ethnic groups within research is not unique to this project. However, this does mean that, because of the small number of participants from the ethnic minority groups, generalisations and inferences cannot be made about specific groups, clinical settings or geographical areas. This is because, in some instances, the findings are 'idiosyncratic' in that they represent the views of one or two individuals.

A further issue that must be considered as a serious limitation is the inclusion and exclusion criterion relating to 'English speaking'. The criterion severely curtailed the potential to recruit a large number of individuals from some of the minority ethnic groups. Because of the cost of employing translators and not wanting to rely on family members to translate, I made the decision early in the investigation to recruit participants from ethnic minority groups who were reasonably 'fluent' in the English language. This meant that a great number of individuals were prohibited from participating in this study and means that the results may not reflect the total population at large. In addition, the matter of acculturation must be considered since some of the participants were classified as British, having been born in this country. Therefore the perceptions and understanding expressed may not accurately reflect the 'purist' views of that particular cultural or ethnic group regarding spirituality and spiritual care.

Non-respondents and non-participants

Thought must be given to the views of non-respondents and non-participants in the investigation. The notion of self-selection into the research on the basis that an individual had an interest in the subject needs discussion. Measures were taken to monitor the numbers of individuals who were not completing a questionnaire and their reasons for this. Charge nurses were asked to keep a record of the number of questionnaires distributed and returned along with some indication of numbers of individuals who refused and why. Capturing the views of these non-participants could have impacted on the overall findings in that their perceptions of spirituality may have been at a variance with those who participated. This methodological concern was managed through the process of theoretical sampling, where individuals were recruited on the basis of their potential to expand the emerging theory.

Access

The issue of access to both patients and nurses warrants detailed discussion because it was by far the most frustrating and, at times, disheartening process that I had to mange and negotiate. The trials and tribulations associated with gaining access to organisations are not unique to nursing. Horn (1996, p. 551) presents the problems she encountered when conducting research within the police force, cautioning access as a 'precarious process, which may never be successful with some individuals, and which can be renegotiated or revoked at any time'. Flick (1998) suggests that organisations need to be accessed at different levels, these being institutional and individual. This is evident in the following quotation (Flick, 1998, p. 56)

> When researching institutions... this problem becomes more complicated. In general, different levels are involved in the regulation of access. First, there is the level of persons responsible for authorizing the research: in case of difficulties, they are held responsible for this authorization by external authorities. Second, we find the level of those to be interviewed or observed, who will be investing their time and willingness.

The quotation implies that the entire area of access may be problematic and difficult in that the researcher may have several layers of management and bureaucracy to contact and negotiate with to be granted permission before the research can proceed. Therefore I will provide an account of the layers of management, process and bureaucracies encountered.

Institutional access

In order to gain access to patients and nurses there was a need to gain approval from the Local Research Ethics Committees (LRECs) and from the Trusts' and Hospice's own Research and Development Departments and nursing management.

On reflection, it seems that both the LRECs and the Trusts worked in close collaboration. For example, if one examines issues surrounding access in all three areas, almost all worked alongside the LREC, demonstrating interdependence with each other. This is evidenced in the correspondence (Appendix 2)

Issues associated with access by area

■ Area I

Area I (hospice) would not give full access and approval to undertake the study until LREC approval had been obtained, despite the institution having its own Ethics Committee. Once LREC approval had been gained, the director of nursing services allowed full access to undertake the study.

■ Area II

In Area II the Trust would only consider an application that had been fully completed and processed through the appropriate Research and Development channels, including a need to obtain signatures from finance managers, and consent from consultants (80) who were willing to allow their patients to be involved in the study. This point warrants further discussion, because all the consultants whose patients could potentially be recruited into the study were contacted and authorisation from them in the way of a signed 'ethics form' needed to be secured. With respect to accessing nurses, the application and documentation needed to be supported and signed by the Director of Nursing.

After receiving authorisation from the Director of Nursing (Area II) access was simultaneously obtained by liaising with all Unit Nurse Managers (whose wards would be included in the study). These individuals were approached and permission was sought to present the proposed research at one of their unit meetings to generate ward managers' awareness of the nature and purpose of the research. By undertaking this activity, although costly in terms of time and travel, it allowed contact to be made and explanations to be given concerning the charge nurse's role in identifying and selecting patients for the study. Also with reference to Area II, the Equal Opportunities Training Adviser assisted in the identification of staff from different ethnic groups who might be willing to participate in the research.

■ Area III

Area III would not consider an application before LREC approval had been awarded. After the study had been approved by the LREC the appropriate documentation/forms could be completed and processed at Trust level. One interesting and noticeable difference in Area III was that consultants were not required to approve of their patients' involvement in the study. Conversely, all Nurse Managers whose wards/specialities could possibly participate in the study again needed to be spoken to and visited in order to gain approval and an indication of their willingness to participate in the study.

At times, the endless form filling, constant telephoning, emailing people to book appointments, and travelling considerable distances (140 miles) to meet-

Table 4.11 Summary of duration between initial contact and final approval.

	Initial contact	Final approval	Duration (months)
Area I (Hospice)	36740	36878	5
Area II (LREC)	36816	37151	12
Area II (Trust)	36737	36844	5
Area III (LREC)	36737	36864	6
Area III (Trust)	36871	37102	8

ings, only to find that upon arrival they had been cancelled or rescheduled, was very disheartening. This type of situation was extremely frustrating and annoying, testing my patience, endurance and ultimately my commitment to the study. These bureaucratic and managerial 'hoops', while necessary, severely prolonged the processes in relation to gaining access.

It can be seen (Table 4.11) that from initial contact or submission of completed forms, the average length of time for processing applications in LRECs ranged from 6–12 months, while the Trusts took between 5 and 8 months. Acknowledgement must be given to the fact that final approval did not necessarily mean 'immediate access'. The researcher still had to attend meetings and discuss the nature of the research with Unit Managers and repeat the entire exercise with charge nurses or ward managers. For a more detailed outline of issues pertaining to access and the correspondence that took place please refer to Appendix 2.

Individual access

After authorisation had been gained, from all levels of the institutions, this meant that access had been granted allowing recruitment to proceed. Individual access entailed the nurse or patient indicating that they would be willing to participate in an interview by signing a section within a questionnaire that had been distributed by the ward manager. After willingness to participate had been expressed nurses were contacted by telephone and the patients were written to (see Appendix 5), usually a week in advance of the telephone contact. Differences between nurse and patient access (recruitment) were due to the fact that an information sheet had to be posted to the patients prior to the patients confirming their willingness to proceed in the study. The format of the information sheet is discussed under ethical considerations.

Summary points

- This section explored several important issues in relation to obtaining the study sample.
- All the stages involved in this process from identification, approaching each of the groups to obtaining access at institutional and individual levels were described.
- Several limitations were presented in terms of representativeness and recruiting individuals from diverse ethnic groups.
- Obtaining the correct sample was important because having the correct range of participants would ultimately determine the overall quality of the data and the eventual theory.

Data collection

Introduction

This section presents the processes and stages involved in data collection. The areas covered are design of the interview schedule, conducting the pilot study, and highlighting the changes made in light of the findings. The processes involved in conducting and recording the interviews will be explored. A rationale for the three phases of data collection will be provided, covering such issues as questions and memo writing.

Activity 4.4 Data collection and analysis

- What do you think would be the best way of ascertaining participants' understandings of spirituality?
- How might you capture these and present what you have captured?

Theory behind interviewing

Interviews were chosen as the preferred method of data collection. The rationale for this selection over other approaches such as questionnaire and observation is that they enabled the voice of key stakeholders to be expressed and heard. Pontin (2000, p. 291) describes a major benefit of this method of data collection thus: 'Interviews are a particularly useful way of finding out about people's perceptions or opinions on specific matters'.

The decision to use interviews for data collection seemed appropriate for achieving the aim of the investigation, which was to discover a diverse group of individuals' perceptions and opinions surrounding the concepts of spirituality and spiritual care. The use of an interview would enable in-depth exploration of the topics with each participant. Thus, as the investigation was conducted and data emerged, the direction of the interview could be revised to ensure the development of categories and themes. In addition, the use of face-to-face interviews was deemed more appropriate for discussing such a sensitive and personal dimension of people's lives.

Interviews

A total of 53 in-depth interviews were undertaken with the three target groups: HCPs, patients and the public. Interviews were conducted between March 2001 and July 2003. The length of interviews ranged from 18 minutes to 66 minutes, the average length being approximately 38 minutes. Interviews were carried out in a range of locations, usually in an office off the ward or in the patient's own home. Interviews were recorded, with the participant's prior consent (in relation to HCPs this was gained verbally, while for patients and the general public written consent was obtained at the outset of the interview and witnessed by a third party). All interviews were recorded using a Sanyo Digital Voice Recorder (Model ICR-B100) and a Sony Cassette Recorder (Model TCM-20DV) as backup, using high quality cassettes to assist in listening to the recordings when transcribing. The digital voice recorder proved invaluable in that it allowed files to be downloaded into the memo-scriber software that was installed on my own personal computer. The quality of sound was far superior to the standard cassette tape, which made transcribing a little easier.

Design of interview agenda (schedule)

Interviews were all carried out adhering to a prescribed format or interview agenda (Table 4.12). The benefits of using this approach were that it allowed

Table 4.12 Interview agenda.

Firstly, I would like to thank you for consenting to participate in this research study. It is very much appreciated. Before proceeding with the interview I would like to give you a brief overview of how the interview will be conducted.
As you are aware from the introductory information on the small questionnaire you completed and returned, this piece of research is part of studies leading to a higher degree, which I am undertaking at Leeds Metropolitan University.
I am not here to interrogate you but to explore with you your understanding of a concept and how you might be addressing this concept within practice (life).
The interview will consist of a series of questions that I will ask. I might also ask you to explain or expand upon points as the interview progresses. The interview will be recorded and I might also make some written notes – so do not be alarmed if you see me writing during the interview (I will show you these notes at the end if you wish).
The nature of the subject we are discussing is personal and sensitive. Therefore you are under no obligation to disclose information that you feel is too personal or that you do not want to talk about. If at any point you would like to terminate the interview you can do so without any fear of recrimination.
I must stress that your identity will remain anonymous. However, some of the information from the recording may be used to inform the overall research report, but still your anonymity will be maintained.
You have been selected to participate in this interview because I was interested in some of the responses you gave on your questionnaire.
Before we proceed are there any questions that you would like to ask?

me to explain the nature and purpose of the interview 'statement of purpose' (Oppenheim, 1992, p. 71).

The agenda allowed me to introduce myself and break the ice by developing a rapport, making a connection with the participant before commencing the interview. It allowed both parties time to settle and compose themselves before the interview commenced. In relation to the participant, it afforded them the opportunity to look at their questionnaire and information leaflet to refresh their memory. Importantly it allowed them time to ask questions, should they feel the need.

Throughout the interview process I made field notes which acted as an *aide memoire*. These notes, recorded throughout all stages of the interview process, assisted me in developing my own awareness as an interviewer, providing valuable reflections and critique of performance. Another advantage of these field notes was that interruptions or events that occurred during an interview could be documented, providing me with a rich contextual detail and thus aiding recall during the transcription and analysis phases. Table 4.13 provides an example of a completed interview schedule, providing details of an interview, processes, disruptions and reflections. Reviewing and reflecting critically upon the information documented on the interview schedules, especially issues relating to my performance, assisted me in developing my self-awareness and skills as an interviewer.

A series of questions were used as prompts or probes to guide the interview, ensuring that emerging themes, categories were addressed. Therefore, the interviews could be classed as 'in-depth focused interviews'. Having the

Table 4.13 Example of interview schedule.

Interview Schedule

Respondent No: 10

Interview No: 3

Date: 17/4/2001

Time: 15.00–15.55 (late starting, participant indicated that they would need to complete interview before 16.00

Venue: Area 1 (Counselling room)

Duration: 40 minutes

Comments/observations made during interview
Both seemed to adopt an open and relaxed posture, plenty of eye contact throughout, and leaning forward when responding. Interviewee seemed to have some trouble with some of the questions? Long pauses between responses – after a long period of silence kept looking to me for prompts, support. Occasionally they struggled to articulate what they thought.

Initial reflections after interview
Found this a tough interview. Felt I interjected too much. Will talk to Keith about this, ask them to review transcript, my questioning. Could have explored some issues in a little more depth. Didn't know how to manage/handle some of the long pauses. Need to consider asking about 'moral relativism' consider including a scenario around witchcraft or the occult to test some of these ideas out.

Quality of recording not very good on listening, hope I can transcribe and hear it when analysing.

questions helped to focus the direction of the interview, ensuring that the same areas were covered with all the participants. However, as the data were analysed, the questions used were derived from the emerging themes and categories, or used to check out emerging theoretical memos or ideas, in keeping with a grounded theory format.

Reflecting upon the interview process

Reflecting upon the interview process revealed that this can be broken down into three distinct phases (Table 4.14). It must be stressed that this three-phased approach to the research was not planned at the outset of the investigation. As the investigation proceeded, the investigation seemed to fall neatly into this framework more by accident than design.

Each phase assisted in the development and refinement of the quality of the data, allowing me to challenge and test the emerging themes and categories and the core category. Adoption of this phased approach ensured that I was able to achieve maximum saturation of all the categories by testing these at different intervals throughout data collection, using theoretical sampling to identify a wide range of suitable individuals to test out or validate core categories and themes.

Another important benefit was that as data collection progressed, and my confidence at conducting interviews grew, I was better equipped to manage

Table 4.14 Three-phased approach to interview process.

Phase	Number interviewed	Purpose
Phase I	22	Piloting of methods, and testing the theoretical constructs of spirituality and spiritual care, and assumptions that these are universally understood and recognised.
Phase II	18	Verify components of spirituality and spiritual care as represented in existing health care literature, checking out the emerging categories and themes, especially the differences in understanding of spirituality between the three groups.
Phase III	13	Validated the findings of Phase I and Phase II by producing a model of spirituality and spiritual care that accurately reflects individuals' diverse perceptions and understandings of spirituality and spiritual care.

and facilitate the interview process. This again ensured that emerging themes were covered and tested. It also meant that there was less reliance upon predetermined questions, allowing the participants' responses to guide the interview process and the areas to be explored. The phased approach also allowed me time to constantly compare and contrast emerging themes with existing conceptual and theoretical ideas surrounding spirituality within the literature.

Reflective question

- Why is it important that a pilot study is conducted prior to the commencement of the main investigation?

Phase I (Pilot study)

Aims

The aims of the pilot study were to test out the processes and instruments to be utilised in the main investigation. Further, the pilot study would enable me to gain valuable experience in the field, especially with reference to conducting interviews and developing my skills in the management and facilitation of some of the other key processes that this investigation entailed such as contacting individuals, forwarding information leaflets and arranging dates for interviews that were mutually convenient.

The practice and benefits of undertaking a pilot study are well documented (Morse and Field, 1996; Burns and Grove, 1997). With regard to the use of grounded theory, the pilot study enabled me to have a trial in the collection and analysis of data, developing my self-confidence as an analyst by introducing me to the techniques and procedures to be employed.

Methods

The pilot study provided me with an opportunity to test out the questions/probes (Table 4.15) and to develop and evaluate my skills in conducting an interview. Phase I involved mainly patients and nurses from Area I. The rationale for choosing Area I was that this was the first organisation to grant full approval and allow access to nurses and patients. At an economic level, this

Table 4.15 Questions for interviews with nurses during Phase I.

- Can you describe the type of care you provide to your patients?
- I am interested in the word 'holistic' that you have used. Can you explain what it means a little more fully?
- You mention the word 'spiritual'; Can you tell me what the word means for you? Could you give me your understanding or interpretation of the word?
- On the questionnaire you completed you indicated that spirituality was.... Can you share your thoughts and reasons with me?
- How do you attempt to provide spiritual care for your patients; for example, are there any specific care interventions that you would undertake?
- Do you think that spiritual care is different from other forms of essential nursing care? (By essential I mean what would be seen as good nursing practice.)
- Could you provide me with any examples of spiritual needs you have assisted your patients to meet?
- Do you feel that you are able to satisfactorily meet your patients' spiritual needs?
- The terms 'spirituality' and 'spiritual care' seem to have become fashionable – could you give me any reasons or possible explanations why this might be?

was the organisation nearest to where I resided. Therefore it would negate the need for long costly journeys across Northern England.

Findings of pilot study

While conducting the pilot study some difficulties were encountered especially surrounding the term 'spirituality'. To establish whether this was unique and specific to a single area I approached the other two acute areas. Therefore, one medical ward within each of Areas II and III was asked to participate. The main aim of Phase I was to try to establish whether nurses, patients and representatives from the major world religions understood what was meant by the words 'spirituality' and 'spiritual care', and to establish whether they had given any consideration to such concepts.

Phase I involved a total of five patients, five representatives from different world religions and 12 nurses. The pilot study was invaluable in that it brought to light several areas that warranted close attention. The five patients who were interviewed had great difficulty in answering the questions associated 'directly' with the word 'spirituality'. When discussing the statement that individuals had selected to indicate their understanding of spirituality, the majority viewed spirituality synonymously with religion. This is best illustrated in the following example:

P: Never has interested me, even in illness, it's never interested me has religion. It has done nothing for me. It did nothing for me mother and she died a horrible death.
R: So how you view this term spirituality is it's about religion? So you wouldn't see it in any other terms?
P: To me it's just religion. *P13 (Male patient, I)*

Reflection suggested that the sources of the problems might be, firstly, using the word 'spirituality' and secondly, my inexperience and anxieties at conducting and managing interviews addressing such a personal and sensitive subject.

Changes made in light of the pilot study

The following issues emerged during the pilot phase of this investigation. Firstly, the findings caused me to stop and evaluate the entire direction of the study in terms of the quality of the data obtained. Secondly, through the use of constant comparative analysis and reflexive exercises I decided, after discussion with my supervision team, that perhaps the solution would be to change the questions used in the interview.

The main difficulty experienced was not to do with the interview instruments, but more to do with the quality of the data being obtained when interviewing patients. On reflection, and through the continued analysis of the transcripts, it emerged that some of the patients and individuals from different world faiths struggled with the concept of spirituality. These issues are discussed in greater detail in Chapter 5. It was felt that sufficient data had been obtained that demonstrated that there were emerging two discourses – professional and public – that surrounded the understanding of spirituality. In light of the significant findings, the pilot study was referred to as Phase I. This phase contributed to the overall findings of this grounded theory investigation, forming a platform for conducting the second phase of the investigation.

Phase II

This phase involved the checking out of emerging themes, especially in relation to the disparity that existed between the way that nurses, patients and individuals from different world faiths viewed the term 'spirituality'. Sampling became more focused, involving relational and variational sampling procedures. This was essential during 'axial coding' to ensure that all the differences and similarities emerging in the data analysis were scrutinised, highlighting negative cases and giving an account of the variation existing within and across the participant groups.

A concern that I had was how to explore the term 'spirituality' more fully with patients to gain a fuller and richer understanding. It appeared that the properties and categories emerging associated with perceptions of spirituality were similar across the patient groups. However, there was a major disparity between patients and individuals from different world religions when compared against the nursing groups. To explore these disparities I felt there was a need for me to revise the format of the questions. This would ensure that I had explored all possibilities and avenues validating the differences in the data. It would also enable me to test out the assumption in nursing and health care literature that there are specific components or attributes of spirituality that are universally recognised and understood.

Having given this area careful thought I decided to explore the published research to see whether there were any published examples of the questions that had been used within their investigations. I did identify three studies that provided examples of the questions they used (Harrington, 1995; Cavendish *et al.*, 2000; Hermann, 2001 and, retrospectively, Taylor, 2003). I also established that many of the qualitative studies reviewed did not ask a specific or direct question incorporating the word 'spirituality'. The area of spirituality was always referred to 'indirectly' by examining attributes or components of spirituality as presented in health care definitions; for example, meaning and purpose, relationships (Clark *et al.*, 1991; Clark and Heidenreich, 1995). Clark *et al.* (1991, p. 71) justified this approach on the basis '... the term "spirituality" was avoided to eliminate bias toward a Judeo-Christian perspective'.

During the search I did come across one piece of research (Ross, 1997) that seemed to address my concerns. After discussing the questions used with the author I obtained a copy and permission to use them. These questions were modified and used in conjunction with some of the statements I had developed in my earlier research (McSherry, 1997; McSherry *et al.*, 2002b). These questions were used throughout Phase II of this study (Table 4.16). It was anticipated that this 'structured' approach would lead to the generation of a richer and fuller theory. It would also establish whether the existing theoretical approaches to spirituality were recognised with different groups.

Table 4.16 Questions used at the commencement of Phase II.

- People seem to have different ideas about spiritual things. What do you think of as spiritual matters/things?
- What do you think people's needs in this area might be?
- During your stay in hospital have you had any spiritual concerns? Or during your life have you ever experienced any spiritual concerns? Can you describe these?
- Do you think that spiritual things are only about going to church or place of worship for the religiously inclined or is it more than that?
- What are your thoughts or ideas about a belief or faith in a God or Supreme Being? Would this be important to your understanding of spiritual things or not?
- What are your thoughts concerning the need to forgive and a need to be forgiven in life? Do you think of forgiveness as a spiritual matter or not?
- Would you say that there is a need to finding meaning in the good and bad events of life? What gives your life meaning? Do you think of this as a spiritual matter or not?
- Have you any thoughts or opinions around nurses enabling patients to find meaning and purpose in their illness?
- Would you say that it is important to have a sense of hope as we go through life or not?
- Would you say that you are at peace within yourself? Do you think having a sense of inner peace is anything to do with spiritual things or not?
- Would you say those areas such as art, reading, poetry, listening to music adds anything to your life or are important to you? Are these areas anything to do with spiritual things or not?
- Would you say that personal friendships, relationships are important to you or not? Would you consider this to be a spiritual thing or not?
- Are there any particular beliefs, values, or morals that have shaped the way that you live your life?
- Do you think the way one conducts one's life here and now is anything to do with spiritual things or not?
- Do you think that nurses can help patients attend to spiritual matters by listening to and allowing you time to discuss and explore your fears, anxieties or troubles?

Table 4.16 (*continued*)

- Would you say that nurses can provide spiritual care by arranging a visit by the hospital chaplain or the patient's own religious leader if requested?
- Do you think that nurses can help patients to meet their spiritual concerns or spiritual needs by spending time with them and giving support and reassurance especially in time of need?
- Do you think that some nurses can help you to meet your spiritual concerns by showing kindness, concern and cheerfulness when giving care? Still working on this question.

Phase III – Validation

The aim of Phase III was to ensure that all categories generated throughout Phase I and Phase II were fully saturated and that any remaining theoretical questions or theoretical gaps were tested and explored so that the resulting theory was fully developed. This phase enabled the testing out or validation of the two main central themes.

Initially I had intended only to interview three groups: nurses, patients and representatives from the major world religions. However, detailed analysis of the transcripts and the emergent themes led to the recruitment of members of the allied health professions (with the exception of doctors) who were perceived to be involved in the provision of spiritual care. Furthermore, the variation that existed between the two central themes: 'professional discourse' and 'public discourse' generated a need to test out some of the professional assumptions surrounding spirituality with the general public, resulting in the recruitment of some members of the general public into the study.

Summary points

- This section described the process and stages involved in data collection.
- The areas covered included design of the interview schedule, the significance of a pilot study, and demonstrating the changes made in light of the findings.
- The three phases of data collection were described, presenting the types of questions and areas to be explored.

Data analysis

It is recognised that the central feature of grounded theory, and the one that distinguishes it from other forms of qualitative research, is the use of the constant comparative method – a method that ensures the quality and rigour of the theory produced. Using grounded theory meant that data collection and analysis occurred simultaneously throughout. Data analysis commenced after the first interview and ended only after 'theoretical saturation' of all themes and categories had occurred. This entire process lasted approximately 28 months.

Activity 4.5 Data analysis

Look at Table 4.17 and read through the excerpts of transcripts. Highlight any points within each transcript that you feel are important.

How might you start to make sense of the points you have highlighted?

In keeping with other researchers who have utilised grounded theory, analysis was undertaken at two levels: 'overview analysis' (a form of 'macro-analysis') and 'line by line analysis' or 'micro-analysis' (Glaser, 1978; Wainwright, 1993; Strauss and Corbin, 1998).

Three steps or levels of coding were used. Level I – or substantive (open) coding assisted in the identification of concepts, properties and dimensions (Table 4.17). Level II – axial (theoretical) coding – is a technique introduced by Strauss and Corbin (1998). This type of coding was about relating and making links between and across categories, subcategories and participant groups. An example of axial coding is provided (Box 4.1) demonstrating how axial coding was used in the identification of the category 'Definitions of spirituality'.

Selective or Level III coding was used in the identification of a core or overarching category.

Overview analysis involved me listening to every interview time and time again to sensitise myself to any ideas or themes that might be present. This approach also assisted in theoretically sensitising me to any theoretical possibilities that may exist in the data. This overview analysis was not a one-off activity but was constantly employed alongside other levels of analysis. By undertaking this 'macro' approach to managing the data I was able to sensitise myself to all the data, ensuring that I did not miss out any broad themes (the bigger picture), which could occur if I only undertook 'micro-analysis' (Strauss and Corbin, 1998).

Table 4.17 Examples of micro-analysis and how this led to the formation of a category.

INT: So (name) in relation to this word spirituality?	INT: So (name) in relation to this word spirituality?
R: Yeah	R: Yeah
INT: What would that word mean to you?	INT: What would that word mean to you?
R: Well first of all spirituality exists within everyone whether you believe in God or not. To me personally it would be to overall, look at the patient overall and address their needs to the way that they would see it! For example when we go on to the wards being religious ministers we don't go on with our hats on as being religious ministers but we go with an open mind and an open view that here's a patient and we are going and work around the patients and not go we've come as so and so! Err for example an eighteen-year-old may well be interested in football!	R: Well first of all spirituality exists within everyone whether you believe in God or not. To me personally it would be to overall, look at the patient overall and address their needs to the way that they would see it! For example when we go on to the wards being religious ministers we don't go on with our hats on as being religious ministers but we go with an open mind and an open view that here's a patient and we are going and work around the patients and not go we've come as so and so! Err for example an eighteen-year-old may well be interested in football!
INT: Yeah	INT: Yeah
R: Err talk about Manchester United, Liverpool you've got football there or cars or anything of that sort! So we go with looking at the patient's agenda rather than going in with our own and err basically that's how we view things and my view of it would be to look at the needs of the individual patient... (Interruption two)	R: Err talk about Manchester United, Liverpool you've got football there or cars or anything of that sort! So we go with looking at the patient's agenda rather than going in with our own and err basically that's how we view things and my view of it would be to look at the needs of the individual patient... (Interruption two)
INT: What you seem to be implying then is you would try to connect with that person, at a level of understanding that or something that would interest them as a means of making a connection, trying to enter into a dialogue with them?	INT: What you seem to be implying then is you would try to connect with that person, at a level of understanding that or something that would interest them as a means of making a connection, trying to enter into a dialogue with them?
R: Exactly, absolutely! Err you'd obviously let us say it's not going in with your own agenda but working around the patient and at their level.	

INT: If I can take you back you mentioned the word spiritual R: Yes (knock at the door) INT: What would your understanding of that word be? R: Well I think it means different things to different people! As far as I'm concerned em it's not necessarily about their religious needs! I think everybody has a soul in my view so everybody has spiritual needs em and I feel that you know our role is to respect whatever they may be. And that is so when patients are admitted to us we sort of say have you got any spiritual needs that you are aware of that we need to be aware of and then we can accommodate that! And basically then it's down to expressed need as to what we would do form then on. INT: Yeah	INT: Like we said earlier one word that seems to be gaining fashion in healthcare is this term spirituality, could you explain what this word might mean to you? Or how might you define that term? Or would you even identify with the term? R: I was gonna say it's not a term we use in Buddhism as such! But em I know of eternity and that sort of view point they do don't they is a large element! Em it's a hard word to define actually (laughing) it's just a difficult word to define! INT: So as a Buddhist if you came into healthcare R: Yeah INT: As a patient and the nurse or some other practitioner sat down with you and said R: Yeah INT: I'm just wanting to assess your spiritual needs or...
R: It may be that they want half an hour a day to meditate they don't necessarily have to be religious but they may need a period of time where they need to be on their own to reflect on whatever! And I feel we have a duty if we are treating them as a whole to sort of respect those needs?	R: Yeah, yeah INT: How would that make you feel? Would you be able to identify with that term or would it be meaningless? R: Em to some extent I could but I think people have a certain image of it that isn't Buddhist in a sense! I mean I'd probably think it is how to develop your high potential or how to develop your potential in a positive way! I'd say it's that aspect of it! INT: That would be your Buddhist approach to spirituality? R: Yeah, yeah! yeah, yeah I would say it's a bit nebulous the word but it's, it's looking at how you can develop you highest potential!

An example of how the process of micro-analysis led to the development of a list of potential codes and properties for the category titled 'definitions of spirituality'.

Definitions of spirituality

Not a term we use	About religion
Difficult word to define	Holier than though (negative connotations)
Eternity	Sister – C of E man (religious leaders)
How develop potential	Exists in everyone
Positive	Believe in God or not
Spiritualist	Address patient's needs patient's agenda

Box 4.1 Axial coding – definitions of spirituality across participant groups

PROPERTY	Religion	Ghosts	No idea	Existential	Inner self	Spark	Universal	Spiritualism	Inner strength	Good
GROUP										
Nurses										
Acute				X	X	X	X		X	X
Pall				X	X	X	X		X	X
Patients										
Acute	X	X	X					X		
Pall			X				X		X	
Religious belief	X			X			X			X
Non-religious belief	X									

Micro-analysis or line by line coding was undertaken. This was a very time-consuming activity. Glaser (1978, p. 55) indicates the essential nature and need for this activity:

> Coding gets the analyst off the empirical level by fracturing the data, then conceptually grouping it into codes that then become the theory which explains what is happening in the data.

By adopting this micro-analysis I was able to break down, examine, compare, contrast, conceptualise and categorise the initial data (Table 4.17). This approach was essential in capturing the complexity and subjectivity associated with the concepts of spirituality and the provision of spiritual care. As data analysis progressed different levels of coding – open, axial and selective – were utilised to form categories and locate properties. These, as Strauss and Corbin (1998) indicate, are the characteristics of categories. After the initial open – line by line or substantive – coding, all coding procedures where employed simultaneously to integrate and refine the theory. By using 'axial coding' it could be argued that, during data analysis, I was following the Strauss school of grounded theory. I must stress that 'axial and selective coding' became an intuitive process in that while listening and analysing transcripts, notes would be made on the transcript reminding me to check back over another piece to check out a theme or the properties of a category.

To deepen and direct the analysis I continually asked questions of the data, as outlined by Glaser (1978, p. 57)

1. What is this data a study of?
2. What category does this incident indicate?
3. What is actually happening in the data?

These questions focused my attention on the data and helped me transcend my own preconceived ideas about the nature of spirituality, enhancing my theoretical sensitivity. The questions forced me to remain true to the data, forming properties and categories that truly reflected the data and ultimately the reality of the participants.

Reflective question

- Imagine you are a researcher exploring the area of spirituality! What observations might you record when you were out collecting data?

Table 4.18 Procedural memo (interview questions).

I know there look to be a lot of questions in Phase II – however, if the patient provides sufficient response to the first three questions then some of the remainder may not be used or appropriate?
The refocusing of questions will fit the constant comparative method of theory generation. This is because I am responding firstly to the properties, themes emerging from the analysis of the patients' transcripts. Secondly, reviewing the literature surrounding spirituality and the provision of spiritual care indicates a dichotomy exists between patients and nurse perceptions which needs exploring in more depth. Thirdly constantly comparing with patients, nurses, from different areas of practice, cultural religious backgrounds will ensure premature saturation does not occur. Hopefully by using the revised questions throughout Phase II I will be exhausting all avenues.

Memo writing

Throughout the data analysis and indeed the research process I wrote three types of memo. One version focused specifically upon the coding process while the second addressed or explained variations in the emerging theory. The third type recorded procedural (Table 4.18) and directional aspects of the study. Occasionally the different types of reflective memo were so much integrated that it was difficult to distinguish one from another. These memos helped me to record my feelings, highlight decisions made, and record thoughts surrounding conceptual or theoretical ideas emerging in the analysis and how these might be related to existing conceptual, theoretical arguments in existing literature.

Transcribing and data analysis

Transcribing was by far the most time-consuming part of the study. On average I was taking between 10 and 14 hours to transcribe a single interview. Obviously this process was influenced by two factors: length of interview and quality of the recording. I had proposed to undertake all the transcribing myself. However, after transcribing 20 interviews and discussing the economic constraints with my supervision team we decided that it would be acceptable for me to enlist the services of a professional audio-typist. However, before any tapes were forwarded I ensured anonymity of the participants by deleting any identifying material. I also explained to the typist the need for strict confidentiality. This decision did save me valuable time. However, it did prove costly. A further issue did arise: checking the quality and accuracy of the transcription. Therefore I had to undertake a form of quality control and revise transcribed interviews accordingly. However, this process was much speedier than having to transcribe the entire interview.

Reflection on decision to pay for audio-typist

The rationale for employing the services of an audio-typist was to enable me to focus more upon data analysis. However, this decision was to prove problematic in that the first audio-typist would leave out large sections of conversation, or worse, transcribe their interpretation of what was being said, not what was actually said. Quality control was very important in this instance. I found myself having to retype or substantially edit some interview transcripts before detailed analysis could be undertaken. If I had not immersed myself in data collection and analysis this could have had a disastrous consequence on the overall findings of this investigation.

Time between interviews and analysis

Another factor that might have impacted upon the overall credibility of this investigation is the time delay between interview and data analysis. In the ideal world this should occur simultaneously. However, because of other commitments, there were occasions when there were considerable delays between the actual interview and data analysis, particularly at a micro-level. At times it felt like I was undertaking a retrospective analysis or an analysis of secondary data. However, prior to undertaking any data collection, all previous interviews were scanned, familiarising myself with interesting materials, and re-immersing and reminding myself of the emerging categories and themes so that the theory could be further substantiated. These apprehensions surrounding data collection and analysis emerge from a deep-rooted desire to adhere to a purist, paternalistic view of undertaking a grounded theory investigation – wanting to get it right! Strauss and Corbin (1998, p. 295) provide reassurance, advocating flexibility, not purism, in the process:

> We advise students not to worry needlessly about every little facet of analysis. Sometimes, one has to use common sense and not get caught up in worrying about what is the right or wrong way. The important thing is to trust oneself and the process.

This quotation indicates that grounded theory is a flexible methodology that can be adapted to meet the needs and personal situation of the researcher. Further, the underlying principle is not to worry anxiously over process but to adapt the methodology to meet one's own circumstance. In the end I had to trust my own instinct regarding analysis and the advice provided by my research supervisors.

Volume of data

The sheer volume of data generated in this grounded theory investigation was vast, and at times almost unmanageable. The length of transcripts and the richness of data meant that on occasion 'you couldn't see the wood for the trees'. It was like going around in circles. The solution to this problem was that once categories began to emerge, and their properties developed and the theory formulated, not every transcript was analysed line by line. Strauss and Corbin (1998, p. 281) endorse this practice '... not every single bit of data has to be analyzed "microscopically"'. This practice alleviated many anxieties and enabled in-depth analysis of all the phases of the investigation. Linked with the volume of data was the quality of the recordings. In some instances audibility of recording was very poor, resulting in some sentences or phrases within the final transcripts being left blank. This meant that interpretation and meaning could have been distorted. However, this problem was managed by the practice of having two recorders, since both recordings were used to check the participant's response.

'N Vivo' Software

An attempt was made to use 'N Vivo' (Richards, 1999) to assist in the management and analysis of the transcribed interviews. From the outset this software proved difficult, requiring a large amount of time to acquire the necessary skill to operate the program. Despite persistence and constant practice, I still struggled to master the software. I decided to revert to manual methods of data analysis using flip charts, index cards and notebooks to record emerging concepts and theoretical ideas. However, the potential gains and benefits of using this software in the storage, coding and retrieval of information cannot be underestimated. The amount of effort and energy involved in mastering this software was contrasted with the time that could be spent on analysis. Therefore I made the decision not to use the software. Possibly the main limitation was in relation to acquiring an overall perspective or 'bird's eye view' of how the different properties and categories were integrated across all the groups and participants. I did not have the expertise or proficiency to derive this information from the software, although I am sure that the software does have the potential to run such procedures.

Summary points

- This section has described data analysis indicating the types of analysis that would be utilised in the development of theory, for example 'micro' and 'macro' analysis.
- The role that asking questions plays in conjunction with memo writing was recognised as central to the identification, development and saturation of properties, themes and categories.
- Some of the practical difficulties associated with transcribing and the use of computerised software in data analysis were illustrated.

Ethical issues

Activity 4.6 Ethical issues

All research raises ethical questions. From what you have read in this chapter write down what you feel are the main ethical concerns for this qualitative study.

You can then make comparisons with the issues presented here and the ones you have identified.

Introduction

This section summarises the ethical issues associated with undertaking this grounded theory investigation. Firstly, there is an outline of the steps taken to gain ethical approval. Secondly, some of the major ethical implications of conducting the investigation are described, such as consent, confidentiality and support. A great deal of thought and consideration were given to this dimension of the investigation because it is probably the most fundamental area. This is because the subject matter of the investigation is deeply personal, making one acutely aware of the potential to create anxiety and discomfort for some of the participants, who are being asked to reflect upon their lives while living with illness, disease and, for some, the prospect of facing death, which made them very vulnerable.

Ethical approval

The process of obtaining ethical approval, as described, was quite long and protracted. Initial forms were submitted on August 2000 and final approval from the three Local Research Ethics Committees was not gained until September 2001. To maintain the anonymity of the areas these forms have not been included.

Once recruitment commenced it soon emerged that the proposed method of recruiting patients and nurses to the study was problematic, as indicated. Therefore a common approach was adopted and applied within all areas. This minor change in methodology meant that approval needed to be sought from one trust (Area II). This delayed proceedings further and formal approval of amendments was not given until 18 September 2001.

Concerns raised by Local Research Ethics Committees

Both committees raised methodological concerns about the sampling procedures that were going to be utilised in the research. The LREC from Area III raised further concerns surrounding the vulnerability of patients and support mechanisms that could be provided. For a more detailed appreciation of the correspondence that took place between me and the LREC, refer to Appendix 2.

Consent

The area of consent was of particular importance and all institutions involved required that written and informed consent be obtained from all patients who were willing to participate in the study. The LRECs and the Trusts had specific formats that they wanted in relation to the design and presentation of the patient consent form. Therefore two consent forms were developed, addressing and incorporating the specifications requested by each of the LRECs (Appendix 3). This made the process of gaining consent a little more difficult in that I had to ensure that I was using the correct consent form when collecting data in the different Trusts.

The notion of patients giving informed consent meant that a patient information leaflet had to be designed and distributed to all participants prior to confirming and undertaking an interview (Appendix 6). The information leaflet was written and presented in a format that was accessible to patients having a 'Flesch Reading Ease' of 60%, indicating high readability. The information leaflet was designed around questions or concerns that prospective participants might have around their involvement.

The information leaflet meant that patients had the opportunity to read and decide whether they wanted to continue their involvement in the study. This mechanism worked well in that all the patients who had agreed to be involved in the research had read the information leaflet provided and consented to participate in the study. Several patients who, while in hospital, had expressed an interest to be involved in the research by signing a questionnaire, exercised their right to withdraw when contacted by the researcher after having read the information leaflet and being more informed about what participation would entail. Despite there being no need to justify their withdrawal, all gave reasons for this; for example, readmission to hospital, did not feel well enough, had been diagnosed with cancer, or simply did not want to be involved any longer.

Vulnerability and support

Consideration had to be given to the personal and sensitive nature of the concept under discussion and the impact that such discussions might have upon those who participated in this research. It could be argued that patients are a vulnerable group, given that they are or have been in receipt of health care and nursing care for an acute, chronic or life-threatening illness. The fact that many of the patients had been hospitalised or been receiving outpatient care meant that they may have felt obliged to participate in the research study for fear of reprisal or recrimination if they did not. Therefore I went to great lengths to ensure that patients, and indeed all participants, had every opportunity to withdraw from the study without giving any justification for doing so if they so wished. In the case of patients this was reinforced by indicating that the withdrawal or termination of an interview would have no repercussions on the standard of care that they received. This information was explained several times: in the information sheet, on the consent form and the interview schedule.

The major aim for me as a researcher was to ensure that everyone who participated in the study felt informed and was knowledgeable about their role and what would be involved if they participated in the study. Information was given verbally and in written format (to patients). Participants were also advised that they could speak to the nurse in charge about the nature of the research. As indicated earlier, all 'charge nurses' involved in the recruitment of patients had been fully briefed as to the nature and purpose of the study. My contact details were placed on all correspondence to participants. This included my work and home telephone details.

One recommendation by the LREC was that patients should have access to support if required following an interview. It was acknowledged that the researcher was available and able to offer immediate support to individual participants who might become emotionally distressed. However, it was felt necessary to build in a safety net for participants, especially if patients should feel a need to discuss an issue some time after their interview. With this point in mind, all information leaflets contained contact details for a trained counsellor who had agreed to provide support to participants if the need arose. Similarly, all participants were informed at interview that should they want to discuss an issue in more detail or require additional support then I could be contacted. They would be given the contact details of a counsellor who would provide ongoing support. Interestingly, none of the participants took up the request for additional support. This is an observation that reflects the experience of Thomas and Retsas (1999), who used grounded theory to investigate the spiritual dimension of people with terminal cancer.

Confidentiality and anonymity

All participants were assured that all information provided during the course of their involvement in the research would be treated and handled in strictest confidence. An explanation was given before proceeding with the interview that anonymity would be maintained by reinforcing that no identifying features would be used. All participants were reassured that no identifying features would be made known to anyone other than the researcher. To achieve this, all participants were given a management code. This code was referred to throughout the study; only the researcher knew the meaning and significance of the code. However, all participants were advised that excerpts from the tape recording transcripts might be used to illustrate or support emerging themes and categories, and might be used to inform the overall thesis.

Storage of data

All identifying information related to non-participants and participants was stored in a locked filing cabinet. This included questionnaires, letters of correspondence, tape recordings and interview transcripts. I kept the filing cabinet locked at all times and it was only opened when I needed access to information for transcribing and analysing. In relation to electronic data, all storage files were coded and given passwords, so that only the researcher could access them. Similarly, I ensured that all transcripts were nameless and given a code, thus ensuring anonymity. If opening or using a file I ensured that the file was closed and the computer was shut down when I left a room. These practices are in keeping with the recommendations made by the Data Protection Act.

Destruction of transcripts

Participants were informed that tape recordings, both digital and manual, would be kept for the full duration of the research and six months after its completion. After this time they would be destroyed, to be totally erased digitally and deleted from the computer and manual recording. All information pertaining to non-participants and participants obtained would be destroyed by incineration.

Raising spiritual awareness

A major ethical concern was that by interviewing individuals about the concept of spirituality and spiritual care I was asking people to reflect upon an aspect of life that they had perhaps never previously considered or, in some cases, did not want to consider. I was asking people to reflect upon personal events, some of which might have been painful and difficult. In reality, there was the potential and danger of opening up 'Pandora's Box'. This notion was immediately evident and reinforced by nurses interviewed during Phase I of the study, some of whom indicated that it was a major barrier to nurses addressing the spiritual dimension with patients. This is illustrated in the following two transcripts.

Participant 1 (Nurse, I) said:

> ... You know not many people can do that Wilf. Or would want to get into that area because it can be very painful especially around here, it can be very painful. You know when people are opening their Pandora's Boxes, you know, and the divulging of lots of things that, you know, are their worries or whatever is happening in their life.

Participant 3 (Nurse, I) indicated that she would use avoidance than rather dealing with a spiritual need:

> ... not having the answers that patients want to hear, so rather than dealing with that you don't do it! ... Using avoidance rather than, you know, I think, yeah, possibly using avoidance rather than actually dealing with it.

Another issue related to the notion of spiritual awareness was that, through questioning, I might indeed change people's understandings of the concept, not intentionally, but just through the process of consenting to and participating in an interview.

Ongoing reflection and analysis upon the interview process revealed that the first of these two ethical concerns did not occur. Individuals during the course of an interview would say 'I don't want to answer that question any more!' or 'Can you ask me another question?', thus moving on from a personal, sensitive issue. Through the interview process I learned that it was the participant who ultimately controlled the level and depth of disclosure. In all the interviews conducted only two patients became upset: the first while providing an account of a very distressing situation involving her young child, and the second when talking about the loss of a partner. During these instances the interview was temporarily suspended, but after being allowed time to recompose and with support and reassurance both wanted to continue with the interview.

With reference to the second ethical concern, this issue did seem to emerge. I became acutely aware of this happening despite offering reassurance and explaining that it was not one of the purposes of the research to change participants' perceptions or understanding. However, despite attempts to reassure, it seems that just by taking part in this study some participants' perceptions of spirituality may have been changed in that they were being asked to think about a concept that previously they had not considered or given little thought to within their lives. I observed during Phase I and Phase II of the research, which involved testing out some of the conceptual and theoretical dimensions of spirituality as displayed in the nursing literature, that this process did occur. Some nurses and participants would end their interview by indicating how they were going to go away and read, develop their knowledge or even practice with regard to this area. This finding implied that some of the participants felt that they had limited knowledge in this area or (possibly of more concern) that the questions asked and the responses they provided led them to believe or feel inadequate, unprepared. This implies that some participants found the interview demanding and challenging.

It was observed that some participants would answer a specific question and then follow this by the phrase 'No I don't believe that but I can see that now!'. Two examples from nurse transcripts illustrate these ethical concerns.

Example 1 (*P3, Nurse, I*):

> I think views are individual aren't they? In what you think it's about. But you're going to make me go away and read an awful lot more I think!

And example 2 (*P6, Nurse, I*):

> But I'm going to go away and I'm going to really try. I'd like to be able to go and assess a patient's spiritual needs or look at auditing it on the unit. I think that's something that this has actually made me more aware and I think we need to be looking at auditing spiritual issues and have we met them!

These issues were discussed with my supervision team and it was agreed that there was nothing that could be done to guard against this. It was a consequence of participating in the research study. However, I did look at the wording and 'phrasing' of the questions to try to establish whether these or my delivery of them were the source of the problem. But analysis of the transcripts indicated that this did not always occur and was more to do with the individual's reactions than the nature and structure of the questions.

Evaluation (validity and reliability)

The question of reliability and validity in qualitative research is a source of many debates and still remains a contentious issue (Avis, 1995; Sandelowski, 1993; Strauss and Corbin, 1998; Cutcliffe and McKenna, 2002). It has been argued that the transferability of these concepts from quantitative to qualitative methods is not straightforward; neither is it acceptable. It would seem that in qualitative research these two positivist and scientific canons have been refashioned and replaced by other terms or standards – rigour, trustworthiness, dependability, transferability and reproducibility – which seem to fit the epistemological differences surrounding quantitative and qualitative approaches.

Glaser and Strauss (1967, p. 238), when discussing the application of grounded theory research, provide four 'requisite properties' for establishing the quality of the theory produced. The theory should '*fit*' the substantive area in which it was developed. The theory should be '*understandable*' by those within the substantive area. The theory should be '*general*' in that the theory produced is flexible, allowing its application to a wide range of situations. The theory should also be general in the sense that it will allow reformulation if it is found not to work. Finally, they introduce the notion of '*control*', which refers to the management of situations and forces that may impact upon a theory when it is being applied. These four 'requisite properties' seemed self-explanatory and it seemed that the measure or degree to which these were achieved was not established by the grounded theorist but by those who were applying or using the theory generated.

Glaser and Strauss (1967) in their original work infer that the quality of any grounded theory can only be established retrospectively, that is when the theory is being applied or tested in the substantive area for which it was developed. Strauss and Corbin (1998) in their work seem to provide a template for the critiquing of grounded theory studies (Table 4.19).

The seven criteria listed address all the methodological processes that are central to the undertaking of grounded theory. However, this activity does not necessarily need to be undertaken retrospectively or, more to the point, when the theory is being applied, for the quality of it to be established. It could be that these criteria are an elaboration of the 'requisite properties' provided in the original work of Glaser and Strauss (1967).

Closer analysis of these criteria suggest that the aim of evaluation within grounded theory is to establish whether the theory produced is applicable, in that it is practical and useful to the substantive area in which the theory was produced. Therefore, the theory, whether formal or substantive, must be derived from the context in which the investigation was undertaken, highlighting the conditions – positive and negative – in which it was created. In reality, the theory must be recognised by those within the area under investigation. With this point in mind, after Phase I of the investigation had been completed, I presented the main findings at a seminar where many of the professional participants (and representatives from other disciplines, e.g. chaplaincy and social work) from one of the substantive areas were present. In addition, two

Table 4.19 Evaluative criteria (Strauss and Corbin, 1998, p. 269).

1. How was the original sample selected? On what grounds?
2. What major categories emerged?
3. What were some of the events, incidents, or actions (indicators) that pointed to some of these major categories?
4. On the basis of what categories did the theoretical sampling proceed? That is, how did theoretical formulations guide some of the data collection? After the theoretical sampling was done, how representative of the data did the categories prove to be?
5. What were some of the hypotheses pertaining to conceptual relations (i.e. among categories), and on what grounds were they formulated and validated?
6. Were there instances in which hypotheses did not explain what was happening in the data? How were these discrepancies accounted for? Were hypotheses modified?
7. How and why was the core category selected? Was this collection sudden or gradual, and was it difficult or easy? On what grounds were the final analytic decisions made?

nurse participants from the same area agreed to independently review their transcripts and that of a patient to verify the extent of agreement with the theory presented.

Reflection on evaluation

It is hoped that, during the generation of this grounded theory and in the writing of this book, I have provided enough transparency and explanation to enable those reading it to establish whether the 'requisite properties' and the 'evaluation criteria' have been met.

Reflexivity

Reflective question

- Do you think it is important that the researcher should declare his or her own personal account of spirituality

Introduction

A central characteristic of qualitative methodologies is the notion of reflexivity. This section answers the question 'What is reflexivity?', describing the epistemological importance of reflexivity for this investigation. The section presents my own personal account of spirituality. This personal declaration is relevant because the reader is made aware of any potential bias that may have inadvertently infiltrated the investigation.

What is reflexivity?

In an attempt to increase knowledge and understanding of reflexivity, several general research texts were reviewed to establish what constituted reflexivity and its relevance to qualitative methods. Pillow (2003) argues that the concept has not really been defined or explained adequately within the literature and is, therefore, open to interpretation. Thinking that reflexivity was a term used predominantly by qualitative researchers, more specialised qualitative research texts were scrutinised (for example Morse and Field, 1996; Creswell, 1998; Denzin and Lincoln, 1998) in an attempt to identify an operational definition. Again the concept was either absent or addressed superficially. Carolan (2003) and Woods (2003) suggest that trying to locate a precise definition of reflexivity is not something new and this may be especially so within the discipline of nursing.

The concept of reflexivity

Several definitions of what constituted reflexivity were located. For example, Flick (1998, p. 6) describes reflexivity in the following context:

> Unlike quantitative research, qualitative methods take the researcher's communication with the field and its members as an explicit part of knowledge production instead of excluding it as far as possible as an intervening variable. The subjectivities of the researcher *and* of those being studied are part of the research process. Researchers' reflections on their actions and observations in the filed, their impressions, irritation, feelings and so on, become data in their own right forming part of the interpretation, and are documented in research diaries or context protocols.

Malterud (2001, p. 484), writing in the Lancet, describes reflexivity as:

> An attitude of attending systematically to the context of knowledge construction, especially to the effect of the researcher, at every step of the research process.

These quotations imply a need for the qualitative researcher to reflect openly and honestly upon all experiences (feelings) that are encountered, actions taken or decisions made. These 'reflections' contribute significantly to the overall quality and transparency of the data, and ultimately the theory generated, in that they reveal subjective dimensions of the research process that may be dismissed or overlooked but that may have a significant influence on the study. For example, openly declaring my feelings, attitudes, frustration, and inadequacies encountered throughout the different phases of this research study will undoubtedly add valuable insight (providing a three-dimensional picture), locating me at the centre of the study. This type of reflexive exercise is important because it helps to locate the researcher within the investigation so that any bias in the form of undesirable or hidden skewness may be accounted for (Malterud, 2001, p. 484).

Levels of reflexivity

Porter (2000, p. 142) states that 'good research' necessitates the researcher to use reflexivity at three levels. Firstly, researchers should present the theoretical framework in which they are operating by including disclosure of values and commitments. Secondly, there should be a declaration of how personal factors and personal biographies may impact upon the investigation. Thirdly, the researcher should present and reflect upon the research methods used and the context in which the research is conducted. Throughout this investigation I attempted to address these levels which clarify decisions made, emotions and feelings experienced thus making the entire research transparent.

Epistemological importance of reflexivity

The epistemological relevance and importance of the concept of reflexivity within the qualitative paradigm is that this process will enhance the rigour of the investigation. Within the quantitative paradigm constructs such as reliability and validity account for the effects that a researcher may exert either intentionally or unintentionally upon the research process (Woods, 2003). As indicated, the primary purpose of reflexivity is to enable researchers to locate themselves within the research study. It is recognised within qualitative research that the researcher cannot be divorced from his or her own socially constructed world which may have been shaped through encounters with varied institutions and life experiences. Therefore reflexivity allows the researcher to openly declare or identify any beliefs, values, attitudes or experiences (preconceptions) that may infiltrate, potentially biasing the study. In reality, 'reflexivity' acts like a quality control, a means of ensuring the general quality of the investigation.

Another important function of reflexivity is that this process can assist the researcher to resolve conflicts and tensions that may arise within the different roles, for example researcher and practitioner (Carolan, 2003; Woods, 2003). This was particularly important for this investigation because I had to be mindful that my primary role was as a researcher investigating perceptions of spirituality and not that of a nurse or spiritual counsellor.

In summary, Woods (2003, p. 4) highlights that 'reflexivity' may add to the rigour of a qualitative study by establishing, 'credibility, transferability, dependability and confirmability' – what could be termed the four 'canons' for evaluating the overall quality of the qualitative research process. With the above consideration in mind, the next section provides a personal account of the institutions, forces and experiences that have shaped my worldview and, ultimately, my understanding of the concept of spirituality.

Personal account

There are two main reasons for undertaking this research. The first, personal, one is that I want to continue to expand and extend my academic potential. The second is professional in the sense that, throughout my practice and educational experiences, I have been extremely conscious that spirituality or the spiritual dimension is often a hidden and understated aspect of health care. There are many examples from my own practice that illustrate the point I am making (McSherry, 2006). One in particular has been very profound in establishing this interest:

> Peter was a 72 year old man, who was admitted to hospital with chest pain and diagnosed as having angina since his ECG showed no acute changes. Peter was a practising Roman Catholic and he found meaning and purpose in his beliefs. Peter had been in hospital overnight and he had not seen his wife. Nevertheless, she knew about Peter's admission and was due to visit as soon as possible. In the afternoon on the following day Peter was due to be discharged when he developed sudden severe central chest pain and collapsed with a cardiac arrest – resuscitation was attempted. During the resuscitation Peter's wife arrived unexpectedly on the ward. Unfortunately she did not see Peter before he died. Immediately following Peter's death his wife asked if the Catholic priest had been informed of his admission and whether he had received the sacraments. Inspection of the nursing records shed no light upon the matter – nothing relating to religious denomination, religious practice had been documented. (McSherry, 1997, pp. 14–15)

The lessons I learned from this experience were many in relation to identifying our omissions and limitations within practice: for example, record keeping and documentation or the lack of any structured holistic assessment. However, the biggest lesson was that a patient-centred, individualistic approach to care was needed. Further, I realised that the rhetoric of 'holism' at that time was purely that, a language and philosophy to which the health care system in which I worked paid lip service. The system in which I worked and socialised was predominantly medically orientated. This critical incident revealed that nursing focused on the physical at the expense of other important dimensions, such as the psychological, social, and spiritual. This critical incident highlighted the 'failures' and limitations of the biological model and scientific paradigm that seemed to leave little room for these other fundamental aspects of the patient. As Piles (1990, p. 37) asks: 'Had the science of nursing overshadowed the art of nursing?'.

This incident led me to question my own practice and evaluate the preparation I had received as an undergraduate nurse in relation to the 'spiritual dimension'. I must stress that my initial thoughts were to explore how 'religious' beliefs and practices were important to patients. However, the more I delved into the subject, my direction changed and the 'spiritual dimension' came into focus. This reflective process soon revealed that while I had received excellent preparation in the biological, psychological and social dimensions, little or no emphasis had been placed on such concepts as culture, religious beliefs or 'spirituality'. These concepts were only briefly addressed within loss, death and bereavement lectures.

My spiritual orientation

It is extremely difficult to give an exact and precise definition or account of what I personally feel spirituality to be because of the deeply private and sensitive nature of the subject. It is not easy to articulate aspects of life that are possibly beyond definition and common language. I also feel that this is a difficult exercise because I am revealing intimate, joyous and painful aspects of my own humanity and spirituality for public scrutiny.

It is never easy to introspect and reflect on matters that sometimes I, or indeed we, try to suppress or hide – not wanting to confront, perhaps because of the emotions that could be generated or memories relived, the hidden demons which sometime plague us. Despite these discomforts associated with introspection and the recalling of some painful events I will try to provide a frank, honest, truthful and vivid account of the events that have shaped my spirituality – ultimately who I am as a person. In this process I will hopefully provide a personal account of what I believe spirituality to be. I will also highlight some key life events that have occurred during this investigation that I feel have impacted upon my experiences as a researcher.

When trying to outline all the factors that have influenced and formed my spirituality it is difficult to know from which point to start. Logically it would be right to state that my spirituality has been formed and nurtured throughout my life span continuum by many social, domestic and familial experiences. I have been raised in a council estate by working class parents, my mother being a seamstress and my father a coal-miner. I was not accustomed to many of the material luxuries that wealth or class brings. However, as a family we received a great deal of love and stability, which in hindsight are probably the greatest gifts parents can provide for any child. Apart from the social factors that shaped my life and attitudes, there was the question of religious belief – being educated in the Roman Catholic Church or a Christian tradition. My life has been both positive and negative, involving many key individuals such as parents, family, friends, teachers, priests and institutions such as schools, church, and health care settings.

Death of my father

One major event that had the profoundest effect upon me was facing family illness and the subsequent death of my father from stomach cancer aged 48 when I was still a teenager. This loss resulted in a great deal of personal anxiety and depression after not really confronting the loss of a parent. The death of my father resulted in me not expressing my emotions and thoughts (bottling every thing up), which eventually led me to suffer from reactive depression at the age of twenty. This period of my life was possibly the darkest but most productive in the sense that I became more aware of who I am as a person – a spiritual enlightenment or, using a Christian phrase, my 'Damascus'. After this event I returned to my faith (Roman Catholicism) after many years of professing to be an atheist. Upon reflection, this could have been a form of security, a fear of facing issues around my own mortality. Irrespective of which view is adopted, this episode in my life made me more aware of my own spirituality, albeit at that time within a formal religious framework. This experience also made me question my relationship with other people, witnessing a decline in the egocentrism of youth and seeing the importance and value of family and friendships.

I do not think that I can provide my definition of spirituality in a sentence or two. Personally I feel that spirituality is a conglomeration of many issues, some interpersonal, some transpersonal and others transcendental in origin. Working from this premise I can categorically state that my spirituality is associated with a belief in God or a Supreme Being, making me aware of the existence of a transcendental, metaphysical dimension – a dimension that is mysterious and complex, but not divorced from my own physical, temporal world because spirituality infiltrates all elements of my existence, seen and unseen, in a mysterious manner, bringing stability, meaning, purpose and fulfilment to my life.

Major forces and institutions

The main influence that has shaped my spirituality is the Catholic schooling system that preached the teachings and doctrines of the Roman Catholic Church. I have been exposed to this tradition with its customs, practices and sacraments since birth and on into childhood and latterly into my adult years. Therefore, my spirituality is rooted in the beliefs and teachings of Jesus Christ. These teachings have guided and shaped my life and indeed my attitude towards others especially those less fortunate than myself. I have always tried to live by the maxim – *do unto others as you would have done unto yourself.*

Having a deep faith formed within the Roman Catholic tradition means that I am very conscious of the need for reconciliation and forgiveness. This is something I believe important to my own spirituality and personal growth. No one is perfect. Church history tells us that the perfect man was born and humanity crucified him on a cross. This highlights that society and the world is full of imperfection. Therefore, we all have our own personal flaws and weaknesses to contend with. Working from this premise spirituality is about experiencing the need to forgive and be forgiven.

Roles and experiences

After leaving school I was fortunate enough to undertake several roles before entering nursing. Firstly, I was a Senior Air Craftsman in the Royal Air Force (RAF), working as a Painter and Finisher. When I left the RAF I went into post-16 education, undertaking a 'pre-nursing course'. After completion of this programme I worked as an Auxiliary Nurse caring for older people, before leaving to become a Seminarian in the Catholic Church which I did for several years. Upon leaving seminary I entered Higher Education (HE), reading for a Bachelor of Science (Honours) in Nursing Sciences. All these institutions and diverse experiences have shaped my worldview and my understanding of spirituality, health and illness.

Being a husband (to Mandy) and a father of two children (Stacey, 15, and Matthew, 13) means that I have had to try to balance the commitments to my family, current and past employers and my research. This has been very difficult, and at times, practically impossible. I must stress that if it had not been for my family's love, support and tolerance during this study, I am sure that the research would not have been completed.

Recent bereavement

I must also acknowledge that halfway through this study my mother died suddenly on 4 May 2000 at the age of 73. This loss resulted in me becoming more aware of my own spirituality and mortality, sensitising me to the needs of others. The fact, that technically, I was now an orphan, needing to go it alone in the world, made life difficult. At that time I wanted to stop all my academic endeavours, but with love, reassurance and support from my family, children and two brothers the sadness and depression faded and I managed to persevere with the study.

Economic and personal barriers

As already implied, another major factor that has hampered the study is the economic constraints imposed by other commitments, i.e. family and work. I have been aware of a pressing need to try to maintain some semblance of normality in life, which at times can be lost when one is so actively involved in the research process. I had learned major lessons from my previous research involvement, and the need for maintaining a sense of proportion in all things.

By far the biggest limitation on this investigation was having insufficient time to become fully immersed in the research process. Trying to do the investigation on one day per week was almost impossible. This meant that I had to utilise my own time, which placed considerable strain on personal relationships. These personal factors, combined with a major bereavement in the middle of data collection, were emotionally demanding and exhausting. Another personal factor that may have subconsciously influenced the investigation is my own perceptions of spirituality. This section describes the forces and life events that have shaped my understanding of spirituality. However, it is proposed that the reflexive processes instituted minimised any personal bias entering the investigation.

Summary points

- This section has provided an overview of the concept of reflexivity, highlighting the important and central role that it plays in enhancing the rigour of qualitative research.
- The section demonstrates how reflexivity entails the researcher to review the theoretical, personal and methodological processes so that any intentional or unintentional bias that could infiltrate the investigation is declared.

Conclusion

This chapter has provided a detailed account of all the methodological processes encountered while undertaking this study. The reasons for choosing grounded theory as the preferred qualitative method have been explained. By presenting all the different stages involved in the research process this has offered insight and transparency into the decisions made and the actions taken, thereby enhancing the quality of the investigation.

References

Anderson, A. (1991) Use of grounded theory methodology. *ABNF Journal*, Spring, 28–32.

Avis, R. (1995) Valid arguments? A consideration of the concept of validity in establishing the credibility of research findings. *Journal of Advanced Nursing*, **22**, 1230–9.

Baldacchino, D. (2002) Spiritual coping of Maltese patients with first acute myocardial infarction: a longitudinal study. *Unpublished PhD Thesis*, University of Hull, England.

Baker, C., Wuest, J. and Stern, P. N. (1992) Methods slurring: the grounded theory/phenomenology example. *Journal of Advanced Nursing*, **17**, 1355–60.

Backman, K. and Kyngas, H. A. (1999) Challenges of the grounded theory approach to the novice researcher. *Nursing and Health Sciences*, **1**, 147–53.

Benton, D. C. (2000) Grounded theory. In: *The Research Process in Nursing*, 4th edn (ed. D. F. S. Cormack). Blackwell Scientific, Oxford.

Bulmer, H. (1971) Sociological implications of the thoughts of George Herbert Mead. In *School and Society* (eds. B. R. Cosin, I. Dale, G. M. Esland and D. F. Swift). Routledge & Kegan Paul, London.

Burkhardt, M. A. (1991) Exploring understandings of spirituality among women in Appalachia. *Doctoral Dissertation*, University of Miami, Florida.

Burkhardt, M. A. (1994) Becoming and connecting: elements of spirituality for women. *Holistic Nursing Practice*, **8**(4), 12–21.

Burns, N. and Grove, S. K. (1997) *The Practice of Nursing Research Conduct, Critique and Utilization*, 3rd edn. W. B. Saunders, Philadelphia.

Carolan, M. (2003) Reflexivity: a personal journey during data collection. *Nurse Researcher*, **10**(3), 7–14.

Carson, V. B. (1989) *Spiritual Dimensions of Nursing Practice*. W. B. Saunders, Philadelphia.

Carter, D. E. (2000) Quantitative research. In: *The Research Process in Nursing*, 4th edn (ed. D. F. S. Cormack). Blackwell Scientific, Oxford.

Cavendish, R., Luise, B. K., Horne, K., Bauer, M., Medefindt, J., Gallo, M. A., Calvino, C. and Kutza, T. (2000) Opportunities for enhanced spirituality relevant to well adults. *Nursing Diagnosis*, **11**(4), 151–63.

Chenitz, W. C. and Swanson, J. M. (1986) *From Practice to Grounded Theory*. Addison-Wesley, Reading, MA.

Clark, C. and Heidenreich, T. (1995) Spiritual care for the critically ill. *American Journal of Critical Care*, **4**(1), 77–81.

Clark, C. C., Cross, J. R., Deane, D. M. and Lowry, L. W. (1991) Spirituality: integral to quality care. *Holistic Nursing Practice*, **5**(3), 67–76.

Cobb, M. (2001) *The Dying Soul Spiritual Care at the End of Life*. Open University Press, Buckingham.

Corbin, J. (1997) *Qualitative Health Research*, **7**(1), 50–4.

Coyne, I. T. (1997) Sampling in qualitative research. Purposeful and theoretical sampling; merging or clear boundaries. *Journal of Advanced Nursing*, **26**, 623–30.

Creswell, J. W. (1998) *Qualitative Inquiry and Research Design*. Sage, Thousand Oaks.

Cutcliffe, J. R. (2000) Methodological Issues in grounded theory. *Journal of Advanced Nursing*, **31**(6), 1470–84.

Cutcliffe, J. R. and McKenna, H. P. (2002) When do we know that we know? Considering the truth of research findings and the craft of qualitative research. *International Journal of Nursing Studies*, **39**, 611–18.

Denzin, N. K. and Lincoln, Y. S. (1998) *Strategies of Qualitative Inquiry*. Sage, Thousand Oaks.

Draper, P. and McSherry, W. (2002) A critical review of spirituality and spiritual assessment. *Journal of Advanced Nursing*, **39**(1), 1–2.

Draper, J. and Draper, P. (2003) Response to: Watson's Guest Editorial 'Scientific methods are the only credible way forward for nursing research', *Journal of Advanced Nursing*, **43**, 219–20. *Journal of Advanced Nursing*, **44**(5), 546–7.

Field, P. and Morse, J. (1985*) Nursing Research: The Application of Qualitative Approaches*. Aspen Publishers, Rockville, MD.

Flick, E. (1998) *An Introduction to Qualitative Research*. Sage, London.

Garfinkel, H. (1967) *Studies in Ethnomethodology*. Prentice Hall, New Jersey.

Glaser, B. G. (1978) *Theoretical Sensitivity: Advances in the Methodology of Grounded Theory*. Sociology Press, Mill Valley.

Glaser, B. G. and Strauss, A. L. (1965) *Awareness of Dying*. Aldine, Chicago.

Glaser, B. G. and Strauss, A. L. (1967) *The Discovery of Grounded Theory*. Aldine de Gruyter, New York.

Glaser, B. G. and Strauss, A. L. (1968) *Time for Dying*. Aldine, Chicago.

Haber, J. (1994) Sampling. In: *Nursing Research Methods, Critical Appraisal, and Utilization* (eds. G. LoBiondo-Wood and J. Harber), Chapter 12. Mosby, St Louis.

Harrington, A. (1995) Spiritual care: what does it mean to RNs? *Australian Journal of Advanced Nursing*, **12**(4), 5–14.

Harrison, J. and Burnard, P. (1993) *Spirituality and Nursing Practice*. Avebury, Aldershot.

Henery, N. (2003) Constructions of spirituality in contemporary nursing theory. *Journal of Advanced Nursing*, **42**, 550–7.

Hermann, C. P. (2001) Spiritual needs of dying patients: a qualitative study. *Oncology Nursing Forum*, **28**(1), 67–72.

Holloway, I. and Wheller, S. (1996) *Qualitative Research for Nurses*. Blackwell Science, Oxford.

Horn, R. (1996) Negotiating research access to organisations. *The Psychologist*, December, 551–4.

Johnson, M., Long, T. and White, A. (2001) Arguments for 'British Pluralism' in qualitative health research. *Journal of Advanced Nursing*, **33**(2), 243–9.

Kearney, S. (1994) Spirituality as a coping mechanism in multiple sclerosis: the patient's perspective. *Unpublished dissertation*, Institute of Nursing Studies, University of Hull, England.

Kendall, J. (1999) Axial coding and the grounded theory controversy. *Western Journal of Nursing Research*, **21**(6), 743–57.

Malterud, K. (2001) Qualitative research: standards, challenges, and guidelines. *The Lancet*, **358**, 483–8.

McCann, T. V. and Clark, E. (2003a) Grounded theory in nursing research: Part 1 – Methodology. *Nurse Researcher*, **11**(2), 7–18.

McCann, T. V. and Clark, E. (2003b) Grounded theory in nursing research: Part 2 – Critique. *Nurse Researcher*, **11**(2), 19–28.

McCann, T. V. and Clark, E. (2003c) Grounded theory in nursing research: Part 3 – Application. *Nurse Researcher*, **11**(2), 29–39.

McSherry, W. (1997) A descriptive survey of nurses' perceptions of spirituality and spiritual care. *Unpublished MPhil Thesis*, University of Hull, England.

McSherry, W. (2006) *Making Sense of Spirituality in Nursing and Health Care Practice*, 2nd edn. Jessica Kingsley, London.

McSherry, R., Simmons, M. and Pearce, P. (2002a) An introduction to evidenced-informed nursing. In: *Evidenced-Informed Nursing a Guide for Clinical Nurses* (eds. R. McSherry, M. Simmons and P. Abbott), Chapter 1. Routledge, London.

McSherry, W., Draper, P. and Kendrick D. (2002b) The construct validity of a rating scale designed to assess spirituality and spiritual care. *International Journal of Nursing Studies*, **39**(7), 723–34.

Mead, G. H. (1934) *Mind, Self and Society*. University of Chicago Press, Chicago.

Morse, J. A. and Field, P. A. (1996) *Nursing Research: The Application of Qualitative Approaches*, 2nd edn. Stanley Thornes, Cheltenham.

Muir Gray, J. A. (1997) *Evidence-based Healthcare: How to Make Health Policy and Management Decisions*. Churchill Livingstone, London.

Murray, R. B. and Zentner, J. B. (1989) *Nursing Concepts for Health Promotion*. Prentice Hall, London.

Narayanasamy, A. (2001) *Spiritual Care: a Practical Guide for Nurses and Health Care Practitioners*, 2nd edn. Quay, Wiltshire.

Narayanasamy, A. (2004) Commentary on MacLaren, J. (2004) A kaleidoscope of understandings: spiritual nursing in a multi-faith society. *Journal of Advanced Nursing*, **45**(5), 457–62. *Journal of Advanced Nursing*, **45**(5), 462–4.

Narayanasamy, A. and Owens, J. (2001) A critical incident study of nurses' responses to the spiritual needs of their patients. *Journal of Advanced Nursing*, **33**(4), 446–55.

Norton, L. (1999) The philosophical bases of grounded theory and their implications for research practice. *Nurse Researcher*, **7**(1), 31–45.

Oldnall, A. S. (1995) On the absence of spirituality in nursing theories and models. *Journal of Advanced Nursing*, **21**, 417–18.

Oldnall, A. (1996) A critical analysis of nursing: meeting the spiritual needs of patients. *Journal of Advanced Nursing*, **23**, 138–44.

Oppenheim, A. N. (1992) *Questionnaire Design, Interviewing and Attitude Measurement*. Print Publishers, London.

Piles, C. (1990) Providing spiritual care. *Nurse Educator*, **15**(1), 36–41.

Pillow, W. S. (2003) Confession, catharsis, or cure, rethinking the uses of reflexivity as methodological power in qualitative research. *Qualitative Studies in Education*, **16**(2), 175–96.

Polit, D. F. and Hungler, B. P. (1999) *Nursing Research Principles and Methods*, 6th edn. Lippincott, Philadelphia.

Pontin, D. (2000) Interview. In: *The Research Process in Nursing*, 4th edn (ed. D. F. S. Cormack), Chapter 24, Blackwell Scientific, Oxford.

Porter, S. (2000) Qualitative research. In: *The Research Process in Nursing*, 4th edn (ed. D. F. S. Cormack), Chapter 12. Blackwell Scientific, Oxford.

Porter, S. and Carter, D. E. (2000) Common terms and concepts in research. In: *The Research Process in Nursing*, 4th edn (ed. D. F. S. Cormack), Chapter 2. Blackwell Scientific, Oxford.

Reed, P. (1992) An emerging paradigm for the investigation of spirituality in nursing. *Research in Nursing and Health*, **15**, 349–57.

Richards, L. (1999) *Using 'N' Vivo in Qualitative Research*. Sage, London.

Ross, L. (1997) Elderly patients' perceptions of their spiritual care: a pilot study. *Journal of Advanced Nursing*, **26**, 710–15.

Rumbold, B. (2002) *Spirituality and Palliative Care*. Oxford University Press, Australia.

Sandelowski, M. (1993) Rigor or rigor mortis: the problem of rigor in qualitative research revisited. *Advances in Nursing Sciences*, **16**(2), 1–8.

Sheldon, L. (1999) Grounded theory: issues for research in nursing. *Nursing Standard*, **12**(52), 47–50.

Smith, K. and Bailey, F. (1997) Understanding grounded theory: principles and evaluation. *Nurse Researcher*, **4**(3), 17–30.

Stern, P. N. (1994) Eroding grounded theory. In: *Critical Issues in Qualitative Research Methods* (ed. J. M. Morse). Sage, Thousand Oaks.

Strauss, A. and Corbin, J. (1998) *Basics of Qualitative Research*, 2nd edn. Sage, Thousand Oaks.

Stoll, R. I. (1989) The essence of spirituality. In: *Spiritual Dimensions of Nursing Practice* (ed. V. B. Carson), Chapter 1. W. B. Saunders, Philadelphia.

Swinton, J. and Narayanasamy, A. (2002) Response to: A critical view of spirituality and spiritual assessment by P. Draper and W. McSherry (2002) *Journal of Advanced Nursing*, **39**, 1–2. *Journal of Advanced Nursing*, **40**(2), 158–60.

Taylor, E. J. (2003) Nurses caring for the spirit: patients with cancer and family caregiver expectations. *Oncology Nursing Forum*, **30**(4), 585–90.

Thomas, J. and Retsas, A. (1999) Transacting self-preservation: a grounded theory of the spiritual dimension of people with terminal cancer. *International Journal of Nursing Studies*, **36**(3), 191–201..

Walter, T. (1997) The ideology and organization of spiritual care: three approaches. *Palliative Medicine*, **11**, 21–30.

Walter, T. (2002) Spirituality in palliative care: opportunity or burden? *Palliative Medicine*, **16**, 133–9.

Walton, J. (1997) Spirituality of patients recovering from an acute myocardial infarction: a grounded theory study. *Unpublished doctoral dissertation*, University of Missouri-Kansas City.

Wainwright, S. P. (1993) Getting a second chance: a grounded theory study of the transformational experiences of liver transplantation. *Unpublished Master of Science Dissertation*, King's College, University of London, London.

Watson, R. (2002) Scientific methods are the only credible way forward for nursing research. *Journal of Advanced Nursing*, **43**(3), 217–18.

Wells, K. (1995) The strategy of grounded theory: possibilities and problems. *Social Work Research*, **19**(1), 33–8.

Woods, L. (2003) Getting it right. *Nurse Researcher*, **10**(3), 4–6.

CHAPTER 5

Delving into the evidence

Introduction

This chapter presents and discusses the main findings of this grounded theory investigation. It explores the themes and categories that emerged during the analysis of the three phases of the study outlined in Chapter 4. The chapter verifies how each phase added to and developed the emerging theory. Each phase will be explored in depth, relating the findings to theoretically sampled literature comprising anecdotal, theoretical and empirical sources. Literature was used to clarify or substantiate positions raised and to aid theory development and refinement.

Reflective question

- When reading the findings of a qualitative study, how would you expect the results to be presented?

Overview of findings

In keeping with a grounded theory method, all the results will be supported by raw data, thus providing a rich contextual background against which essence and meaning can be established, keeping theory development rooted in the data. The section is presented using the following format. Firstly, it is in keeping with the 'funnel down' approach advocated by Glaser (1978, p. 131):

> To set out the general nature of the core variable and then funnel it down to a theory on a specific process or problem that is associated with one property of it is very effective.

The core category titled *'Assumption versus expectation'* and its two associated properties – professional discourse and public discourse – are outlined. The core category was labelled because it would seem that health care is in danger of professionalising spirituality in terms of language and practice, thus making a generalisation about what the term means for diverse groups and what their needs in this area might be without asking them. Furthermore, the core category and its associated properties were constructed because they explain and pull together all the categories created during the three phases. In addition, the core category was able to accommodate the variation that existed within categories and between participant groups (Strauss and Corbin, 1998).

Secondly, the findings of the three phases are presented in detail. In Phase I the assumption that spirituality is universally recognised and understood was explored with the participants. It was found that there was considerable variation in the way that HCPs and patients understood the concept and that they had different expectations in terms of receiving spiritual care. These notable disparities led to the identification and creation of the core category and its associated properties mentioned above. The name 'professional discourse' accounted for those findings that may have led to the spiritual dimension being recognised and understood within health care, for example the desire to provide holistic care and the findings pertaining to education. In contrast, the term 'public discourse' reflected patients' real expectations and fears in terms of understanding spirituality and receiving spiritual care. Phase I also led to the construction of five subcategories, labelled definitions of spirituality; diverse perceptions of spirituality; provision of spiritual care; socialisation of the spirit; and drivers. These subcategories provide a detailed account of how spirituality is perceived by the diverse groups, offering insight as to why variation in understanding and expectation may occur.

In Phase II, participants' understanding of spirituality and spiritual care were further explored by testing out some of the components considered important aspects of spirituality within health care such as relationships, forgiveness and creativity. Analysis led to the formation of two further categories – spiritual narratives and subconscious awareness of spirituality – thus expanding the theory. Phase III drew upon the findings of Phases I and II, resulting in the testing of the recurrent themes that had been identified in all the phases of the investigation. This phase led to the creation of the 'Principal Components Model' for the advancement of spirituality and spiritual care. The section describes how the model may be used to assist development in health care practice, education and research.

Explanatory notes

Because of the vast amount of data generated it is impossible to include excerpts from all the transcripts that led to the formation of properties, categories and the core category. A table of all participants involved in each of the three phases is provided within each section and the reason for theoretical selection indicated. In addition, the tables provide important demographic detail surrounding each of the participants. The following codes will be used when integrating excerpts of transcript:

P = Participant
R = Researcher

Participants were allocated a number which is used for identification purposes, ranging from P1 to P53.

Nos. 1–22 participated in Phase I
Nos. 22–40 participated in Phase II
Nos. 41–53 participated in Phase III

Where further clarity or additional detail is required, this is provided in brackets; for example when comparing and contrasting different groups the following examples are provided: *P1 (Nurse, I)* and *P13 (Patient, I)*.

The Roman numerals I–III indicate the area from which participants were recruited.

Core category – assumption versus expectation

'Assumption versus expectation' was an overarching theme that continually emerged throughout data collection and theory development. This became the 'core category' because it had relevance for all the participant groups, providing an explanation for all the categories in that it could account for variation and it had the power to pull together all the categories. This category became central to the development of this investigation at a very early stage. Strauss and Corbin (1998 p. 146) write:

> A central category has analytic power. What gives it that power is its ability to pull the other categories together to form an explanatory whole. Also, a central category should be able to account for considerable variation within categories.

The core category was named *'assumption versus expectation'* because analysis revealed a dichotomy between what nurses regarded as 'spirituality' and how this was viewed by patients and the public. The nursing and, it must be added, the wider health care literature makes assumptions regarding patients' and the public's perceptions of spirituality and, indeed, what these needs might be. This mismatch between professional assumptions and patient/public expectation became more apparent as the investigation progressed. The following transcript is an example of an 'us' (Professional) and 'them' (Patient) mentality. This is illustrated metaphorically by the nurses or other HCPs being on one side of the fence and the patients being on the other:

> P: Again there's difficulty on, on, the patient's side as well isn't it? When you actually explain about spiritual care as we've said before, you'll get you may get you know, em and again, I'm not you know sort of saying all patients are like this, some patients will say 'woo, woo', 'spirituality'. And they think it's, you know, sort of holding hands in a séance. And, and it frightens them, it frightens patients. Em and so they don't want to address it. At, at, especially at times, when they are vulnerable, they feel vulnerable any way, I think people coming in [*short pause*] ... and I think, so it's the way we explain to patients. So the knock-on effect of that, we've got to understand what were talking about [*giggle*] and what were trying to get across, so we can actually speak to patients and what they will, you know, they don't have to have the label spirituality when they are talking to us there actually passing on, you know spiritual or it won't be put in those terms, about themselves about, their you know, their life and their philosophy on life. They are already talking about it; sometimes again, I don't want to keep repeating this. It's sticking labels on people and making things fit into things, that's you know it, it, instead of [*long pause*] .... I don't know, I don't know, I keep getting back to this blank page and it would make it very difficult. *P1 (Nurse, I)*

Subsequent phases of the investigation together with ongoing analysis of the data along with the 'technical' literature tested out the strength of the 'core category'. This testing out or refinement established that a dichotomy exists in the way that some groups of patients, representatives from the major world religions and the general public perceive spirituality when contrasted against the health professions.

For many participants the concept of spirituality, as used and defined in health care, was an alien term that did not feature in their language or vocabulary. A number of participants within the patient and general public groups had never heard of the word nor given any 'conscious' consideration to the meaning of this concept within their own lives. Conversely, the majority of the HCPs participating, with the exception of one physiotherapist and one occupational therapist, attempted to define spirituality, readily recognising this as an important yet often neglected dimension of their role. The evidence emerging from this inquiry would support the hypothesis that health care may have unwittingly and perhaps unconsciously fashioned a form of spirituality that is not readily recognisable by all groups within a pluralistic society. The two properties of the core category were named 'professional discourse' and 'public discourse'. These two discourses, while associated with the same phenomena, are very distinct in terms of the language and descriptors used to define spirituality and the assumptions and expectations in relation to receiving spiritual care.

Professional discourse

Identifiable within the nursing and health care literature is a growing unease with the 'blanket' application of the concept of spirituality across all groups and sections of society (Draper and McSherry, 2002; Kellehear, 2002; MacLaren, 2004; Narayanasamy, 2004). Visible in this investigation is a realisation that the 'language' surrounding spirituality which has been developed within health care was not recognisable or familiar to some groups. This growing awareness by researchers and academics substantiates the proposition that a professional discourse and dialogue have been constructed that may not be readily recognisable by patients. This was certainly a major and recurrent theme throughout all three phases of this investigation. A polarisation of views was obvious, with some of the patients not sharing the same language, or not having the fluency or articulation of nurses and the other allied health professionals regarding what constitutes spirituality. Similarly, there were variances in opinion between professionals' and patients' expectations in terms of spiritual care. The following examples of transcript illustrate these points. In the first example, the nurse demonstrates a fluency and familiarity with the concept of spirituality:

> P: I would say it is our very soul. It is who we are. Spirituality is different for everybody. Everybody has spiritual needs, some people say they have no religious beliefs, but I still believe they have a spiritual side to them. *P25 (Nurse, III)*

The next example, taken from a patient's transcripts, supports the hypothesis that some patients may not have given any real consideration to the concept of spirituality, meaning that they had no preconceived ideas about receiving spiritual care:

> R: You have not really heard of the word spirituality?
> P: No, not at all! *P22 (Patient, III)*

The same patient:

> R: Do you think nurses should be involved with this area?
> P: Well I don't know, I think they have got enough on their plates doing what they do, without being involved with that! I mean, quite honestly, they are run off their feet as it is.

The professional discourse is evidenced by three characteristics:

1. Firstly, there has been the creation of a shared language and dialogue surrounding the nature of spirituality that seems specific to the culture of health care.
2. Secondly, the manner in which the allied health professions, in particular nurses, have sought to provide spiritual care, suggests that there was a professional and, to a lesser degree, a managerial expectation that this dimension should be formally assessed and addressed within practice.
3. Thirdly, there is an indication from the data that the educational preparation of all allied health professionals, particularly nurses, may be constructing and perpetuating the dichotomy between patient expectations and professional assumptions in terms of how spirituality may be perceived within a pluralistic society.

It must be stressed that this professional discourse, while being tangential to patients, does not mean that the concept is to be ignored and all the pioneering work undertaken during several decades discarded. Narayanasamy (2004) argues that the danger of focusing solely upon the divergent views associated with the language of spirituality for professionals and patients is that the importance of the concept may be diminished. He writes (Narayanasamy, 2004, p. 463):

> To be dismissive of the significance of spirituality in health care on the grounds that patients do not use similar languages to those of spirituality researchers amounts to professional patronization and imperialism.

While this is an important observation, it must be stressed that it is not just researchers into spirituality who are constructing this language. As I argued in Chapter 2, professional and political agendas have resulted in many of the allied health professions being 'forced' to focus on the 'spiritual dimension' of patients without any real explanation of what the concept means and little guidance of what constitutes spiritual care. If nursing and all the allied health professions, including medicine, fail to acknowledge and investigate the disparities surrounding the assumptions that are made regarding the language and understanding of spirituality then we do not only run the risk of 'professional patronization and imperialism' (Narayanasamy, 2004, p. 463), but also of discrimination and alienation.

Consequences of a professional discourse

The acknowledgment of a professional discourse within the health care literature demonstrates a positive desire to 'deconstruct' (to gain deeper understanding) and to expand insight into spirituality so that future strategy and policy are shaped not only by bureaucrats and civil servants but by all stakeholders, particularly the providers and consumers. Reflecting diversity of dialogue in terms of understanding spirituality will ensure that the term has relevance and significance for all, presenting a more balanced discourse. Drawing attention to the professional discourse is not to dismiss or minimise the importance of the concept for individuals. On the contrary it reinforces and 'cements' the importance of spirituality for health care by raising awareness of potential dichotomies. The adoption of an 'ostrich mentality' to the management of these deliberations will not advance practice or achieve any resolution. In fact, such avoidance will be disadvantageous on the grounds that it will suppress future innovations. Failure to capture the vocabulary and articulation of patient groups in terms of perceptions of spirituality, whether they use the word or not, is not to devalue or suggest that the word is redundant. The process of elucidation of the term will ensure that future reforms in practice and education reflect these diverse representations of spirituality. Taylor (2002, p. 3) refers to this as establishing common ground highlighting how this 'common' understanding will be helpful in elucidating the concept.

In addition, I do not think that arguing over whether patients identify or recognise the term is an attempt by researchers and academics to make the term obsolete! On the contrary, the danger is if this type of conceptual development is not embraced and contested but ignored. Failing to engage and challenge conceptual developments associated with spirituality will undoubtedly result in the perpetuation of a theory of spirituality that is weak and underdeveloped, lacking conceptual and theoretical credibility, because it will not reflect the voice of service users. Furthermore, an inherent danger is that academics may institute a schism and accept *carte blanche* that patients do not have to articulate what spirituality is for it to have relevance for practice. This would be condescending because it would result in the perpetuation of a paternalistic model of spirituality and spiritual care, a transgression against the emancipation of patients in directing care and research in this area.

Key points

- The professional discourse is substantiated in the desire to establish 'spirituality' as a fundamental and central dimension of health care.
- The properties of this category reflect a familiarity with the concept and the aspiration to raise awareness of this within the spheres of practice and education.
- The following subcategories were evident within the transcripts of the majority of nurses and they also had significant meaning for the other allied health professionals: *Mantra – holism; Recognition of spirituality; Universal application; Existentially driven; and Educationally shaped.*

Mantra-holism

A question posed to all nurses and [a different variation of the question to] patients was:

> R: Can you describe the type of care that you seek to provide to your patients?

Almost all of the nurses responded with the phrase 'holistic care' or a synonym: 'total patient care'. With respect to the hospice, several of the nurses responded with 'specialist palliative care'. These phrases were used with some frequency, like a mantra. The phrase was communicated in an automated manner, like an innate intuitive response. This is evident in the following transcript:

> P: Well [*short pause*]... it's a new word – 'holistic' that business, em, that describes it in a modern way, but, I always put it as total care really! Patient, family, extended or anybody around em [patient] who needed support and all aspects of care really because if a patient is worried about something that isn't have to do with physical, well say with the illness, still as an impact on, on, em, the patient's improvement! *P5 (Nurse, II, Intensive Care Unit)*

The term 'holistic' was subsequently broken down by nurse participants to include the dimensions: physical, psychological and social. Several of the nurses would add 'spiritual' without any prompt, demonstrating recognition of the importance of this dimension within the individual. This finding is supported by Hilton (2002, p. 33), who stresses:

> Holistic health practice involves caring for the physical, psychological, social and spiritual needs of patients, all of which affect a person's health status

This approach and the one exhibited by many participants achieve holism via a reductionist model. With the participants there was no description of how all dimensions of the individual are interrelated or connected. Interestingly, the notion of providing holistic care was identifiable in all specialities of nursing represented. It did not matter from which area of practice a nurse originated; the vast majority recognised the importance of 'holistic practice':

> P: It's caring for all their needs whatever they may be and that can include the spiritual needs, whatever, it's seeing them as a whole and it's not just the limb that we are repairing. It's actually addressing all issues, you know, social issues etc within, you know, the care that we provide. *P12 (Nurse, III, Surgical)*

In addition, the term 'holistic' was qualified or extended by some of the nurses adding the terms 'individualistic' or 'patient-centred care'. This implied that the individual patient and his or her family were central to the philosophy of holistic care and not the opposite, the nurse imposing a paternalistic and professional dominance in terms of authority.

The transcripts presented in this section reveal that treating the patient holistically could be achieved through a conscious process. There was recognition that 'holistic' care would be more beneficial to patients and this could be orchestrated within practice. In qualifying the term 'beneficial' in this context, holism appeared to be used against the notion of ritualistic practice and a form of medical reductionism, where the focus was predominantly upon the initiation or completion of physical tasks such as bed baths. One nurse referred to this activity as reverting to type. The nurses recognise the inability of the medical model to explain subjective aspects of human nature. Maslow (1971, p. 29) acknowledged this limitation:

> Of course, though the medical illness model is necessary (for tumours, bacterial invasion, ulcers etc.), it is certainly not sufficient (for neurotic, characterological, or spiritual disturbances).

These points are supported in the following account:

> P: The care that we provide, as I say Wilf, when we talk about holistic, sometime we pay lip service to that actual concept. Huh mm, and hopefully not here, but when I look through my nursing career and other areas that I have worked, I think it is still physically predominated and

> the psychosocial – spiritual – whatever, is an add on bit and still the physically is still looked on as you know. If you talk to nurses, oh make sure the bed baths are done d.d.d.d. [*Meaning the same attitude can be applied to other physical tasks*] and, that's what actually, you know, we are wanting to get away from here. *P1 (Nurse, I)*

Eleven out of the 12 nurses participating in Phase I judged 'holistic care' to be a positive and liberating concept that directed and determined the quality of care they provided. One nurse provided an alternative response that was divergent from the rest of the nurse participants:

> P: ... the key word holistic but I am not really carried away with that. Because I think as a nurse sometimes you're, em, a person as well and some of my expectations, my expectations are given over to them. I'd like to think that I would be treated as this person the 'whole person'. And that my needs and wants, but I might be a bit pushy, but I don't always side with the family, if it's not what the patient wants. But you say holistic but I don't think that it is! I do think individuals, patients to the best they can it's their wants and needs. *P20 (Nurse, III)*

For this nurse, the holistic approach seemed to undermine the role of the individual in determining their own care especially where the concept of holism embraced family. This nurse felt that holistic care could not be provided impartially because ultimately their own beliefs and values would determine the priority of an individual's wants and needs.

The majority of the nurses interviewed during the course of Phase I indicated that a holistic philosophy was integral to patient care because this approach to care delivery recognised that patients were made up of several important yet, seemingly discrete dimensions, all of which warranted careful and equal attention including the spiritual. Detailed analysis reveals that the noun 'holism' appeared in preference to the adjective 'holistic'. Holistic practice seemed to recognise the voice and concerns of patients, valuing them as individuals with diverse needs and wants. The mantra of holism implied concern for the individual, seeing them as someone who holds a central part in the orchestration of their care.

Recognition of spirituality

Analysis of the transcripts in Phase I revealed that many of the nurse participants recognised the concept of spirituality as being important both personally and professionally. As indicated, this dimension was expressed as an 'integral' aspect of holistic care. Several of the nurses mentioned spirituality or 'spiritual' without any prompting or probing. Others would arrive at a definition by another route, for example personal beliefs or faith, often subsumed under religion or religious affiliation. Irrespective of how the nurse drew attention to the concept, there was a conscious awareness of the importance of this constituent of health care, especially in relation to maintaining a person's self-identify and sense of well-being. Recognition of the concept is illustrated in the following quotations while talking about holism:

> P: Looking at the holistic care of the patient including the psychological, physical and spiritual. *P6 (Nurse, I)*
>
> P: Well obviously the spiritual side of things, cos, I know, I know that, I think everybody's got a spiritual side of their nature that's my belief... *P8 (Nurse, I)*

When discussing the concept of faith:

> P: Em... it's not just looking at the patient and symptoms and their illness but looking at, em, their social needs, everything, em, you've got, em, any particular faith, it's, it's everything, em, not all people have faith, a strong faith, em [*long pause*]... and that!... *P3 (Nurse, I)*

Recognition and, to a lesser degree, familiarity with the concept was exhibited in the language of nurses describing spirituality. This was reinforced during Phase III when other allied health professionals were interviewed. Almost all of the allied health professions recognised and described spirituality as a multifaceted phenomenon comprising several layers of meaning as opposed to a singular layer of meaning espoused by many of the non-professional groups.

An example of multifaceted approach to spirituality offered by a nurse:

> P: Well, as I said before, everybody has a soul. So everybody has a spiritual pathway in order to enhance their own souls. Em and I feel personally that's the purpose of our existence, you know, is to, is to develop our spiritual qualities. And that can be via the way we behave, the way we are to other people, or may be the way we have religion or you know, how we pray to God etc., etc. [*Demonstrating familiarity with the constituents of spirituality*] and all that is part of developing our spiritual qualities! So to me the spiritual side of people is not meaningless, it is a very important aspect of our own development. *P12 (Nurse, III, Surgical)*

In contrast to a single layer approach offered by a patient:

R: One word that seems to be used quite a lot now in health care is spirituality, if I was to ask you what that meant, how would you describe it?

P: I have not a clue. I really don't know what it means. To me it is just about religion. I don't know how you describe it quite honestly. That's why when you rung up I thought to my self, I don't know what I am going to say to you, because I don't know what it means. *P22 (Patient, III, Surgical)*

This finding validates a great deal of international research acknowledging that health professionals perceive spirituality as an essential element of their role. The findings affirm that many members of the allied health professions are acutely aware of the spiritual dimension within themselves and the importance of this dimension for some service users.

Universal application

A popular belief held by many of the nurses and, it must be added, one of the patients interviewed during Phase I was a conviction that spirituality applied to all individuals. For many of the nurses spirituality was more than just pertaining to the religious and pious. It applied to all people – believers and unbelievers (Cawley, 1997). In fact, many of the nurses and, indeed, patients were opposed to 'religiosity'. Spirituality as a concept was applied universally to all people whether the term was used directly or indirectly. This is evidenced in the following transcripts:

R: What you seem to be implying then is there are certain components of spirituality that could be universally applied to all individuals?

P: [*interjects before I'd finished signalling strength of feeling*] Yeah I'd go with that, I'd go with that! But it is quite difficult to argue and impossible to prove but I would certainly agree with that very strongly! *P4 (Nurse, II, Manager)*

R: And from what you seem to be saying you would suggest that, that applies to everybody irrespective...

P: Absolutely everybody! Because I believe everybody has a soul so therefore spirituality applies to everybody! *P12 (Nurse, III, Surgical)*

This patient felt that spirituality was present in all individuals:

P: I think everyone has spirituality but the majority of us have it at very low level. *P14 (Patient, I)*

The patient's sentiments are echoed by this nurse who did not like the term 'spirituality' but still felt that there was something deep within each person:

> P: So I aren't that comfortable with spirituality, but everybody has an inner something, I don't know what it is, what ever drives you and what ever drives me is totally different. *P20 (Nurse, II)*

However, when the principle of 'universality' was extended, via a scenario, to include groups of people whose beliefs and spiritual practices could be categorised as being unconventional in the sense that they could be perceived as going against the norm of what people consider morally and socially acceptable (for example, people who practiced the occult or witchcraft), the concept of universality became precarious. It was clear that many nurses had not thought of spirituality in this way. It was a case of universal application with some reservation and constraint. One patient felt that spirituality was able to distinguish between good and evil:

> P: And spirituality tells you when you're on sacred ground and the negative side when you are on evil ground, it speaks to you, you, can sense the vibrations. Right! *(P14, Patient, I, Pagan)*

The notion of good and evil in terms of spirituality provoked some interesting responses. One nurse (P4, Area II) indicated that he felt it was an oversimplification to talk about good and evil, heaven and hell, and that, basically, we all have the capacity to do good and bad. He did not feel that attending to someone whose spirituality was expressed through the occult or Satanism would prevent him from attending to patients' needs on the basis that 'we are asked to provide care to all sort of people from all sorts of backgrounds'. This demonstrated a tolerance and an acceptance for the management and facilitation of diversity. It also reinforced the notion of universality in the sense that spirituality may be expressed and held in different forms.

Equally, one nurse felt that this type of situation would need to be managed sensitively, bearing in mind the restriction of her professional registration:

> P: That's sort of like your cultural and your spiritual coming together.... Now, I would say because somebody's... spiritual needs as such, that may not be morally right to me! But may be that I am C of E may totally disgust them? But I think... there'd have to be explanations and may be this is... you'd have to fall back on your restrictions of your registration, etc. and what you are doing and because of the fact that there are other patients there that, you know, you cannot... put those, erm, type of, erm, spiritual needs you cannot enforce those on those other patients as well, so you're looking.... So, erm, you would have to

> actually address it sensitively, but I think what you would probably do is make arrangements for them to actually go and do that else where, you wouldn't stand in their way, you would sort of like, so well I can help you get to a certain place, I can help you go there and I can arrange for you to come back! Or you can help them indirectly in those types of ways! *P6 (Nurse, I)*

Generalisations cannot be made, but it would appear that some nurses do believe spirituality to be a universal phenomenon in that it resides in all people, good and bad. It would appear that there is a great deal of transference or crossing over between dimensions such as the social, cultural and spiritual. There is also a realisation that the meeting of particular religious or spiritual needs may be constrained by the nurse's own moral position and by adherence to the 'Code of Professional Conduct' (NMC, 2002, pp. 3–4). Yet analysis of the same implies that a nurse should not discriminate between good or bad:

> You are personally accountable for ensuring that you promote and protect the interests and dignity of patients and clients, irrespective of gender, age, race, ability, sexuality, economic status, lifestyle, culture and religious or political beliefs.

Taken literally, the code implies that no moral distinction be made and, in addition, nurses should be actively upholding and promoting the interests of their patients, irrespective of whether a patient's beliefs are different from the norms and practices of that particular society.

Existentially driven

A major theme identifiable within the professional discourse is a realisation that spirituality is primarily concerned with existentialism, which is the need to find meaning, purpose and fulfilment in one's life. The definition of meaning and purpose offered by Elkins *et al.* (1988, p. 11) captures many elements exhibited in the nursing transcripts:

> The spiritual person has known the quest for meaning and purpose and has emerged from this quest with confidence that life is deeply meaningful and that one's own existence has purpose. The actual content of this meaning vary from person to person, but the common factor is that each person has filled the 'existential vacuum' with an authentic sense that life has meaning and purpose.

The following two transcripts illustrate this observation:

> P: I believe there's something but I don't know what it is! But I feel that I am a very spiritual person! I enjoy living, I enjoy getting up in the morning and that's what makes me wan' a come to work! Get home, look after my family, be there, be where I am. And I think that's what spirituality is for me! *P2 (Nurse, I)*

> P: It's what's important to me at this time in my life, em [*nurse pauses before completing the response*]... I'm sort of happy with how my life is going with what I'm actually achieving at work, family things like that! And it makes me feel whole! *P3 (Nurse, I)*

The existentialist approach to spirituality is a major defining attribute of spirituality within the health care literature. This finding is not unique to this investigation. Harrington (1995, p. 8), when asking nurses to describe their understanding of the term spirituality, established that some nurses related it to: '... the uniqueness of the person. Embraces belief, meaning, direction in life'.

This is an interesting comparison, given that Harrington's investigation was conducted in Australia and this investigation in the UK. The fact that this finding features in two studies conducted on opposite sides of the world suggests this to be a universal phenomenon. This raises the question 'Why does existentialism feature so prominently in nurses' understanding of spirituality?'. This might best be explained at two levels. Firstly, conceptually and theoretically there has been an increase in publications that highlight 'existentialism' as an important ingredient of spirituality (Frankl, 1987; Burnard, 1988a; Elkins *et al.*, 1988; Shelly and Fish, 1988; Carson, 1989; Greenstreet, 1999; McSherry, 2000; Narayanasamy, 1999a, 2001). Secondly, it would appear that nurses and allied health professions become sensitised to 'existentialism' through professional and practice encounters.

Many of the nurses interviewed were acutely aware of the need to support patients, carers and families facing very traumatic and difficult situations, such as loss of physical health or facing death. Some of the nurses articulated that their involvement in such issues expanded their understanding of life, making them appreciate and value their own part in the world. It was as a form of 'enforced introspection'. An intriguing point was that some of the nurses felt very strongly that enabling individuals to find meaning and purpose in their illness or hospitalisation was not part of their professional role. This seemed very much dependent upon the individual patient him- or herself. It was almost a conscious realisation on the nurse's part of the potential for coercion. This is evident in the excerpt from a very detailed scenario provided by one nurse who suggested that the patient had to be supported in her decision and care shouldn't be taken over:

> P: Wanting to achieve things and she wanted to achieve these things and that was our role, was not to take over and say, woo [*stated patient's name*] I don't think you're well enough to go to pictures, I don't think

> you should really, you know. Why put them dampers on that... if it's unrealistic, you know, were not going to lie to her but she's still got to see to fail and she wanted to go to the pictures and she went to pictures and she thoroughly enjoyed that day. *P1 (Nurse, I)*

The findings of Harrington's (1995) research in conjunction with this investigation lead me to believe that the notion of spirituality being existentially driven is not just an isolated case or that it applies only to westernisation. In this inquiry many of the nurses, when selecting a statement on the recruitment questionnaire that best described their understanding of spirituality, chose item two: 'Spirituality is concerned with finding meaning, purpose and fulfilment in life'. This was in stark contrast to the patients, the majority of who selected the statement 'I do not know what is meant by the term spirituality'. This finding insinuates that philosophically and epistemologically many of the nurses viewed existentialism as an important constituent of spirituality. Yet, when some of the nurses were asked about the genesis or nature of this relationship they were unable to articulate why they felt that issues such as meaning, purpose and fulfilment were important to their understanding. This is evident in the following transcript where the nurse struggled to provide a coherent account:

> R: Why fulfilment?
>
> P: Because... but, that, that's, that's how I see, that's how I see it has being, is that fulfilment, that, em, that's, how that person, how you perceive things are, that are because of what... what you feel fulfilled in life, what you have achieved etc.... I just think it is a very good word... to, to describe how, some how spirituality and fulfilment seem to go together! *P6 (Nurse, I)*

In summary, many of the nurse participants felt that existentialism and spirituality were two interrelated concepts. A possible explanation for this view might be that these aspects of spirituality – meaning, purpose and fulfilment – are disseminated as important components of spirituality within health care literature and, more latterly, through educational programmes. Further, nurses and other allied health professionals may become more existentially attuned through direct exposure and involvement in situations where they are supporting individuals who are facing changing situations for example a diagnosis of terminal cancer.

Educationally shaped

A further strand pertaining to the development of a professional discourse arises within the context of education. Several of the nurses indicated that formal education, for example attending courses or workshops, or informal education (undertaking self reading and reflection) had positively enhanced their perceptions of spirituality. This is evident in the following illustrations:

> P: I am guilty of thinking of spirituality as being religion. At some point over the last few years I haven't! That's changed because of educational, you know, having, em, going to, eh, workshops etc.... well not workshops, em, having sessions. *P6 (Nurse, II)*
>
> P: Erm, it wasn't until about erm, a few years ago that I personally thought about that there was a difference, and I thought I was ignorant of the fact that they were two different things, but now I see them definitely not as two different things, but as erm, erm, oh, what's the word, they're not too separate things, I mean there isn't a black and white erm, but what I mean is a very strong connection about somebody's religious affiliation or whatever branch they go to God and their own spirituality you know but I've only defined that lets say over last few years.
>
> R: And what is it that's led you to believe that?
>
> P: A lot of it's been to do with working here [*Area I*]. And, em, at the same time that I realised all this, I, er, went to our minister at the church I go to that, I've belonged to since I was three, and I said 'do you know I've been coming here since I was three and I don't really know what it's all about?' [*Laughing*] *P8 (Nurse, I)*

It must be stressed that not all education or continuous professional development was viewed optimistically. On the contrary, two nurses recruited from within Area II (geographical area with rich ethnic diversity) felt that 'cultural' and 'spiritual' training days were counter-productive. One nurse felt that these types of days did not advance the cultural and diversity agenda because, rather than focusing upon significant issues such as racism and working with diversity and conflict, the courses just appeared to promote stereotypical images of particular religious or ethnic groups. Secondly, these types of training appeared to make nurses more conscious of disparity, hampering their dealings with patients by removing the intuitive, instinctive elements of their practice. This is reflected in the following accounts.

> P: ... we have these, kind of a cultural awareness days, a kind of cultural training, you have to go on these cultural awareness day. I was sent on one recently. I haven't done one for a few years and it's the same old stuff. This is a Sikh and this is a Jew! And quite actually, surely, we have got beyond that now! Surely we should be talking now actually about what is racism? And I think we should be getting underneath that and exploring our own ideas rather than sort of, you know, talking

about differences that people have?... I think, you know, some people can actually kind of, you know, produce cultural barriers by teaching about differences... [*long pause gives emphasis to remainder of the point*] is a bit uneasy really. *P4 (Nurse, II)*

P: We were sent on spiritual awareness courses and they were fairly patronising because I have learnt things that made me change because of that knowledge and I think, that then somebody else has that lost. I now know, that an Asian man objects to a woman touching him. Now I have never ever felt that I had done wrong, nobody has ever pulled away from me, and now I am wary of it, I don't do it. [*Short pause*]... An example is taking somebody to theatre and I would hold anybody's hand, I would hold your hand, and I did, they didn't pull away, but you know, I knew they weren't comfortable and it came into my head about this business but I just went with him, but then he had to return to theatre for something further, and I said I won't tell if you don't and he reached out for my hand. Maybe, if I had just held his hand the first time, without thinking about it. *P20 (Nurse, II)*

The notion that all the health care professions should be instructed and formally educated and thus 'informed' about matters pertaining to spirituality, in my opinion, requires careful planning. The introduction of poorly constructed modules and programmes may be more detrimental than helpful. I say this because the experiences of some of the nurse participants revealed that the educational methods adopted will be crucial in determining the effectiveness of such instruction. In addition, a purely academic approach to the concepts may fail to incorporate the diversity of opinions that exist within the population at large.

An adjunct to 'educationally shaped' is the notion that nurses throughout the course of their interactions with patients should be prepared to enlighten patients regarding the concept of spirituality. Taylor (2003, p. 589) advocates this 'Nurses need to be prepared to educate patients and caregivers about why they practice holistic care. Furthermore, patients and caregivers can misinterpret what defines spiritual care'. This notion of 'informing' was especially evident within the hospice. This is reflected in the following excerpt:

P: I think it, it, again it's that communication. It's those, you know, sort of those boundaries that say, when they're saying, woo, I'm not into spirituality but you say, what you are actually talking to me now is about spiritual issues. *P1 (Nurse, I)*

Justification and legitimisation for this within hospice and palliative care originates from a deep desire to do things right for and by the patients. Nurses seem to be guided by the belief that you only have one chance to do things right, leaving little room for error or mistakes.

The findings support the ongoing international debate about how best to educationally prepare health care practitioners to attend to their patients' spiritual needs. The result of this category adds a further twist to the debate, recognising an urgent need for academics, educators and practitioners, all working within health care to listen and engage with the 'public discourse' that is often overlooked and neglected in the debates surrounding spirituality. Adopting a more humanistic, phenomenological approach to researching and teaching spirituality (Elkins *et al.*, 1988) may serve to prevent the perpetuation of a 'scientism' (Dawson, 1997) which is perceived to be one of the catalysts fuelling the creation of a professional discourse.

Public discourse

The public's perceptions of spirituality were largely based on the old traditional form (discussed in Chapter 2, Part I) which is founded upon religious and theocentric descriptors in that a large proportion of patients, religious participants viewed spirituality synonymously with religion. It emerged that some patients and representatives from four of the major religions did not relate to, or identify, with the concept of spirituality in that the 'concept' did not feature in their vocabulary. Interestingly the findings of this investigation suggested that several of the patients, and some of the representatives from the major world religions, did not have any expectations regarding the provision of spiritual care by HCPs. The public's perceptions and expectations pertaining to HCPs attending to the 'spiritual dimension' of some participants appeared foreign to their cultural, religious practices. These views are evident in the three subcategories: 'expectation and realisation', 'treatment versus care', and 'fears and apprehensions'.

Expectation and realisation

The nine non-nurse participants interviewed during Phase I did not have any real expectations regarding spirituality and the provision of spiritual care. This discovery supports Taylor (2003, p. 589) who observed 'Some do not expect anything overtly related to spirituality or religiosity to be within the purview of nurses'. Analysis of the transcripts demonstrated that patients were totally realistic and complementary in terms of how they perceived the quality of the care that the staff had provided. The majority of the patients commented in terms of the qualities of the carers or described how the focus of care was upon physical and medical interventions. This is evident in the following:

> P: Well it's a very relaxed care you know! Em, and always.... Em, they're out to please yeah, and you know, their desire is to make you feel more comfortable. And this is one thing I do appreciate. Em, I don't know what else you can say about it? *P11 (Patient, I)*

One patient felt that he was not in receipt of any care while attending the hospice, seeing attendance as purely a recreational activity:

> P: I don't get any care. *P13 (Patient, I)*

The following comments highlight that staff working in the acute sector would not know how to provide spiritual care and that the priority was on physical tasks:

> P: No they don't know how to do it! They've got enough on with the patient and what the patient needs and that one, wants four lots of pills per day, he wants feeding, he wants his bed making and make sure he doesn't go pissing down the corridor! *P14 (Patient, I)*

And when the same patient was asked:

> R: Do you think it should be their responsibility to care about your spirituality?

this triggered a very strong response:

> P: No! No, No!

This patient's perceptions of the spiritual care in the hospice provide a useful comparison:

> P: Hospice, are quite separate, they know about spiritual needs because they've been through it themselves! [*Laughing*] *P14 (Patient, I)*

It seemed that some of the patients did not feel that nurses had the time to be providing spiritual care:

> P: Well I don't know, I think they have got enough on their plates doing what they do without being involved with that, I mean quite honestly they are run off their feet as it is. *P22 (Patient, III)*

These limited findings reveal that some patients had no predetermined expectations in relation to the provision of spiritual care. Further, the trend was that many patients had no idea of what constitutes spiritual care. Many patients did not make reference to spirituality or spiritual care. The emerging theme was that patients seemed realistic in terms of what care can and cannot be accommodated while in the hospice and the acute sector. Some patients also described and appreciated that the context in which care was provided was instrumental in determining the level of support and help that they received, which ultimately determined their overall perceptions of the standard and quality of care.

Treatment versus care

An interesting comment raised by one patient who had experience of care within both sectors, acute and hospice, was a distinction they made between 'care' and 'treatment':

> P: You get care in hospice because you are important to them and there are fewer numbers. In a hospital you are getting medical treatment plus a bit of food. I say, if you say to somebody, hey nurse I haven't got me glasses can you bring me, how about a glass of water, I'll bring you one. *P14 (Patient, I)*

The patient went on to say that in the hospice he would have a glass of water provided before he even asked.

The excerpt implies that the care setting, whether hospice or acute sector, may well be instrumental in determining patients' expectations and perceptions of care. Further, it seems that the focus of the acute sector is about the condition and its treatment, while in the hospice the focus appears to be upon the individual as a person and not the medical diagnosis. This finding, although based upon the views of one individual, was verified by hospice nurses, again some of whom had experience of working in both sectors. They highlighted dissatisfaction with the organisation and focus of care in the acute sector in comparison to their experiences of working within a hospice setting.

Fears and apprehensions

It became apparent that some individuals had strong fears and apprehension in relation to the concept of spirituality. This was noticeable in some of the patient transcripts and was verified in the nurse transcripts. The extent of this fear and apprehension is communicated in the following examples:

> P: ... some patients will say, woo, woo, spirituality and they think it's you know sort of holding hands in a séance and, and, it frightens them it frightens patients, em, and so they don't want to address it. *P1 (Nurse, I)*

> P: Eh ...I think, I think, I see spirituality. I don't mind, you know, how it is quoted here [*interview*] but there was during my cruise through life. These spiritualists that were a bit overpowering and that I don't want! And that is why, you know, when I got your letter that you were coming I was undecided. Because if you had got deep into it like that I would probably have exploded and told you where to go. [*Laughing*] *P11 (Patient, I)*

These excerpts suggest that there are strong emotive powers attached to the word 'spirituality' that determine some patients' perceptions of spirituality. These powers may reflect an individual's previous life experiences and associations. The excerpts also reveal, despite all the literature suggesting that attitudes towards spirituality have changed, that misunderstandings and misconceptions still surround the word, causing apprehension when the term 'spirituality' is used. The apprehensions may originate from a fear of proselytising and from the false impression that spirituality is linked synonymously with religion (Allen, 1991). The data indicate that these perceptions are not only restricted to older adults because some of the younger participants expressed similar fears and apprehensions. It suggests that there are still strong connotations associated with the word 'spirituality' that may stem from its historic discourse.

Phase I

Introduction

This phase was designed to establish the authenticity of the word 'spirituality' as used within health care and, more specifically, the nursing literature. The notion that the term 'spirituality' is universally recognised and understood within nursing is an assertion that requires verification and confirmation. I am very much aware of the pioneering work of several eminent academics from a wide range of disciplines. Their published 'classical' and 'seminal' works allude to the fact that humankind does have a sense of the sacred, holy, transcendent, and mystical elements (James, 1902; Otto, 1950; Smart, 1969; Maslow, 1970; Hardy, 1979). This awareness is often referred to and described under the term 'religious experiences'.

Hardy (1979, p. 131) in his work the *The Spiritual Nature of Man* concludes:

> It is one thing to talk about 'the spiritual nature of man' meaning that side of his make-up which, if not always leading him to have what he might call religious feelings, may at least give him a love of the non-material things of life such as natural beauty, art, music, or moral values; it is quite another matter to talk of the very nature of spirituality itself. Who would be so foolish as to imagine or pretend that he could make such a definitive pronouncement?

Hardy suggests that there may be a distinction between the religious and the spiritual. Furthermore he suggests that establishing a definitive answer about spirituality may be ambitious, contentious and very presumptuous. With regard to health care, and more specifically, nursing the approach has not been so much to verify 'religious feelings' but to assume and postulate that all people are aware of, and in touch with '*the very nature of spirituality itself*'. However, it would seem that within health care there has been a growing realisation to check out the validity of this universal application and acceptance with diverse cultural groups (Burkhardt, 1991; Harrison and Burnard, 1993; Kearney, 1994; Draper and McSherry, 2002; Swinton and Narayanasamy, 2002).

The results of Phase I revealed that individuals' perceptions and understandings of spirituality are diverse. The discourses surrounding the development of one's spirituality and the manner in which this may be expressed are complex and ultimately dependent upon the individuals' own experiences, perceptions and socialisations. In reality, an individual's spirituality is shaped and formed by a number of intrinsic and extrinsic factors. This finding supports the words of Lie (2001, p. 183): 'Every individual has a name, a complex history, and a personality formed out of a multi-cultural environment'.

During Phase I a total of 22 participants were interviewed (Table 5.1). At this stage of theory development open sampling was used (Chapter 4) and participants were selected not so much on the basis of furthering emerging categories, but to start the process of checking out the theoretical credibility of existing positions and arguments surrounding the construction and use of the term 'spirituality'. The rationale for using open sampling was to allow the development of broad categories that would account for the possible similarities and variations that may exist across a range of different groups. Open sampling would assist in the identification of properties and the development of categories that might support, refute or develop existing conceptual and theoretical positions associated with spirituality and spiritual care.

Analysis using line by line open coding allowed each of the transcripts to be broken down thus allowing similarities and differences to be established. This microanalysis enabled me to group properties of a similar nature into categories. This attention to detail allowed 'discrimination and differentiation' among the categories to be undertaken (Strauss and Corbin, 1998, p. 102). The process was very tedious and time-consuming, but rewarding in that it provided a rich and deep insight into the thoughts and feelings of the participants. As discussed, the detailed analysis allowed the conceptualisation of the core category 'assumption versus expectation' and its associated properties. Besides, five subcategories were created that offered insight and expansion of the emerging theory (Table 5.2). The properties of each category were derived from some of the key words and phrases provided by the participants. Therefore, coding could be termed '*in vivo*'.

Phase I – Subcategories explained

> **Activity 5.1 Emerging categories.**
>
> Spend some time reflecting on Table 5.2 examining the structure and presentation of the emerging categories. Ask yourself the following question:
>
> Do the categories and their properties appear to make sense?

Introduction

This section presents a detailed analysis of the five subcategories developed during Phase I of the investigation. Each of the categories and their properties will be presented and discussed. Both 'technical' and 'non-technical' literature was used in the creation of these categories. Familiarity and sensitivity to the existing literature aided the analytical process. Both technical and non-technical' literature, such as draft government reports and reflective diaries, added a rich contextual background against which hypotheses could be formulated and tested. Both forms of literature supplemented field notes and data, stimulating analytical thinking relating to the properties thus broadening the emerging dimensions. These were initial considerations and the categorisations and

Phase I

Duration: 23 January 2001 – 18 February 2002
Total length of interview transcript: 13.6 hours
Length of interviews: 18 minutes to 57 minutes – average 37 minutes 20 seconds.

Table 5.1 Participants included in Phase I of investigation.

No.	Age	Gender	Religion	Practising	Group	Area	Date interviewed	Reason for theoretical selection
1	42–49	Male	No	NA	Nurse	I		No religion and male
2	42–49	Female	C of E	No	Nurse	I		Religion and female
3	34–41	Female	C of E	No	Nurse	I		Worked part time, Enrolled Nurse
4	34–41	Male	Quaker	Yes	Nurse	II		Manager Area II – with religious belief; Acute Trust medical speciality
5	50–57	Female	RC	Yes	Nurse	II		Manager, education, ICU, RC Acute Trust
6	34–41	Female	C of E	No	Nurse	I		Charge Nurse specialist palliative care
7	50–57	Female	No	NA	Nurse	I		No religious belief – age range
8	50–57	Female	Methodist	Yes	Nurse	I		Strong religious belief
9	34–41	Female	C of E	Yes	Nurse	I		Develop emerging categories/properties
10	34–41	Female	C of E	No	Nurse	I		Develop emerging categories/properties
11	> 82	Female	C of E	Yes	Patient	I		Patient perspective, age/religion, spirituality only involves religion
12	34–41	Male	Bahai faith	Yes	Nurse	III		Bahai faith, charge nurse, surgical background
13	66–73	Male	No	NA	Patient	I		Patient, male, no religious belief, atheist, didn't know what was meant by the term spirituality
14	66–73	Male	Pagan	Yes	Patient	I		Religious belief

Table 5.1 *(continued)*

No.	Age	Gender	Religion	Practising	Group	Area	Date interviewed	Reason for theoretical selection
15	26–33	Male	Muslim	Yes	Chap	II		Islamic perspective
16	26–33	Female	Muslim	Yes	Chap	II		Islamic perspective
17		Male	Hindu	Yes	Chap	II		Hinduism – perspective
18		Male	Sikh	Yes	Chap	II		Sikhism – perspective
19	> 82	Male	No	NA	Patient	I		Age, no religious belief, did not understand the term spirituality
20	42–49	Female	C of E	Yes	Nurse	II		Medical speciality 26 years experience
21	42–49	Male	Buddhist	Yes	OT	II		Buddhism perspective (Occupational Therapist)
22	74–81	Female	No	NA	Patient	III		Elective Surgery, same area as interviewee 12, no idea about the term

Table 5.2 Emerging categories.

Core category	Central categories	Subcategories
Assumption versus expectation	**Professional discourse** Mantra – holism Recognition of spirituality Universal application Existentially driven Educationally shaped	**Definitions of spirituality** Synonymous with religion Religiosity/religious influences Belief in a god Supernatural forces/ghosts and ghouls Connectedness Essence and core **Diverse perceptions of spirituality** Religious variation Individually focused Community awareness (obligation) Commonalities
	Public discourse Expectation and realisation Treatment versus care Fears and apprehensions	**Provision of spiritual care** Qualities of carer Hierarchy of care Spiritual assessment nurse led or expressed need Spiritual care deficits Integrated spiritual care **Socialisation of the spirit** Maternal influences Moral principles Innate spirituality **Drivers** Managerialism Professionalism

significant properties underwent further refinement and testing resulting in the destruction and reconstruction of the theory throughout Phase II and the development of a model in Phase III.

Definitions of spirituality

All the participants in this phase were asked to describe what they understood by the terms 'spirituality' or 'spiritual'.

> R: As part of defining holism you've also indicated this word spiritual? What does the word spiritual mean to you?

Detailed analysis of all the transcripts, and in particular the responses to the above question, revealed that definitions of spirituality were diverse and the language surrounding the concept elaborate and convoluted. Defining spirituality for some individuals meant the integration and assimilation of several layers of meaning, these being personal, theist, existential, philosophical and mystical. This finding is similar to the categories outlined in other grounded theory investigations (Burkhardt, 1991; Harrison and Burnard, 1993; Kearney, 1994; Harrington, 1995) and qualitative research (Hay and Hunt, 2000) addressing 'spirituality'. This category contained five subcategories which participants indicated as constituting spirituality. The subcategories were named: 'synonymous with religion' (subproperty religiosity/religious influences); 'belief in a God'; 'supernatural forces/ghosts and ghouls'; 'connectedness' and 'essence and core'. Each of these subcategories will be discussed.

The review of the nursing literature suggests that spirituality is a multifaceted dimension involving a number of key elements (Murray and Zentner, 1989; Reed, 1992; Cawley, 1997; Harrington, 1995) such as personal beliefs, values and creeds. Elkins *et al.* (1988) and, more recently, Taylor (2002) present several components or manifestations of spirituality embracing, for example, transcendence, existentialism, and connectedness. Taylor (2002) provides a useful categorisation, suggesting how spirituality may be manifested through several needs: relating to self, others and the transcendent. She also suggests that these needs may vary between and within groups.

There is also recognition that spirituality or the spiritual dimension may consist of several levels or layers of meaning. This is evident in the work of nursing authors such as Stallwood (1975), demonstrating that spirituality is at the core of our human existence permeating and influencing all other dimensions of our nature, physical and psychosocial. The model highlights how the human person functions as a dynamic whole (McSherry, 1997). Stoll (1989) offers a two-dimensional (dualist) approach describing a horizontal (the individual's role in the material world or the physical reality) and a vertical (the notion of transcendence, relationship with a metaphysical omnipotent being) dimension. Reed (1992) maintains that spirituality concerns 'existentialism', and 'relatedness' for example the individual may experience 'spirituality' at different levels: intrapersonally (within themselves) interpersonally (outwith themselves in their dealings with others) and transpersonally (in relation to an awareness of a higher power or superior being). Goddard (1996), on the other hand, describes spirituality as 'integrative energy' presenting spirituality in nonpartisan and nonreligious terms and emphasising the universality of the concept.

More recently, Narayanasamy (1999b), reviewing the work of Hardy (1979) and others, for example Hay (1994), revisits the notion that there is growing evidence to support the biological basis or origin for spirituality. This biological basis is based on the evolutionary principle of 'biological survival value'. This work has now been extended by the emergence of neurological work (Newberg *et al.*, 2002) and neuro-theology, a science concerned with the identification and labeling of specific areas within the brain that are associated with the manifestation of a sense of transcendence.

Irrespective of which model or approach one subscribes to, the bases of such models are often anecdotal or theoretical. However, there is a growing amount of empirical work focusing upon religious experience. Yet, because of the emphasis upon 'religious experience' in the general population, its application and relevance to health care may be limited. Oldnall (1996) also suggests that theories and concepts derived from the echelons of academia are difficult to transfer and apply to practice and the real world. In reality, concepts, theories and latterly models associated with spirituality may be subjective and contentious. This is especially so when they are universally applied to all people. However, the properties identified and presented within this category indicated that participants did provide a diverse range of definitions, some of which support the philosophical, conceptual and theoretical models outlined.

Earlier it was argued that historically spirituality was developed within a religious discourse, providing the word with a heritage, language and vehicle for expression (Bradshaw, 1994; Narayanasamy, 1999a; Pattison, 2001). In recent years the word has become dilute, 'eclectic' (Cobb, 2001), and associated with a range of meanings and interpretations, resulting in a separation, fragmentation and, it could be argued, a disassociation from the historical links and connotations. These two polarisations or extremes were evident in the transcripts of participants who viewed spirituality either as having a singular layer of meaning relating to religion or to supernatural forces, and those whose understanding of spirituality had several layers of meaning, for example a sense of awe and wonder at creation or even a oneness with the universe.

Comparisons suggest many patients and representatives from the major world religions other than 'Christian' adopted a singular or unilateral approach to spirituality, while many of the nurses believed spirituality to be multilateral and multidimensional. This finding supports the suggestion that there is no real authoritative definition (Narayanasamy, 2001). The finding reinforces the idea that spirituality is uniquely determined and defined by the individual depending upon their unique and personal world view (Martsolf and Mickley, 1998). This category contained six properties (Table 5.2). These properties reflect the historical and modernistic views of spirituality. Although explored in isolation, some of the properties are interconnected and repetitious. Some participants' definitions were constructed by drawing upon several of these properties. This category gives credence to the construction of 'a taxonomy of spirituality' presented in Chapter 2.

Synonymous with religion

There is a realisation within nursing that religion and spirituality are interchangeable or synonymous (Simsen, 1985. 1986; Harrison and Burnard, 1993; Narayanasamy, 2001). Religion has been defined within health care as (Murray and Zentner, 1989, p. 259):

> A belief in a supernatural or divine force that has power over the universe and commands worship and obedience; a system of beliefs; a comprehensive code of ethics or philosophy; a set of practices that are followed; a church affiliation; the conscious pursuit of any object the person holds as supreme.

This definition appears ethnocentric in that is seems to posses a Judeo-Christian bias. However, it does highlight several important features about the nature and structure of some world religions and how these structures may influence the entire foundation, fabric of society at a range of levels morally, socially, politically and ultimately individually (Smart, 1969). My reasons for drawing attention to these structures are that they form the basis of several patients' interpretations of the concept of spirituality presented within this subcategory.

A further argument surrounding and perhaps one of the main aims for addressing the concept of spirituality in the nursing and health care literature has been to dispel some of the myths and misconceptions that surround spirituality and religion (Allen, 1991). The overriding concern in this debate is that spirituality is not just about religion and for the religious. In fact, analysis of the health care literature implies that spirituality applies to all people, believers and non-believers alike (Burnard, 1988b; Cawley, 1997; Bash, 2004). However, what is not clear in this debate is on what premise or empirical evidence this universal application is judged and based. An objective of this investigation is to establish whether the term 'spirituality' is used or recognisable with diverse groups. The construction of the core category affirms that a dichotomy exists between professional and non-professional groups. The dichotomy reveals that many of the nurses were able to articulate and identify the concept, sometimes offering multiple definitions each possessing a large number of defining characteristics. Conversely, patients and representatives from some of the major world religions did not share these characteristics, equating religion with 'spirituality'.

Transcripts revealed that the majority of non-nurse participants in Phase I either struggled to articulate a definition of spirituality or were adamant that the term was concerned with, and unable to be divorced from, religion. This is evident in the following patient responses:

> P: I have not a clue. I really don't know what it means. To me it is just about religion. I don't know how you describe it quite honestly. That's why when you rung up I thought to myself, I don't know what I am going to say to you because I don't know what it means. *P22 (Patient, III)*

> P: Well that's what I thought when I got this letter you know. Well, I thought, well again, were back to religion! You know, I'm Church of England! *P11 (Patient, I)*

> P: Well from national service days I was the only one in the British army with two religions in the pay book. And I had two religions for the simple reason, is, if it was fall out RC's, I used to fall out and go do something else. And, if it was, fall out C of E's, I used to go and fall out [laughing] and they caught up with me in the finish. But say it has never interested me. *P13 (Patient, I)*

When I mentioned the word 'spirituality' to some patients they became very defensive because they felt spirituality equalled only religion. In this situation, insight into spirituality or being able to articulate what spirituality might be implied they could be perceived by me as being a religious person.

> P: Well I'm not religious at all! *P19 (Patient, I)*

These transcripts suggest that patients seemed to share a 'historical or traditional' approach to spirituality either directly or indirectly equating the word with religion. This association implies that the argument that the meaning of spirituality is derived from a religious context and discourse (Bradshaw, 1994; Pattison, 2001) is corroborated within some patient and public groups. This finding contradicts some of the trends in nursing and health care that seem to assume that there is now a shift away from viewing spirituality as synonymous with religion (McSherry, 2000a). Furthermore, the transcripts imply that 'spirituality' *per se* is not universally recognised as a dimension in peoples' lives, especially in the way that it is constructed and portrayed in the nursing literature.

This does not just pertain to individuals from western or Judeo-Christian traditions. On the contrary, individuals from some of the eastern religions subscribe to this philosophy. The following transcript from a Muslim (female) demonstrates how 'spirituality' is associated with religious belief and practices. For this individual religion and spirituality were inseparable, revealing how everyday rituals and practices lead to the development of one's inner self, making a connection with God, demonstrating the synonymous relationship, interconnectedness of religion and spirituality.

> P: The way I see it as a Muslim there is nothing that's secular. There isn't anything!... because things like going to the toilet, getting dressed, there is a prayer that you say before you do anything in a Muslim faith and for me spirituality equals religion. *P16 (Muslim female, II)*

This transcript validates some Islamic writers' perceptions of spirituality and its association with religion. Mayet (2001, p. 172) writes:

> To the health care professional, spiritual care may simply mean that the hospital chaplain takes care of a patient, whilst faith groups may define spiritual care in more specifically religious ways. Islam an all-encompassing faith, considers every facet of human life to fall in the domain of religion. Even simple aspects of daily life like sleeping, visiting the washroom, eating dressing are considered acts of worship when done in a manner prescribed by Islam. Spirituality is defined as the combination of the outer and inner aspects of actions, devotions, giving them their real significance.

This quotation reinforces the views presented in the extract of transcript, mirroring them exactly in terms of content and meaning. Though generalisation cannot be made, it suggests that followers of Islam may struggle to identify with the way spirituality is presented in health care. For some Muslims spirituality cannot be divorced from their religion, since both share closeness and an intimacy that cannot be polarised or separated.

Religiosity/religious influences

Analysis revealed that while individuals viewed spirituality as synonymous with religion and they were tolerant of others' religious beliefs, some participants (predominantly nurses and, it must be stressed, patients with negative experiences of religion) were vehemently opposed to any form of religious practice or religious influence in their perception of spirituality. Some patients also felt that acknowledgment of spirituality within them was tantamount to religiosity. Religiosity in this instance was the commitment to a particular religious framework such as Christianity, Judaism or Hinduism and the adherence to the religious doctrines and teaching of that particular faith community.

MacKinlay (2001, p. 88) makes a useful observation of how the terms 'religion', 'religious' and 'religiosity' are used interchangeably to convey an individual's feelings, attitudes and behaviours towards religious concepts. The interchangeable nature of the words may offer some explanation as to why the majority of participants across all cultural groups identified and appeared comfortable when using the word 'religion' whilst some individuals felt uncomfortable with the concepts of religion and spirituality. The word 'religion' appears impersonal and it is universally recognisable, thereby rendering it innocuous. Interestingly, many patients did not just use the word 'religion' but the term 'religious', making it more personal and value-laden. This term may have provoked more anxiety in that it insinuates adherence to a set of ritualistic practice and, ultimately, a commitment to, and involvement in, a particular religious framework. It may be that these connotations and associations roused such a strong reaction in some patients.

Belief in a god

The previous category explored the relationship and possible associations between religion and spirituality. This category delves into the notion of a god or a deity being central to participants' understandings of spirituality. The idea that spirituality concerns a belief in a god or supreme being (deity) is an established 'truth' in the health care literature and a central tenet in the teachings of some of the world religions. This component of spirituality is central to, and sometimes the foundation of, many people's understandings of spirituality. Indeed, some nursing writers whose work has a Judeo-Christian perspective would argue that striving to serve and develop a harmonious relationship with God is the sole function of life (Stoll, 1979; Shelly and Fish, 1988; Bradshaw, 1994), and, indeed, nursing may well be a means of enhancing or expressing that relationship.

Bradshaw (1994, p. 330) asserts that perhaps some of the uncertainty and ambiguity that surrounds 'caring' and nursing is the 'undermining of the Judeo-Christian foundations of nursing care', central to which is the belief and faith in one God. This type of Judeo-Christian bias fails to acknowledge and engage with some major debates surrounding 'multiculturalism' and 'cultural sensitivity' that are prevalent and gaining momentum within nursing. Recently there has been a proliferation of works providing insight into the religious and spiritual needs of individuals from all the major world religions (Markham, 1998; Sheikh and Gatrad, 2000; Narayanasamy and Andrews, 2000; Orchard, 2001). The main concern raised is that the Anglo-American and Judeo-Christian approach to spirituality alienates and discriminates in that it may not reflect or indeed incorporate the opinions and beliefs of individuals from other religious traditions.

The reason for drawing attention to these debates is that analysis of transcripts reveals that, for some individuals, the belief in a 'god' (however defined) is a composite part of understanding spirituality. This was particularly evident in some of the representatives from the different world religions and Western and Eastern traditions. For example, a Christian nurse stressed the importance of her spirituality being about a personal relationship with God and not adherence to formal religious structures:

> P: It is to do with, partly to do with religion, but I very much differentiate that religion is a very structured formal thing, as opposed to a relationship with God, so that's were I make that differentiation, between spirituality, a lot of people think religion – church but to me spirituality is a relationship with God. P29 *(Nurse, II, Born again Christian)*

However, this was especially noticeable in the Muslim transcripts, where spirituality is intertwined with ones faith in one God, Allah.

> P: ... With the younger generation it's quite changing now, because they are turning to counselling. I mean counselling is another interesting aspect of this, err, it's like do Muslims need counselling? And many would say the older generation would say 'No because we have faith in God whatever happens!' You've lost your whole family, err in a road traffic accident or so and it's like 'that's how God wanted it to be!' 'They were in the wrong place at the wrong time, but it was meant to be like that!' 'What about your needs of the loss of your family?' Well, err, 'God will help me!' That's a typical heavy-minded scenario, where as a younger Muslim refer to counselling and be counselled, err so you've got this scenario also! *P15 (Muslim male, II)*

> P: ...for a Muslim we see spirituality as being inner peace, I would say, and find your self and result of that is the connection with God. The journey of finding yourself and the purpose in life and that for Muslims is that we are put on the earth to praise God and so for us spiritual needs, does equal religious needs. *P16 (Muslim female, II)*

The notion of spirituality being inextricably linked with religion is conveyed by a Hindu describing how the first stages of life are a preparatory state acquiring knowledge so that one's twilight can be spent in the presence of God:

> P: Yes spirituality is pertaining to religion and its principles, so spirituality I'm very spiritual. You know, and in Hindu, Hinduism, we believe in forward, I would like us to identify with the four ways. The first twenty-five years is called the 'Brumcheriarshum', is you look after your health and you study and then after twenty-five years, you may have children, you learn as much as you can, and after the age of fifty you spend more time with God. *P17 (Hindu male, II)*

It must be stressed that not all the religions held the belief in a god. One follower of Buddhism was strongly opposed to the notion of a single god who created the universe:

> P: In Buddhism, what they try and look at is what they call the, em, 'nature and reality', is the way the world exists. And in their scheme of things there is no God, there is no creator God, there's just reality. The main focus is to try and understand what that reality is! And philosophically there aren't any arguments to support God, so they don't em, accept one! *P21 (Buddhist male, II)*

Many of the nurses emphasised that their spirituality was not associated with a belief in God. However, most did understand that for some patients this would be an important aspect of their lives. In addition, many nurses, despite not holding such a belief, would support patients in maintaining their beliefs and religious practices. It is not necessary to enter into philosophical and theological debate about the nature of God for each of the groups. This is not the objective of this investigation. Suffice, this property reinforces that for many individuals their spirituality is concerned with a personal relationship with a god, their God. This relationship provides such individuals with a structure, meaning, purpose and fulfilment in life. This finding reinforces that generalisations cannot be made. Firstly, religion equates with a belief in a god, and, secondly, all people's spirituality will be based on a theistic philosophy. This level of awareness is very important now that allied health professionals are providing care in a multi-ethnic, multicultural and multi-faith society (Henley and Schott, 1999).

Supernatural forces/ghosts and ghouls

During the interview process patients, in particular, suggested that spirituality may be linked to the 'spiritualist movement' or to 'ghosts and ghouls'. Only one nurse participant during Phase I made reference to 'spirituality' as 'spiritualism':

> P: I'm always a bit wary of the way, say, you know, spiritualism, but I, would think my definition is anything that's going to lift your spirits, anything that gives meaning to the day, especially somewhere like here. *P7 (Nurse, I)*

There was some fear and anxiety around this area which is expressed in the transcript. One gentleman provided a detailed and vivid account of how as a child he and his mother had seen a ghost:

> P: So this matron then told my mother, said 'well this house is haunted'... she says and eh, there's just some spirits walking about it and it had been an old vicarage.... Well, yes, – its like, it's like spirits, is like spirituality. But, I've never seen anything in my life, so but em, I know me mother wasn't a nervous women or anything and she just saw this figure pass like and thought it was a nurse but, em, she definitely seen it like! But I've never seen anything in my life. But I'm like that, like I don't know whether there is an after life or not? *P19 (Patient, I)*

The fact that several participants associated spirituality with supernatural forces 'ghostly apparitions' and non-worldly entities warrants further exploration. Within the health care literature little reference is given to the fact that for some individuals 'spiritualism' or an awareness of another supernatural realm plays an influential role in shaping their attitudes towards the concept of spirituality. The lack of credence given to spiritualism, or belief in a supernatural realm within the health care literature may need to be addressed. It would appear that for some individuals this aspect of spirituality provides explanation and a meaning for life and death.

Shirahama and Inoue (2001) identify that ancestor worship was a major theme in their exploration of spirituality among members living within a farming community in Japan. They present a two-dimensional model with vertical and horizontal axes. The vertical is directed towards ancestors and spirits (gods of nature) while the horizontal is concerned with living alongside others in the wider society. This research suggests that there are fundamental differences between Japanese (Eastern) and Western ideas of spirituality. Yet, this approach to understanding spirituality may explain why some individuals perceive 'spiritualism' and supernatural forces as being part of spirituality. Furthermore, if spirituality is to be universally applied then the concept must accept that there will be cross-cultural and intra-cultural differences in interpretation and definition, especially in an ever-changing world.

Connectedness

As indicated earlier, several nursing authors have explored the notion of connectedness as an essential component of spirituality. Reed (1992) discusses how connectedness can occur at several levels: 'intra' within the individual, 'inter' outwith the individual and 'trans' in relation to a higher power. Connectedness was expressed by many individuals as an important aspect of their spirituality. Reed's classification of connectedness provides a suitable template for establishing how connectedness relates to one's understanding of spirituality. The following is an example of how one patient felt a strong connection to creation and the environment.

> P: Now with regards to spirituality. I'm daft about stone, carved stones, erm, because they speak to me. Erm, let me find a single tree, right poor thing's been surviving there for 120 years, but you can talk to him. I've seen all manner of lunatics underneath funny clothes, funny hats, I'm still here but you won't be here next year type of attitude. *P14 (Patient, I)*

It was apparent that many individuals had a sense of connectedness with the outside world and nature. Connectedness was also articulated and expressed in individuals' relationships and dealings with other people. In terms of connectedness, spirituality was described as a force or energy. This energy bonded together all dimensions of the individual, emphasising an attachment with the whole of nature and the wider universe.

Essence and core

Tanyi (2002, p. 507) concludes her review of the meaning of spirituality with an important statement 'The "spirit" the core of human existence – is fundamental to all'. The realisation that spirituality is the essence and core of human existence was acknowledged as a fundamental component by some participants who recognised the existence of a spiritual dimension within themselves. This was expressed in several forms through use of the adjectives: essence, core, and spark and through personalisation using 'me' and 'you'. These phrases suggested that there was awareness that spirituality is not a separate entity residing within the individual or located in an existential vacuum. Quite the reverse, it appeared to be perceived as something inseparable and intrinsic central to the notion of 'self'. This is evident in the following:

> P: ... to me spirituality is what makes me... [*Pause*] feel what makes me... [*Pause*] the, the essence of living! It, it... [*Pause*] makes somebody feel whole, it's the sparkle *P2 (Nurse, I)*

> P: ... to me personally, it's, its part of you, it's what, what makes, you, if you like! *P10 (Nurse, I)*

The use of the words 'me' and 'you' suggests that spirituality is perceived to be the very foundation of one's being and person. For such individuals spirituality is not just concerned with awareness and connection with other people or a transcendental awareness of a higher power, although for some participants, these were crucial to their perceptions of spirituality. These observations imply a profound belief that spirituality is what makes them a unique living volitional being. Interestingly, individuals were unable to qualify such statements or explain why they held this belief. This implies that spirituality is something innate and, possibly, biologically determined.

Neuman (1995) recognises the spiritual variable to be one of the five interacting variables that maintain and preserve the integrity of a person's entire well-being. Curran (1995) describes how the spiritual variable is the major influence of a person and, because of this, it is pivotal to the 'Neuman Systems Model'. Interestingly, the spiritual variable was added to the model in the late 1980s, highlighting how nursing theories and models evolve to meet the changing needs of patients. Neuman (1995, p. 28/29) writes:

> The spiritual variable... is viewed as innate, a component of the basic structure, whether or not it is ever acknowledged or developed by the client or client system.

For Neuman the basic structure refers to factors common to all organisms. The fact that spirituality is perceived to be something at the very core of the human system implies that spirituality permeates all other systems. The findings of this investigation, in conjunction with earlier works on religious experience and spiritual awareness, support the proposition that spirituality is not just something metaphysical, but physical in the sense that it may be innate within the human species.

Diverse perceptions of spirituality[1]

Introduction

It emerged that individuals held unique definitions of spirituality. Comparison among the different groups revealed that definitions of spirituality were

1 Aspects of this section are reprinted from McSherry, W., Cash, K. and Ross, L. (2004) Meaning of spirituality: implications for nursing practice. *Journal of Clinical Nursing*, **13**, 934–41. Copyright 2004 with permission from Blackwell.

'diverse' in the sense that a participant's approach to spirituality could be accounted for and explained within one of the following properties: 'religious variation', 'individually focused' and 'community awareness (obligation)'.

It was apparent that definitions of spirituality are diverse, and that some of the properties emerging support the proposition that spirituality is uniquely defined and ultimately determined by the individual. Yet closer analysis of the transcripts reveals that a purely 'individualist approach' may not be truly representative in that an individual's spirituality may be influenced by much wider 'communal factors'. Evidence for these communal factors was identifiable in such things as adherence to religious doctrines and duties and concern for the environment and one's neighbour. Therefore consideration needs to be given to the gravity and weighting of these communal forces and the impact that these might have upon their interpretation of spirituality. It would be wrong to dismiss these and address them collectively under a broad, all-inclusive, individualistic approach to spirituality. Therefore it was felt necessary to develop a category which addressed and explained these variations that account for diverse perceptions of spirituality.

Reflective question

- Do you think it is important that subsequent research into spirituality reflects the rich cultural, religious and ethnic variation that exists within contemporary society?

Religious variation

Analysis revealed that there were some variations in the way that spirituality was defined between the religious groups and between believers and non-believers. While this finding was significant and saturation did occur, I still feel there is scope for further development. Stern (1994) indicates that underdeveloped categories are no excuse, since data collection should continue until the category is fully developed or discarded. This point was considered, but it did not resolve the difficulty of identifying and recruiting individuals from minority ethnic groups into this investigation. In light of this limitation, this finding cannot be generalised on the basis that some of the world religions were represented by only one individual.

Five representatives from four of the major world religions were interviewed during Phase I. Issue must also be given to the question to what extent individuals were representative of their faith communities. The five participants were all actively engaged in their faith communities and practising their religion. However, just because someone practises their religion does not necessarily mean that their views reflect everyone who subscribes to that particular belief system. Therefore, by nature these findings, while shedding light on how an individual from a particular world religion may view spirituality, will be 'idiosyncratic'.

The following excerpts provide a useful insight into how spirituality is viewed among different Eastern faith groups.

> P: Well first of all, spirituality exists within everyone, whether you believe in God or not. To me personally, it would be to overall, look at the patient overall and address their needs to the way that they would see it. *P15 (Muslim male, II)*

> P: I didn't feel I had enough knowledge about spirituality and as I got into the post and went to training and read up on my subject. I found out things and realised the way people see spirituality, as a Muslim, I probably don't see spirituality in the same way *P16 (Muslim female, II)*

> P: Yes spirituality is pertaining to religion and its principles *P17 (Hindu male, II)*

> P: Sikh religion is secretion of the spirituality. Spirituality is the main thing in Sikh religion *P18 (Sikh, II)*

> P: I was, gonna say, it's not a term we use in Buddhism as such! It's a hard word to define actually, [*laughing*] it's, just a difficult word to define! *P21 (Buddhist male, II)*

The excerpts demonstrate that two participants had difficulty identifying with the word 'spirituality,' struggling to offer a definition, whilst two viewed spirituality as synonymous with religion. Whilst one representative from the Islamic religion provided a definition of spirituality that resembled, or contained elements similar to those provided by some of the nurses (provided in earlier discussion), the majority did not perceive or think of spirituality in the terms or manner in which it is presented within health care definitions.

There were several implications arising from this discovery for health care practice. Firstly, some individuals' meaning of spirituality will be derived and explained by their association with a religious belief. Secondly, there is a strong indication that for some individuals from Eastern faith traditions the concept may not feature in their vocabulary. Thirdly, this finding affirms the theory that diversity in perceiving spirituality does exist between and within different ethnic, cultural and religious groups. In addition, this finding describes how diversity in opinion may stem from cultural and regional variations. In conclusion, this limited evidence substantiates claims that some of the Eastern religions do not possess and are not familiar with the language of spirituality as reflected in contemporary Western health care.

One significant variable that seemed to influence the extent and depth of participants' perceptions of spirituality was religious affiliation. It seemed that those individuals (from Western and Judeo-Christian traditions) who identified, and were active in their religion had a more comprehensive, universal recognition of the term within both themselves and others. These individuals seemed more able to articulate the nature of spirituality besides having a fluency and enthusiasm in their response, something that cannot be communicated in this narrative. These individuals appeared more at ease and less threatened by the term. The following two transcripts illustrate this enthusiasm and universal application:

> P: Spirituality a nice word but we have to define it! I think, everyone has spirituality but the majority of us have it at very low level. I think, it goes back to almost Oestolapithesis when man stood upright. This is noticeable in a photograph of a man and a woman walking over pumice and a child following jumping in their parent footsteps. You can see it on the beach now. That was just a hint that man was becoming human. I think, it was built in strongly to early man almost as a warning signal or a defence signal. He knew or he could sense when he was in danger everyone wanted a bite out of him! And it was this extra sense. It has now been knocked out of us. Our brains are crammed full of rubbish TV, letters, information! *P14 (Patient, I, Pagan)*

And a Christian Methodist nurse provided the following account:

> P: Well, obviously there's the spiritual side of things, cos, I know, I know that, I think everybody's got a spiritual side to their nature, that's my belief right! How they present that, I mean, you can call spirit mood really, sometimes. Well you can raise somebody's spirits or put somebody's spirits down, can't yeah! That's how I, and I'm not talking about mood swings, I'm talking about feeling. How you feel, and a woman can feel so disgusting and horrible, if she wants her hair doing! But you do her hair and her spirits lifted straight away, and that's part of her spirit, and it's how you feel, it's right inside of how you feel and, and but people have different ways of. Everybody's different, that's the thing, everybody's unique aren't they? And different things, erm, provoke, different things, are valuable to different people. So we can look at beautiful painting and be moved spiritually and shed a tear... erm, a rock and roller can hear a legend, rock and roller banging away in the

background, it wouldn't move me, it'd be against my spirits but to him, it would be, ah the best thing since sliced bread, and I can look at a beautiful mountain and a lake, em, oh, that moves me that... *P8 (Nurse, I, Methodist)*

These accounts reveal that perhaps those who have a broad understanding of spirituality arsing from a religious belief are more aware of this dimension within themselves and others. Speculatively this implies that such persons have been introspective, possessing a higher degree of self-awareness in terms of establishing the meaning of spirituality and how this can be nurtured and applied in practice. It must be stressed that it was not only those with a strong religious affiliation who were familiar with the language of spirituality. Conversely, some nurses who indicated that they did not subscribe to any religious belief system recognised this as an important dimension of their lives and were comfortable in addressing such issues with their patients.

Judeo-Christian perspective

One question that may require clarification is what the view of spirituality was in participants who identified themselves with the Judeo-Christian tradition. This question cannot be answered other than at a purely simplistic and superficial level within the context of this thesis. Markham (1998), Bash (2004) and more recently Fawcett and Noble (2004) provide useful insights into spirituality within this tradition. Markham (1998, p. 74) indicates that the Christian will recognise that individuals are not just composed of a physical body but they are made up of a mind – spirit or soul. Christians live in a world created by God and the reason for existing is to worship a transcendent God who is 'the source of goodness, love and beauty'.

The following text, taken from religious leaders within the Evangelical Free (Minister), Roman Catholic (Priest) and Orthodox Jewish (Rabbi) traditions gives significance to, and to a lesser degree corroborates, Markham's defining characteristics:

P: My current understanding is that it's three-fold! The meaning purpose aspect which is most often talked about, is only part of spirituality and I would say that equally at least relationships and I still struggle to find the right word, a sense of transcendence awe, wonder, mystery are also important parts of spirituality and spiritual care. *P42 (Minister, I)*

P: The whole person for a start and it's certainly not exclusive to churches. Because we will often meet people, as you can imagine, who aren't affiliated to any sort of special church, who are terribly spiritual people, but they won't think they were may be!... a very inclusive, takes in a whole lot of things and it should never exclude anybody! *P46 (Catholic Priest, III)*

P: Anything which makes you aware of a deeper purpose in life. Spirituality is also linked with God. As long as God enters the picture you could be involved in the most mundane activity even something which appears to be may be selfish, if God becomes a part of that experience then there is a spiritual dimension to it! *P51 (Orthodox Jewish, III)*

Implicit in these examples to varying levels is the belief in a transcendent being, God, existentialism and the conviction that spirituality is a universal phenomenon. These examples are in stark contrast to the understanding articulated by Eastern traditions. Yet, rather than focusing upon 'difference', it might be more constructive to recognise that there are commonalities in the way spirituality may be perceived among diverse religious traditions. Noticeable in all definitions are the theistic, religious and, to a lesser extent, the transcendent elements. Evident in many of the religious traditions is the notion of service and responsibility for the people, humanity and the environment.

Some cautionary words, the aforementioned works in conjunction with the examples of transcript suggest that there may be a great deal of commonality or a 'homogeneous' view as to how spirituality may be viewed within Judeo-Christian traditions. However, my suspicion is that if one delved deeper and explored the meaning and significance of spirituality within all Christian traditions and denominations then a more 'heterogeneous' picture would emerge.

Recognition of a potential Judeo-Christian bias is emerging in contemporary health care writing. For example, Lie (2001, p. 191) states 'Material on spiritual care emanating from Christian perspectives is widespread', indicating that there has been an absence of other faith communities contributing to or offering their understanding of the subject. However, the argument being levied that contemporary definitions of spirituality in health care are 'Judeo-Christian' must be questioned because the evidence presented here implies that the argument is over simplified in that it does not account for, nor does it reflect, the diversity that may exist at intra-religious and intra-denominational levels.

Key points

- What seemed to emerge in this investigation were striking differences in the way that the concept of spirituality was viewed by different groups of people, nurses, patients and representatives from five of the major world religions!
- I am very much aware that the findings may not be representative of all the groups participating in this study or people who subscribe to a particular religious framework. However, these excerpts suggest that the concept of spirituality (as used in health care) may not be universally recognised, emphasising the need for caution when trying to directly apply the concept to diverse religious groups.
- Again, consideration must be given to the language and terminology that health care is using to define spirituality, because the excerpts reveal that 'spirituality' as a word may not feature in the vocabulary of all religious traditions or groups of people, at least not in the manner in which it is presented within health care.

Individually focused

It was described earlier that some definitions of spirituality constructed within health care focus upon the individual. For example, Murray and Zentner (1989, p. 259) write 'comes into focus when the person faces emotional stress, physical illness or death'. The emphasis in this illustration is the person. In most cases the person is extended to include personal relationships with God, friends and the environment. A major omission in many health care definitions is the failure to acknowledge a 'context'. By this I mean the place or role of the individual within a wider community. Kellehear (2002) suggests that a possible explanation for this on the basis that health care definitions have and continue to perpetuate a terminology of spirituality that is clinically derived. As a clinically derived meaning it embraces the narratives of scientific disciplines such as medicine, psychiatry, clinical psychology. The net effect is that the emphasis is not so much on areas such as health, culture or community, but on crises and problems resulting in possible professional rivalry. This may explain why some of the allied health professions viewed spirituality as an area to be managed. In addition, the perception that spirituality is unique to the individual reflects the holistic philosophy propounded in all health care circles, again reflecting a professional discourse.

The realisation that spirituality is unique and individually determined was certainly visible in the responses provided by many of the allied health professions. This perception of spirituality may be problematic if it is applied unquestioningly to all groups within a pluralistic society. Yet the benefits of introducing an individualised approach to health care cannot be understated in that they have helped to remove the dehumanising and impersonal effects of the scientific medical model. Interestingly, an individualised approach will not explain the importance of community to some participants meaning of spirituality. Kellehear (2002, p. 175) states:

> The fact that knowledge of community can compete with and give context to professional knowledge is seldom given practical recognition or discussion.

This quotation alludes to the notion of a professional and public discourse. It also implies that there is a need for both discourses to have a symbiotic relationship if the spiritual dimension is to have relevance to all.

Community awareness (obligation)

The previous section explored how some participants' perceptions of spirituality were based on an individualistic philosophy. The opposite to the notion of individualism is the concept of collectivism. This finding was called 'community awareness' because it highlighted the idea of service and collective responsibility. Several participants, rather than adopting an individualist approach to spirituality by using words such as 'essence' and 'core', spoke more in terms of service and responsibility for others.

This notion of community awareness was predominantly expressed by representatives from the Eastern religions. For some the notion of service, self-sacrifice and expressing commitment to the wider faith community were very strong elements of viewing spirituality. In fact, in some of these religions this was a religious duty or obligation. These characteristics are illustrated in the following examples:

> P: All of a sudden, you've got the extended family, the immediate family, the extended family and the community coming to see this person!... It's a religious duty amongst Muslims within the community to visit! *P15 (Muslim male, II)*

> P: Spiritual need is the term you should ask somebody from the temple or create a relationship with the local institute of Hinduism to come and

give a helping hand, to the person who is very poorly. To encourage him to get better and God will help them get better. *P17 (Hindu male, II)*

P: I am a Sikh. I work here for the Chaplaincy, so we are here to learn about the people. The Chaplaincy is a very different world. It's a very good on the religion side as well. So I have a little spare time. My life is not good, if I am not doing some good works for the chaplaincy, because I am also involved in the Sikh 'Guthoras' and I do some things within my own community. *P18 (Sikh male, II)*

P: Yeah so really it's looking at how you can develop yourself, so that you can then be of more use to other people, so how you can help them to overcome their own problems and stuff. *P21 (Buddhist male, II)*

It must be stressed that the notion of a community responsibility was also expressed in some of the Western faith traditions. Therefore this finding will have significance to most religious traditions. The reason for drawing attention to this is to demonstrate that within a pluralistic society, in some of the ethnic, cultural and religious traditions the idea of belonging to a wider community, and the responsibilities arising from this association, will be central in shaping attitudes towards spirituality.

Provision of spiritual care

Introduction

This category presents several key properties that impacted upon the way that nurses, patients and representatives from some of the major religions perceived the concept of spiritual care. This category was named 'provision of spiritual care' because it became apparent that the provision of spiritual care was deeply subjective, problematic to define, and dynamic in that it was not a linear process since it involved several variables in the interaction between carer and the cared. The findings also revealed that 'spiritual care' could be influenced by a number of factors: personal, economic/organisational and educational. The properties discussed in this category are 'qualities of carer'; 'hierarchy of care'; 'spiritual assessment: nurse led or expressed need'; 'spiritual care deficits'; and 'integrated spiritual care'.

Throughout the last decade there has been a proliferation of empirical and anecdotal evidence within the health care literature about the nature and structure of spiritual care. The approach adopted in such literature is very prescriptive and dogmatic in that practitioners should be providing spiritual care. Yet little consideration is given to the practical, ethical and emotional costs (Walter, 1997, 2002). Thankfully, because of the issues raised in the work of individuals such as Walter this unquestioning approach is being challenged, signalling a shift away from 'conceptualisations' to exploration of the practical implications. This criticality will hopefully lead to an analysis of the proposed 'properties' of spiritual care within the practice arena. With regard to the findings, analysis revealed several properties that can be accommodated under the category labelled 'provision of spiritual care'. These properties reveal and reflect the concerns of the public in relation to expectation, both professionally in terms of the qualities of the carer and practically, meaning what can be feasibly achieved. This category outlines the factors, anxieties and lengths that professionals will go to in order to provide effective spiritual care. Analysis reveals that all participants' perceptions, either positive or negative, concerning the provision of spiritual care are very much influenced and dependent upon organisational factors, for example the clinical setting and personal factors (such as the personal qualities displayed by the practitioner or patient).

Qualities of the carers

It has been stated earlier that spiritual care is not a linear process but a dynamic one involving personal interaction between the carer and the cared for. For this process to be effective there are certain qualities such as kindness, understanding and sensitivity that must emanate from the carer and the environment in which care is provided. The following transcripts offer a profound insight into the way that patients attending a hospice commented upon the care they received:

> P: Well it's a very relaxed care you know! Em, and always... Em, they're out to please yeah, and, you know their desire is to make you feel more comfortable. And this is one thing I do appreciate. Em... I don't know, what else you can say about it? But this is why I like to come on a Monday because they are. They're kind and understanding! *P11 (Female patient, I)*

> P: And everybody's that nice and the nurses, all the other patients are all friendly and I can't believe how nice everybody is! *P19 (Male patient, I)*

This transcript insinuates that patients may assess quality of the 'care' received against two criteria. The first is the 'general' atmosphere of the clinical setting whether this is welcoming, and comforting. The second is the 'personal' qualities exhibited by individual nurses such as kindness, empathy, listening. It must be stressed that not a single non-professional participant spoke of or made reference to 'spiritual care'.

Focusing upon the first criterion, the 'general' atmosphere conveyed seemed to be perceived differently between the hospice and the acute sector. The patients implied that the focus of attention, whether this was upon the individual or the medical treatment, influenced their perceptions concerning the type of care that they would receive. It was highlighted by some patients that there was insufficient time in the acute sectors for practitioners to be involved in anything other than the provision of physical care. While in the hospice, the emphasis was upon the individual, not the medical diagnosis. This distinction is provided in the following:

> P: When talking about spiritual care in the acute sector quoting 'they're too busy on the medical side...' contrasted against the hospice... 'they give me confidence. I know that I can rely on them for medical information, physical contact, care, you know. And I've got this confidence this boost. I've got a team to look after me. *P14 (Male patient, I)*

The notion of being able to establish patient confidence was a recurrent theme in many nurse transcripts, irrespective of whether they worked in a hospice or the acute sector, for example on an Intensive Care Unit. The ability to establish or develop this confidence within one's dealings with patients was of paramount concern to nurses and patients, ultimately determining the overall quality of interactions and establishing comfort and the feelings of safety and security.

The second criterion, 'personal' qualities displayed by the practitioner, is fundamental in the identification of a spiritual resource person. One gentleman distinguished between 'a really hard nurse' and one that was concerned with the 'spiritual'. This highlighted that 'individual concern' was of paramount importance in differentiating between the nurse who was perhaps medically driven and one that was more 'holistic' in their interaction with patients.

> P: Professional nursing is professional nursing. You can get a really hard nurse who is good at their job! You can get another nurse, who relates quickly to a patient, they are straight into your space, you don't object right!
>
> R: When you say visual indications what would that be?
>
> P: Facial, attitude, body language, erm, her initial few sentences, gives her away. You can tell, whether she's concerned about you as individual and not as a patient. She will probably ask you 'oh what did you do before you came here then?' As an introduction and you will give her

> a few answers and she can work on them, you see spread the tree out before getting to your complaint. She has established herself! Whereas, the hard nurse will come in 'what's all this about pain in your chest we'll sort you out?' You know made the point!
>
> R: Looking at the two illustrations that you've given us. One would say looking at the pain in your chest is medically focused?
>
> P: One's looking at you! Then the pain in the chest! You're, treating the patient not the complaint. The complaint's secondary! If you can't get the patient right, what's the point you know. Confidence, confidence from the patient is worth eighty percent. *P14 (Male patient, I)*

This transcript has undertones of 'spiritual audit', not in the bureaucratic sense but in the idea that patients may well be undertaking their own 'spiritual audit' of 'all staff' to identify a suitable person, someone whom they feel they can trust and who will be sensitive to their spiritual needs. It must be stressed that this may not necessarily be a qualified professional, but the ward 'hostess', i.e. the ward domestic.

A central theme permeating and emanating from both criteria is the use of interpersonal and communication skills in the forming of relationships and in the establishment of an open, friendly, non-threatening culture or caring environment; an environment that supports and nurtures individual's needs. The terms 'good communication' and 'interpersonal skills' were phrases that were repeatedly used by participants, especially nurses when making reference to meeting the spiritual needs of their patients. There was a conscious realisation that 'good communication' would establish a trusting, supportive, environment (Clark *et al.*, 1991), in which patients would feel comfortable and at ease to disclose and discuss their innermost concerns. This finding supports the work of Carroll (2001, p. 91) who found: 'A trusting relationship between patient and nurse had to be present before a patient's spiritual concerns could be explored'.

Reflective question

- What are your thoughts on health care professionals using spiritual assessment tools within their practice?

Spiritual assessment: nurse led or expressed need

This finding sheds light on the use of spiritual assessment within the practice of health care. Analysis reveals that spiritual assessment may be managed either formally or informally. Within this investigation these terms are referred to as 'nurse led' or 'expressed need'. To clarify: 'nurse led' does not imply that spiritual assessment was solely the responsibility of the nurse. On the contrary, several of the allied health professions felt that they had a role to play in this area. However, many felt that nurses were usually the main professional group who conducted formal assessment with patients upon admission.

Several dilemmas associated with spiritual assessment have been documented. McSherry and Ross (2002) draw attention to the types of spiritual assessment, alerting readers to some of the ethical and practical considerations. The drive to justify and quantify almost every aspect of nursing care has led to the development and implementation of a range of spiritual assessment tools, ranging from the direct questioning approach to quantitative assessment based upon spiritual distress indicators. However, the findings of this investigation point out that, while there is a need to ensure that some essential questions are asked as part of the admission process, initially this may be just to enquire whether someone has any specific religious beliefs. It may be that to move beyond this initial level of inquiry is inappropriate in some cases.

The 'nurse led' approach was described as the nurse or allied health professional using some structured spiritual assessment tool, asking the patients a series of questions to establish whether the patient has any religious or spiritual needs. It was indicated that this type of questioning would usually occur during the admission process. This is evident in the following transcript:

> P: When people are admitted, on to the unit, you are only going to get a certain amount of information. It could be that somebody comes in with pain, so that's you're priority, you've got to address that. They are not really going to want to talk about, you know, their philosophy of life and that when they are actually in excruciating pain. So you've got to be, you know, sort of realistic. But that can be built up over a time and things could be ongoing, not just admission written in tablets of stone, and that's how it stays until they actually leave here, in which, you know, which ever way! It's an ongoing thing, you know, and that's because patients will talk to certain people, where they want talk to others and that's just personality. *P1 (Charge Nurse, I)*

Many of the allied health professionals interviewed had some reservation with this approach, for example suggesting a preference for 'expressed need'.

> P: Because everybody is so different and it is so easy to impose what your own ideas of spirituality on to people! Therefore, I feel in something like this, it would have to be driven by the individual, through expressed need and that's really the only way I feel you could do it!
> *P12 (Charge Nurse, III)*

In contrast, the 'expressed need' approach to spiritual assessment involved the individual patient expressing his or her needs and wants. The manner in which such needs were expressed could be verbal or non-verbal. Therefore this process involved the nurse or any member of the health care team using a range of communication, interpersonal and observational skills to establish whether an individual might be displaying cues that may be indicative of a spiritual need. This informal process is integrated within the total package of care offered to the patient, not an additional element. Whether intervention is required would very much depend upon the patient inviting it or expressing a need in this area, allowing and consenting the practitioner to assist them with any spiritual need.

While there are advantages and disadvantages with both approaches it would appear that the care setting is influential in determining the approach used. In the hospice the emphasis was very much upon individuals and identifying all their needs. The nurse led approach was referred to frequently in nurse transcripts and the justification for using this was on the basis of gaining as much insight as possible into the individual's needs. It would be a gross misrepresentation to suggest that the formal approach was managed insensitively on the basis that individuals were confronted directly with a series of questions. This was not the case. The nurses were very much aware of the need to establish a rapport and a dialogue with the patient using observation and communication skills to make the patient feel at ease.

To clarify, those participants who made reference to spiritual assessment suggested that this was structured involving two parts. Firstly, a question surrounding any religious needs and wants was asked. This was usually followed by a second section enquiring about spiritual needs. The latter was often addressed hours or days after admission because of awareness of the potential for intrusion. In reality, the nurses were using a combinational approach to spiritual assessment. Although something was documented on admission, the assessment was continuous in nature and revisited throughout the patient's stay, should a need be expressed either verbally or non-verbally.

The above approach was not adopted in the acute sectors. Many nurses felt uncomfortable with a direct method of spiritual assessment. In fact, many of the nurses indicated that they did not use any direct methods of spiritual assessment, even suggesting that they would not ask any questions surrounding religious or spiritual needs. In the acute sector it seemed that the approach used was for the patient to express and identify any spiritual or religious need upon assessment.

The evidence presented implies that the success of either the nurse led or expressed need approaches to spiritual assessment is that both depend upon flexibility and adaptability. Both forms can be modified to suit diverse care settings and the expectations and care needs of diverse client groups. The evidence implies that practitioners use experience and common sense in the caring relationship rather than relying solely upon bureaucratic aids that may inhibit and distort the art of caring.

Hierarchy of support

The main aim of spiritual assessment is to identify and then support the individual to meet any spiritual need(s), whether these have been assessed formally or expressed by the individual. There seems to be identifiable within the nurses', patients' (and the HCPs in Phase III) transcripts a 'hierarchy of support'. This hierarchy ranged from providing 'general support', to supporting individuals with 'specific or complex' needs (Fig. 5.1). The hierarchy is clearly illustrated in the following transcript:

> P: I actually think that you can help then to achieve their spirituality by sitting (Presence) with them, actually and that's okay, if that's what they want? Em, I don't think, it takes any more than that! I think, if you want to listen to them em... [*short pause*] or if they want to talk (Express) about their spirituality, then that's okay, em, but like anything else I might want to talk about it and I might think crumbs, I don't know anything about this, but it's not, about, necessarily about, what they are saying, but it's about your response to it, and the contact or the qual-

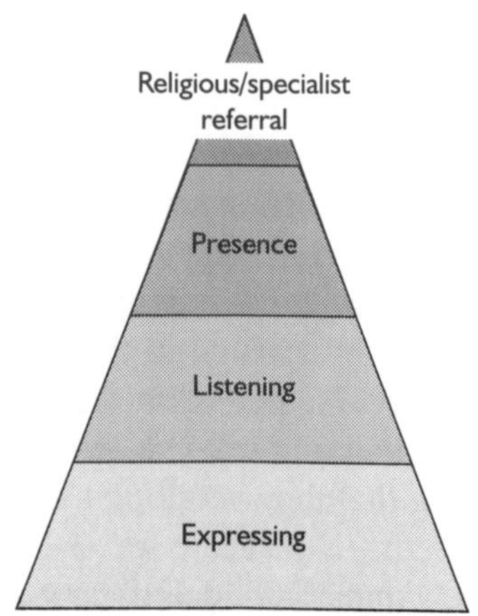

Figure 5.1 Hierarchy of support.

ity of the contact you have with them... [*short pause*] does that make sense? *P4 (Nurse, II)*

At the base of the pyramid would be the term 'expressing', where individuals feel supported to disclose their worries and concerns, or feel confident to request particular resources. This would move on to the next area of support, that staff are 'receptive and listen' to expressed need. At the middle of the pyramid would be 'presence and facilitation'. Staff are able to provide time and give of themselves to assist patients with requests for help. This may involve the nurse or allied health professional liaising with religious and spiritual leaders or even specialist counsellors and practitioners. Towards the top of the pyramid come religious needs and specialist interventions such as counselling.

The nurses and the allied health professions recognised that there may be certain religious rituals, practices, and emotional and psychological problems that may warrant specialist and continued intervention to help patients to meet specific religious and spiritual needs. The pyramid reveals that spiritual support may depend upon several components which, if not present, may inhibit the provision of spiritual care. For example without the first, 'expressing', the others could not occur.

This hierarchy of support operates at two levels: firstly, this may be the order in which individual patients test the water for spiritual care. Secondly, it can be applied to all the allied health professionals in that it describes the types of intervention and the order and sequencing of skills that may need to be used if any form of 'care', including spiritual care, is to be provided effectively. This hierarchy can be superimposed on all types of care, since spiritual care should be integrated and not fragmented.

Spiritual care deficits

This property explores some of the implications arising from nurses and the other allied health professionals when they indicated that they were not able to satisfactorily meet their patients' spiritual needs, for example:

> P: If I said that, I'd be really arrogant! No, I think, as I said, I do fail at times, we all fail at times, I do, I do my best, and I try to, and I try to learn more, so that I can, I can do better if you like. I think, that's the answer, if you keep on learning, but no, I don't think erm, anybody would claim to hundred per cent meet somebody's spiritual need! *P10 (Female nurse, I)*

In earlier work I identified five domains – economic, educational, environmental, ambiguity and sensitivity – from which potential barriers to the provision of spiritual care could emerge (McSherry, 1997, pp. 136–7). These domains mirrored the findings of Ross (née Waugh) (Waugh, 1992; Ross, 1997, p. 145) who provides a detailed illustration of the possible factors influencing spiritual care. The factors are categorised under four broad domains: nurse, patient, other forces and other professionals.

The findings of this investigation corroborate that, despite all the research activity accredited to spiritual care, many of the allied health professions represented in this investigation still highlighted the same deficits. In terms of terminology, I think the term 'spiritual care deficits' is more helpful than 'barriers', which sounds concrete and absolute. The use of the word 'barrier' implies the placing of something consciously and deliberately to obstruct or impede its path. The findings of this investigation revealed that, while some participants highlighted specific deficits that impacted upon the way in which they provided spiritual care, they also demonstrated a strong desire and willingness to redress such shortfalls. In this sense it can be argued that individuals and organisations were not deliberately trying to prevent the provision of spiritual care in terms of awareness, policy or strategy.

Economic deficits refer to organisational and institutional limitations that impact upon the provision of spiritual care. Participants described how insufficient staff, time or personnel resources impeded the delivery of spiritual care; for example:

> P: Just to be able to, if what ever they, well everyone has different perceptions of it haven't they! So, just to be able to discuss any areas they would like to discuss about spiritual things. But it's not an area that comes up a lot, as part of nursing on a surgical ward, it is not as though, we have time to sit down and say, have you got any spiritual concerns?
> *P31 (Nurse, III, Surgical)*

Another economic deficit proposed is the extent and focus of care. If the focus of care is upon the medical management and performing of physical tasks, then the likelihood is that the spiritual dimension will be perceived as having reduced importance. What is not being argued is that spiritual care should take priority over other forms of care. Many nurses argued that, because of insufficient time, the priority of care was often upon the medical and nursing management of a specific illness or condition. Rephrased, physical care took priority over non-physical care. This philosophy was equally relevant for all care settings, hospice and acute. The notion of priority being given to physical care was justified on the basis of preserving life, alleviating pain and controlling other unpleasant symptoms, because, if the patient's attention was focusing upon these, there was less likelihood of the same person wanting to talk about spiritual issues. An interesting question emerged that related to the core category 'assumption versus expectation'. Do patients want their spiritual needs assessing? One nurse was adamant that this is perhaps overstepping the mark and becoming too familiar:

> P: We are not here to take over that person, we are not here to encroach on what they think or do. We are here to cut out their in-growing toe nail or whatever, sometimes and that is what people want, we haven't got that right, to worm our way to that patient's thoughts, unless of course they want us to. We have no right to do that, I would object, I sometimes think we are to familiar with people, we shouldn't expect to be. *P26 (Charge Nurse, III, Medical)*

An educational deficit refers to educational preparedness (Narayanasamy, 1993). This domain included practitioners stating that they did not feel adequately prepared or sufficiently knowledgeable to address the spiritual needs of their patients. Environmental deficits were explained as a lack of privacy. This was often due to limited environmental facilities; for example, availability of a quiet room where patients could be counselled privately.

The published literature alludes to the fact that a major obstacle in the provision of spiritual care is lack of self-awareness (Shelly and Fish, 1988; McSherry, 2000; Narayanasamy, 2001). A lack of self-awareness may manifest itself as an uncertainty or ambiguity surrounding the meaning of spirituality. The result is that such participants exhibited a general lack of awareness of the implications of such meanings for diverse groups of patients and clients. This leads me to conclude that some spiritual care deficits do arise out of ambiguity in the sense that there are still a great many misconceptions associated with the concept. Some participants also expressed fear of mismanagement of a patient's spiritual needs, using direct avoidance so that they would not have to engage with such issues.

Sensitivity as a spiritual care deficit pertains to the use of avoidance or other psychological processes to detach oneself from addressing spiritual issues. In this instance, the nurse or allied health profession would view the entire area as being too personal and, therefore, an area they might refuse to address. The use of such avoidance is provided in the following account:

> P: Yes. It is very easy, looking at our own spirituality, it is very easy to, if someone is critically ill and in an intensive care setting, then to pull away emotionally to view that person, as working on a daily basis, as part of the machinery because you don't want to get involved, because it is tough, if you get psychologically involved with them, it can be very demanding on both of us. *P25 (Nurse, III, Intensive Care)*

Avoidance seemed to be used by practitioners to preserve their own emotional energy because it appeared that many were acutely aware of the emotional cost and burden of becoming involved with an individual at a spiritual level. However, as indicated, some individuals found that coming alongside a patient at a spiritual level enriched their professional role.

The validation of the five spiritual care deficits reveals that there are still some misconceptions surrounding spirituality and spiritual care. Yet, on a positive note, this investigation reveals that nurses and other allied health professionals are supporting and satisfactorily meeting their patients' spiritual needs. In addition, analysis of the five deficits reveals that many practitioners are attempting to redress the imbalance that may exist in their knowledge and practice to overcome such deficits.

Integrated spiritual care

The nurse and patient participants allayed fears about the potential danger of fragmenting spirituality by creating it as a discrete dimension requiring attention by HCPs. A persistent theme that appeared in many of the transcripts during all the phases, particularly Phase I, was the notion of 'integration'. This was evidenced at two levels. Firstly, it was indicated that spiritual care was often 'hidden' in that nurses were providing spiritual care unconsciously during the course of their work and in their dealings with patients:

> R: Would you say that they satisfactorily help you to maintain your spiritual needs?
>
> P: Yes to a large extent but they don't know they are doing it?
>
> R: So they wouldn't articulate it?
>
> P: No, it's through the care and concern. *P14 (Patient, I)*

Secondly, many nurses and, indeed patients, described how they were in receipt of spiritual care but did not label it as such:

> P: They don't actually have the label spirituality, when they are talking to us, there actually passing on, you know, spiritual or it won't be put in those terms, about themselves, about their, you know their life and their philosophy on life. *P1 (Nurse, I)*

This is an interesting observation on the basis that it implies that spiritual care may not be different from other forms of essential care provided by practitioners. The trend in health care seems to establish 'spiritual care' as a discrete set of practices and procedures that must be performed and for which skills such as developing self-awareness, communication, establishing trust and rapport must be developed (McSherry, 2000; Narayanasamy, 1991, 2001). The evidence from this investigation reveals that many practitioners already possess such skills and are utilising them in delivering of general care (including the physical, psychological and social), not under the pretext of spiritual care but routinely in their dealings and interactions with patients. This then raises the question 'Is spiritual care different from essential care?'.

Bradshaw (1994, 1997) recognises the interconnectedness of the caring dimensions:

> Physical care therefore brings with it spiritual care. And spiritual care is inseparable from physical, social and psychological care because it is indistinguishable from the wholeness of care. (Bradshaw, 1994, p. 282)

Participants echoed this view because many of them did not perceive spirituality or spiritual care to be a separate entity. Spiritual care was provided in an integrated manner, not seen as a set of tasks or a procedure to be performed. Some nurses described how they were meeting the spiritual needs of their patients while performing other physical tasks such as bathing, putting on a lady's makeup or doing a patient's hair. Spiritual care was delivered in the course of these interactions. The manner and qualities that the nurse displayed determined how this was perceived by the patient. Such interactions and communications could provide a context, mechanism or vehicle for a patient to discuss matters of a spiritual nature or concern.

Many nurses were acutely aware of the dangers of fragmenting spirituality in terms of assessment and the impact that such actions might have on the development of a nurse–patient relationship. Some nurses felt that spiritual needs could only be assessed once a trusting relationship and rapport had been established. This finding brings into question the suitability of implementing strategies and frameworks for the assessment of spiritual needs. Further, the findings imply that spiritual care is so intimately interwoven within other dimensions of care that it may well be beyond any form of objective measurement in terms of audit.

Draper and McSherry (2002) argue that there exists adequate conceptual vocabulary to support patients in spiritual issues without compounding and adding to the quagmire. Byrne (2002) supports this position, stating that nurses are already involved in the delivery of spiritual care without having the conscious awareness or language to articulate the nature of this experience. This position would imply that we do not need to do anything further to promote spiritual awareness in nurses. While the evidence from this investigation may support such a premise, there is a need to look more closely at the implications of such positions if they were enforced. Swinton and Narayanasamy (2002, p. 159) present an informed and balanced response:

> However until we explore thoroughly the implications of incorporating the language of spirituality into mainstream nursing discourse, we cannot be certain whether we are missing out on something that is vital to our patients, and crucial to the integrity of nursing as a profession.

Therefore, while this finding is interesting and reassuring and cautiously optimistic, because it reveals spiritual care is being provided within the context of integrated care, there is still a great deal of work to be done to establish whether this is the case on a much wider sample and diverse group of people.

Socialisation of the spirit

This category has been labelled 'socialisation of the spirit' because it deals with issues that seemed to have a powerful shaping force upon participants' beliefs and values and ultimately their 'spirituality'. These forces in the main had an affirmative action on the individual; that is, they made the individual more spiritually aware. Conversely, some of the influences resulted in the individual adopting very rigid and inflexible attitudes towards spirituality and religious belief.

Maternal influence

This first property deals with one of the institutional forces that can shape an individual's perceptions of spirituality, namely maternal influences (the mother). Several texts (for example Erikson, 1963; Fowler, 1981; Shaffer, 1999) describe how an individual's identity and ultimately their spiritual self are influenced throughout their lifespan through socialisation and nurturing. Three of the patients (two males and one female) interviewed during Phases I and II of this investigation related their understanding of spirituality to situations in which their mother had acted as a catalyst shaping either consciously or unconsciously their understanding, observation of a situation. These experiences, in which the mother had a central, primary role, had a lasting impression on the individual concerned. For example, one man spoke about his mother's death and, subsequently, how this had shaped his attitude towards religion (spirituality):

> P: Never has interested me, even illness, it's never interested me has religion. It has done nothing for me. It did nothing for me mother and she died a horrible death. *P13 (Male patient, I)*

The other male spoke about spirituality, relating it to an experience he and his mother had encountered together when he was a child ill in hospital. This situation may account for the gentleman believing that spirituality was associated with ghosts and ghouls:

> P: And, eh, my mother came to see me. It was night time, about eight o'clock and they had put us to bed and my mother sat in the room and the building was like a hall with all the doors inside this hall way. And, eh, my mother was sat and all of a sudden she saw what she thought was a nurse pass the door! And eh she shouted and said 'oh nurse I would like to have a word with you'.... About ten minutes later the matron of this home came by and she came into the room and my mother said to her 'oh there's a nurse just passed there, but I shouted to her and went and had a look but I couldn't find her? Got no reply! So this matron then told my mother, said well, this house is haunted... she says and, eh, there's just some spirits walking about it and it had been an old vicarage. *P19 (Male patient, I)*

One female patient described how her mother felt that spirituality was associated with coming back from the dead. However, this young lady did not share the same understanding of spirituality as her mother:

> P: Spirituality, I think it is personal, it depends on what the individual believes, for example my mother believes spirituality to be physic, ghosts and people coming back from the dead. *P23 (Female patient, II).*

The reason why the patient did not share the same understanding of her mother may well be explained by the fact that this individual was educated in the Roman Catholic tradition where the notion of spiritualism is disregarded and, indeed, go against the doctrines and teachings of the church.

These excerpts of transcripts reinforce the notion that an individual's spirituality, in this instance the male's, may be shaped by extrinsic forces that may shape personal beliefs, values and responses to such concepts as religion and spirituality. The limited evidence provided implies that maternal forces, because no paternal examples were presented, can exert a powerful control on one's perceptions of spirituality. This may take the form of imprinting, mirroring of perceptions. Again it is suggested that these forces are so powerful that they are perpetuated throughout subsequent generations and perhaps the wider community. Robinson *et al.* (2003) describe how 'family' is a powerful force in shaping an individual's meaning of life and one can assume their spirituality. The notion of maternal influences was echoed in the transcript of one male patient:

> P: I don't know, but when a child is born, it comes from the mother the father has involvement but it comes from the mother, she is the one that raises it from the little seed to a human being, that is the forces between the two must be very strong. As a force is between my kids and I are strong, [*name*] she sacrificed her life for her kids, she made me suffer sometimes because of the kids, which is quite right. Women have this special spark. *P38 (Patient, I)*

From this perspective it could be argued that historically the mother was perceived as the cornerstone, the central figure of the family, meaning that their beliefs, attitudes and experiences will be extremely influential.

Moral principles

It has long been established within health care that the concept of spirituality may be associated to a person's beliefs, values and moral principles. The formation of this category affirms this association. Many of the participants from all the groups indicated that their spirituality was associated with acting and living life according to specific moral principles and values that directed their actions in specific situations. For some, their moral beliefs and principles had been shaped by adhering to the teachings and doctrines of a specific religion, while for the non-religious participants their moral principles operated around more humanitarian and humanistic codes, for example justice, peace and fairness. This is evidenced in the following:

> P: Well, I should have looked this up in the dictionary really, but what I think about spirituality, is I thinking immediately of religion or beliefs, a code of how you think you should live your life and how others should but a basic code that every Christian or decent human being should work with. *P38 (Patient, I)*

The notion of fairness and justice certainly influenced one patient's perceptions of God. This individual could not reconcile the notion of an all-knowing loving God on the basis of such a God allowing cruelty and atrocity being inflicted upon innocent children:

> P: Well, to tell you the truth, I don't believe in a God because I'm very tender hearted in a way, because when I read about these children that's been attacked assaulted and beaten and all like that, I can't watch it on telly, if it's on telly, because and then I think to myself, if there is a God, why does he allow such things! I mean, little children that can't defend themselves, I think, if he's suppose to be so powerful and that

> and everybody prayers to him, why does he let that happen? *P19 (Male patient, I)*

It was expressed by individuals that spirituality was associated with a code or framework that shaped an individual's attitudes and perceptions towards life generally. The following excerpts demonstrate that this was not unique to one group, but was a recurrent theme in the majority:

> P: I've always, em... I've always, you know, tried to follow me religion and help, I've spent me life trying to help people. *P11 (Patient, I)*

> P: ... I feel that I have moral standards in my life which I work, you know.... I believe in, but I don't think that I need a religious instruction to make me what might be put in inverted commas, being a good person. Eh... mm and so that's what I mean about individuals, that come in here, you know, it is about their beliefs, their understanding, what makes them, them as an individual – what's important to them might not be similar to me but so what! *P1 (Nurse, I)*

These precepts were often based around fundamental beliefs and practices, such as service and charity. Analysis of these transcripts reveals that they are similar to the Christian maxim 'love thy neighbour as thy self' or the humanistic 'golden rule': 'Treat other people as you would like them to treat you' (Narayanasamy, 2001, p. 58). There was also recognition that people's moral principles and beliefs might not always be the same, suggesting a need for tolerance and flexibility. This was especially evident in some of the representatives from the other world religions:

> P: Hinduism as I said is before is a way of life. I don't think love thy neighbour is only for Christianity it is for everybody. I should be ashamed if somebody is in need and he lives next door to me and I don't run to his or her help, then I am not a true Hindu. I love thy neighbour, I want to help the people who are need and this is what's happening. *P17 (Hindu male, II)*

This finding has significance for the all of health care because it suggests individuals have a broad understanding of spirituality in that it is not only shaped by religious doctrines. Some individuals hold beliefs that are shaped by more humanistic philosophies. Furthermore, these limited findings imply that individuals are flexible and accommodating of difference and diversity. These are very important qualities and should be capitalised in the inter-faith and cross cultural dialogues that are currently taking place. This tolerance and flexibility that individuals possess may be indicative of an innate and strong desire to break down deficits/barriers that arise between the diverse groups that live within a multi-racial society.

Innate spirituality

The conception that spirituality is an innate aspect of the human condition, and as such everyone possesses the potential to experience spirituality, was borne out in this inquiry. This was a central and recurrent theme that emerged repeatedly throughout every phase of this investigation. It was evident in all groups of participants, believers and unbelievers:

> P: Yes, most definitely. I think some people refuse to find it or look for it, or not to look, because it is there, to use it. *P38 (Male patient, non-believer, I)*

The notion of innate spirituality manifested itself under two forms. First, *consciously aware* was articulated and viewed as a central part of one's being and make up. Words like *sparkle*, *essence* and *inner* and phrases such as *'it's what makes you, you!'* were used to describe and locate spirituality at the core of the human condition.

> P: I think its different to every person, to me spirituality, is what makes me... feel what makes me be em... the emotional side, the, the essence of living! It, it... makes somebody feel whole. It's the sparkle... *P2 (Nurse, I)*

Therefore, the notion of spirituality having a central location within the individual supports the theory that there may well be a biological explanation for experiencing and expressing a sense of spirituality. The precise mechanism of this relationship between body and spirit is mysterious, and in my opinion, beyond the realm of scientific scrutiny and philosophical explanation. Macquarrie (1972b, p. 46) suggests that the 'spirit' is the 'extra dimension' that distinguishes the human species from the rest of the animal kingdom. This perspective was articulated by one individual who felt that spirituality was indeed biologically determined, describing it as a survival mechanism:

> P: Erm, it, this is noticeable in a photograph of a man and a woman walking over pumice and a child following, jumping in their parent footsteps. You can see it on the beach now. That was just a hint that man was becoming human. I think it was built in strongly to early man almost as a warning signal or a defence signal. He knew or he could

sense when he was in danger everyone wanted a bite out of him! And it was this extra sense. *P14 (Patient, I)*

The second way that the innate nature of spirituality was manifested was through an '*unconscious awareness*' or realisation of the concept. This was evidenced when individuals were asked to comment upon, or provide their understanding of, the term 'spirituality'. Several individuals felt that they did not know what was meant by the word. Interestingly, as the conversation progressed, they began to talk about experiences and philosophies, beliefs they held that had guided their life that would be included in the classification of spirituality. Therefore, while such individuals were unable to articulate an understanding of the word, there appeared to be some innate understanding of dimensions or properties of spirituality that were triggered by my use of the word. This observation suggested that individuals had an unconscious awareness of the meaning of spirituality. This finding has significance because it reinforces the notion that everyone has spirituality (universality). Further, just because the word possesses no significant meaning for them, there is still some unconscious association with the dimension.

Drivers

One of the questions asked participants to comment upon why the concept of spirituality had become fashionable within nursing and health care. Almost all the allied health professions recognised that spirituality and spiritual care were indeed vogue terms, buzzwords. McSherry and Ross (2002) discuss the drivers for nurses' involvement in spiritual care, suggesting that these can be viewed as either political or professional. The themes emerging from this inquiry support this classification. In this investigation the drivers for spirituality becoming fashionable are considered and categorised within the context of two properties: *Managerialism* and *Professionalism.* This category validates and advances the notion of a 'professional' and 'public discourse'

Managerialism

Managerialism in this instance refers to bureaucratic control over the actions and interventions of HCPs. Chapter 2 revealed that there is certainly a political and managerial agenda emerging surrounding the delivery of spiritual care. It must be stressed that the findings of this investigation were not totally opposed to managerial control. Having stated this, some participants implied that involvement in spiritual care was an attempt to shake of the shackles of a scientific, paternalistic control that had infiltrated and removed the 'humanistic' elements of care. Donley (1991, p. 178) recognises the inherent consequence of this:

> High-technology medicine, the insatiable demand for more and better technology, and cost containment have made health care uneven in quality, less human, and very expensive.

Donley highlights two characteristics of managerialism. The first is the insatiable demand for better technology (care) and the second is that this has to be achieved while costs are contained. Excerpts of transcripts demonstrate that nurses were very much aware of a managerial agenda that inhibited spiritual care through the institution of practices that appear to complicate the practice of caring:

> P: ... on that side of the fence, were on this side with all these pathways and all these wonderful intricate things that we look at doing which makes the actual issue of nursing more complicated. *P1 (Nurse, I)*

The 'wonderful intricate things' can be taken to mean assessment, spiritual and general documentation and the implementation of the named nurse system. Some nurses expressed concern about health care being run like a business:

> P: I did hear something that bothered me once, that the Trust and NHS as such are working towards a business type acumen, I remember being quoted Marks and Spencer's. Well, yes, you can take a jumper back to Marks and Spencer's if you wash it and the colour runs. *P20 (Nurse, II)*

This nurse felt that the managerial and business approaches to care failed to acknowledge some of the limitations of this system, stressing the importance of interacting with 'people', not products. An additional limitation of mangerialism is that it has a focus upon process and procedure which may result in the voice and concerns of providers and consumers being overlooked.

Professionalism

One of the main drivers in the desire to establish spirituality at the heart of health care', and more specifically nursing, was the notion of professionalism. The notion of 'professionalising' spiritual care is not new. Dobmeier (1990) listed five benefits to the profession by using the 'nursing process' in addressing spiritual issues. Item 3 was pertinent to the findings of this investigation: '3. Documentation of the nursing process protects nurses from accusations of unprofessional conduct by other nurses, physicians and institutional authorities'. Dobmeier, over a decade ago, recognised some of the potential gains from professionalising spiritual care. It is interesting that, despite considerable activity in this area, spiritual care still features low on the professional and personal agenda of some allied health professions.

It became apparent that there were several points raised by the nurse participants that were indicative of a drive towards professional recognition of the concept. The types of points raised were very broad ranging. For example, several nurses commented upon the positive role that education can play in establishing, and subsequently shaping, HCPs' perceptions of spirituality:

> P: I think, yeah... a, a, a,... I don't know, I think, within may be nurse education and I'm not aware that... or, or... [*Participant was animated and talking very quickly*] [*stutter*]... you know in nurse education, now this may be things that are on their curriculum, I don't know. It may be issues that they are looking at that and that prompts them and, and, and that's good, you know, sort of invest that interest into it. Ehm, it wasn't in mine [*laughing*]... that wasn't part of my nurse training unfortunately. *P1 (Nurse, I)*

Other nurses felt that innovations and strides made in care delivery since the inception of the nursing process were responsible for focusing the attention of the individual not the condition.

> P: I think there's probably a greater emphasises towards that that, we're trying to provide quality care to our patients and that doesn't, you know, they aren't coming as a hip replacement or knee replacement, they are an individual, you know, and that's what we are trying to aim for. And spirituality, as I've said earlier, affects everybody so there's obviously become an emphasis on that aspect because it is part of the individual as a whole! *P12 (Nurse, III)*

Additionally, some participants felt that because of the institution of a more organised systematic approach to care this had resulted in the creation of nursing theory and models that had focused attention on the holistic nature of individuals. Since other dimensions had been attended to in the past, such as the physical and social, it was a logical progression to look at spirituality. In terms of professionalising spiritual care, not all patients felt that this was a realistic goal. This is reflected in the following excerpt:

> P: No [*laughing*] because they're too busy on the medical side so they will have to employ an extra nurse who is skilled in psychology, psychiatry, extra people's needs religious background. *P14 (Patient,* I)

An important driver in terms of professionalism is the notion of meeting the needs of diverse cultural groups. The notion of providing culturally sensitive care and the subsequent attention paid to such issues within health care were responsible for concepts like spirituality becoming fashionable within nursing and wider health care settings. Consideration must be given to the fact that not all the comments provided by nurses in particular were complementary in terms of professionalism. Some nurses felt that nursing in particular had focused on the spiritual dimension firstly because of the vast amount being written on the subject, and secondly so that it could be another feather in their caps, something else that nurses can say they do:

> P: I don't know, is it Steve Wright, you know, who writes all those papers on spirituality in the *Nursing Times*, I don't know, I don't know eh why! Em... [*Someone interrupts interview*]... I don't know, why that em.... In some ways it's like a kind of different debate, isn't about what is nursing? But a perennial debate about what it is nursing? Em, I always feel sometimes that we are justifying what we do? *P4 (Nurse, Manager, II)*

Another interesting point in the desire to establish spirituality as a central and fundamental aspect of health care means that practitioners must be prepared to handle and manage the repercussions of setting themselves as potential guardians or custodians of all things spiritual. This was reiterated in the comments from a nurse manager who disagreed with a managerial agenda on the basis that professionalism had made the concept popular:

> P: I don't think that there is anybody putting pressure on, I don't think they are putting pressure on, I think we put it on ourselves, don't we? Because we've made it fashionable haven't we? *P6 (Nurse, Manager, I)*

Summary points

- This section has presented and discussed the significant findings that emerged during Phase I of the investigation.
- This section has presented and explored the core category 'assumption versus expectation', with its associated properties 'professional discourse' and 'public discourse'. The five subcategories and their properties were detailed and their implications for nursing and health care practice discussed.

Phase II

Introduction

This phase was used to verify the disparities that existed between the different groups regarding the core category and its associated properties that had been constructed. This phase would enable the theory to be refined and tested. I was also conscious that four out of the five patients interviewed in Phase I could be classified as having a very 'traditional' perception and interpretation of 'spirituality' based on historical principles; therefore was this representative of the wider population? In addition, only one patient had been recruited from an acute sector. This under-representation needed to be rectified. Not wanting to close categories prematurely I felt that I needed to explore the area of spirituality more fully to check out the professional and public discourses constructed.

On this occasion, rather than just using the term 'spirituality', I structured the questions around attributes or elements of spirituality as presented within the nursing and health care literature mirroring the subcategory 'Definitions of spirituality'. Sampling became more focused, which could be classified as variational and relational, as participants were selected more on the basis of how they might further develop a category or theme (See Table 5.3). The findings of Phase II were very similar to the categories that had been created in Phase I. Therefore, to avoid repetition only those themes and properties that were disparate from those previously discovered are outlined. Table 5.3 provides demographic details of all the participants recruited into Phase II of the investigation.

Themes and categories

The findings of Phase II were very similar in that the themes and categories developed during Phase I still had meaning, significance and relevance for the majority of the participants. However, two points that warrant further exploration and comparison with earlier transcripts are the notions of 'spiritual narrative' and 'subconscious awareness of spirituality'. These two categories helped to expand the properties of the core category by providing a richer insight into how personal and professional experiences can impact upon one's own spirituality. Similarly, the second category tested out some of the assumptions made pertaining to the components of spirituality presented in the health care literature with the participant groups. The findings suggest that some of the

Phase II
Duration: 12 April 2002 – 21 February 2003
Total number of interview hours: 12.6
Length of interviews: 21 minutes to 66 minutes – average 42 minutes.

Table 5.3 Participants included in Phase II of investigation.

No	Age	Religion	Practising	Group	Area	Date interviewed	Reason for theoretical selection
23	18–25	No	No	Patient	II		Younger person's perspective, spiritual awareness increases with age?
24	34–41	C of E	Yes	Nurse	II		Charge Nurse, practising religion, medical area. Test out assumption that higher grades provide spiritual care
25	34–41	Christian	Yes	Nurse	III		Critical care, practising Christian, male perspective – look at medicalisation and holistic approach
26	42–49	C of E	No	Nurse	III		Charge Nurse, length of service, non-practising. More experienced, more likely to be spiritually aware
27	26–33	No	No	Nurse	III		Worked in same area as interviewees Nos. 12 and 22. Wanted to check out issues of spiritual needs being patient led
28	42–49	C of E	Yes	Nurse	II		Specialist Nurse, 23 years qualified. Check out needs led. Concept of spirituality with someone not practising their religion
29	42–49	Born again Christian	Yes	Nurse	II		Enrolled Nurse who completed both questionnaires – seemed keen to be interviewed
30	18–25	Methodist	Yes	Nurse	III		Recently qualified, fitting younger end of life span approach to spirituality
31	26–33	C of E	No	Nurse	III		Nurse perceptions of spirituality, working in a colorectal surgical ward. Look for similarities and make comparisons between all areas

Table 5.3 *(continued)*

No	Age	Religion	Practising	Group	Area	Date interviewed	Reason for theoretical selection
32	43–41	No	No	Nurse	II		Working in critical care, look at notion of holism, medicalisation. No religion. Good to establish similarities, differences with interviewee No. 25
33	26–33	Jehovah's Witness	Yes	Patient	II		Younger person, with strong religious beliefs. Establish how these have been managed while in hospital. Test out the theory of patient led!
34	42–49	C of E	Yes	Nurse	III		Other nurse interviewed from this ward, suggested I interview this person because she was the one they felt best managed patients' spiritual needs, and who was most consulted in these matters
35	26–33	Roman Catholic	Yes	Nurse	II		Only qualified several months, RC, came to work in Britain from the Philippines
36	26–33	C of E	No	Nurse	II		Only qualified, not practising religion, test out if these areas covered in curriculum, if education helps
37	58–65	No	No	Patient	I		Test out theory that spiritual issues come to focus when individuals have a life threatening illness
38	50–57	No	No	Patient	I		Explore some of the general theory that has emerged from this phase with patient groups
39	58–65	No	No	Patient	I		Was encouraged to interview this patient from staff, because of the beliefs they held. Test out notion that men do not discuss spiritual issues as freely as women
40	66–73	C of E – Christian	Yes	Patient	I		General exploration of themes and categories that have been developed during Phase I and Phase II

disseminated components of spirituality may not be readily recognised as such by patients and nurses.

Spiritual narrative

Throughout Phases I and II several nurses and patients provided detailed accounts of experiences, life events or caring episodes that had had a profound impact upon them as individuals. Indeed, some of the nurse participants implied that engaging with their patients' spiritual issues added richness to their professional roles and lives – this phenomenon I've termed 'professional enrichment'. This notion of spiritual narrative is not new. On the contrary, if one looks at the introductions of several postgraduate theses (for example Waugh, 1992; McSherry, 1997; Baldacchino, 2002), there is a narrative that ignited the researcher's interest in spirituality. Similar narratives or critical incidents are identifiable within the nursing literature; for example, Piles (1990) recalls an incident while working as a faculty member in a critical care unit.

More recently, Narayanasamy and Owens (2000) used critical incidents to explore nurses' involvement in spiritual dimensions of care. The participants were asked to provide details of critical incidents in four areas, description of the nursing situation, identification of need, extent of involvement, effect of involvement. A limitation of this investigation was the inability to validate the written accounts provided by conducting in-depth interviews with the respondents. Narayanasamy suggests that nurses' involvement in spiritual care can enrich their professional role. He concludes that the positive messages derived from the use of such research should be disseminated. Importantly, these narratives support the development of this category because it seems that nurses possess a repertoire of such incidents that may shape their approach to the delivery of spiritual care.

It is suggested that narratives appear to have had a significant and lasting impression on the individuals referred to above, causing them to be more 'spiritually aware' and 'spiritually driven' in the sense that they recognise this need within others. However, there are pitfalls, especially if this activity is not balanced and proportionate. That is, the energy is to be directed and applied sensibly and rationally. Since not all people will share the same fervour, enthusiasm and passion, the margin of error in terms of causing offence is high.

The narratives identified within this investigation appear to fall within the following categorisations. Firstly, as indicated above, there are 'professional' narratives: these are events or critical incidents that have raised the professional's awareness of the spiritual dimension. Secondly, there are personal events or crises, such as bereavement, loss of role, physical illness, disease or disability, that cause the individual to be more introspective. Interestingly, these personal events are not always associated with dreadful events or crises, but quite the opposite. Some individuals highlighted that not everything was bad about illness. These 'personal narratives' (appearing irrespective of stage on the lifespan continuum or gender) made the individual more aware of his or her place within the world and about the finite nature of life. In addition, not all life events such as the diagnosis of a disease resulted in an individual becoming more spiritually aware. Murray and Zentner (1989) imply that spirituality comes into focus when the person 'faces emotional stress, physical illness or death'. This certainly was not the case with several patients who were coping with and living with life-threatening illness, again reinforcing how assumptions cannot be made in terms of how individuals will cope with or react to major life events. The following excerpts support the idea of personal spiritual narrative.

This patient recalled how her newly born child was critically ill, and how this made them more spiritually aware:

> P: One that I can really say that is a spiritual concern is my first daughter when she was born. She was six weeks premature and she nearly died and I was told that if she wasn't off the ventilator after three days, I would have to consider turning it off and just letting her go, and she was baptised on Christmas Eve.
>
> R: So it was a difficult time then?
>
> P: Yes. I was talking to the priest that came to baptise her and he said that he was going to pray for her, at midnight mass, and she started to fight the ventilator and she came off it on Christmas Day. I think that can be classed as a spiritual episode in my life. *P23 (Female patient, Age 18–25, II)*

This patient described how hospitalisation and their illness (Type I diabetes) made them reflect upon life:

> R. Since your illness, since you have been unwell, would you say you think more of spiritual things at that point than at other points in your life?
>
> P: Yes you do, as it is a case of, you don't do it subconsciously, it is as you have more time, you have more time to ponder, when you are at home or out and about doing your own sort of thing, you don't really contemplate things, it is almost like an admission switch, you do it automatically, yet when you are in hospital you have more time to reflect about what you have been doing. *P33 (Female, Age 26–33, II)*

A nurse recalled how her terminally ill aunt's faith inspired and motivated her:

> P: From a personal point of view, I have an aunt who is terminally ill and I have nursed her on the ward with my colleagues for over two years and she was diagnosed terminal, in January. Three times, she has been into the hospice on the brink and she has fought back, she has her faith in the fact that that she is a spiritualist. She goes to a spiritualist church and that might not be good for some people, but it is for her! It is what has helped her through, she has a faith and a belief in spiritualism and that has pulled her through and her determination and her will to live, she is not ready to die and she says, she doesn't want to die yet. *P34 (Nurse, II)*

The third form of 'spiritual' narrative I've termed 'social narratives'. These include events not of a personal nature that have resulted in the individual reflecting upon life at a spiritual level. This was evident in some of the interviews that occurred after 11 September 2001. It must be stressed that some individuals provided examples of both the personal and the social. Wright (2002, p. 24) writes 'nurses do not live in isolation. We and the people we care for may have been changed by September 11 – were you?'. There is a notion of change driven by some social event, whether on the catastrophic scale, like September 11th, or whether it was recalling an encounter with some youths who acted on some advice that the participant had given years earlier. These events made the participants reflect and ponder at a deeper level. This is evident in the following excerpts from two men living with the chronic debilitating disease 'Parkinson's':

> P: I caught five young ruffians stealing adhesive tape from my displays outside the shop. Each one had hidden some tape in a muddy towel, they said they had been swimming in barmy drain. [*Transcript shortened*]... I marched them into the shop and asked them if they wanted me to call the police or their parent. They kept telling me over and over how sorry they were. At this point my heart melted... and I sent one of them for ice-creams all round. I gave them a stern lecture... and let the matter rest.
>
> About ten years later a tall smartly dressed young man... entered the shop and said. 'You don't remember me do you?' He recalled the incident ten years previous... he thanked me for the lecture (and the ice-cream) he said from that day on his life had changed for the better. He said he worked hard at school and progressed to a good job in management. We shook hands and as he walked out of the door I felt very humble and I thought to myself what a wonderful world. *P37 (Patient, I)*

This transcript supports the concept of an integrated narrative in that there is a realisation that personal and social narratives make one think at a deeper level:

P: Yeah! I mean, apart from what hits you personally when my wife died and then my mam and dad you know. Apart from that, that really focuses your mind on those things. Then the next thing that really makes me focus is big national events, like that! It is not that I don't bother about other people about the average 'Jo Soap' in the public, it isn't, is it, but it brings it in to your mind again, the amount of evil in the world, and the amount of good as well. When you hear the response of every nation, just ordinary human beings, when you hear the response to that it is reassuring in away. *P38 (Patient, I)*

Ezzy (2002) describes how 'illness' narratives can take on many different forms, being categorised as 'linear' or 'polyphonic'. Linear narratives are characterised by a well-integrated story where there is optimism for the future. Polyphonic narratives are characterised by inconstancies, focused on the present and more comfortable with uncertainty about the future. Analysis of the narratives suggests that both types of narrative were used by some participants of this investigation. Kirsh (1996) discussed the benefits of a narrative approach in addressing spirituality in occupational therapy practice. Spiritual narratives enable individuals to gain understanding, an insight into what may provide meaning and purpose in one's life. Latterly, Robinson *et al.* (2003) talk about the therapeutic benefits of allowing individuals to recall and explore the meaning of their spiritual narrative.

In this investigation the conception of spiritual narrative was not specific to HCPs. On the contrary, this category had relevance and meaning for all the participant groups. It also explains how individuals may construct their understanding of spirituality based on personal, social and even professional experiences. The narratives are reformulated and utilised in the construction of one's own personal view of the world and one's existence within it.

Reflective question

- Do you think individuals have to be consciously aware of the concept of spirituality for it to have any meaning or significance in their life?

'Subconscious awareness of spirituality'

Phase I supported the notion that spirituality was a multifaceted phenomenon that was individually determined. Further, the emerging theory sustains the premise that spirituality was comprised of religious, theistic, existential and transcendent elements. This finding reinforces Narayanasamy's (2001, p. 3) view that spirituality is an abstract concept embracing religion, meaning of life, love, humanity, inner peace, tranquillity, meditation, relationships, individuality and personal worth. A limitation of Phase I was the inability to check out with participants whether they did perceive any of these components to be part of spirituality. If they were not, then how were these characteristics perceived by individuals?

Throughout this phase individuals were asked to comment upon some of the descriptors of spirituality outlined above (detailed in Table 4.15), including relationships, forgiveness, inner peace, morals and creativity, in the sense of listening to music or reading poetry. The vast majority of patients, and indeed some of the nurses, did not perceive all of these descriptors as being part of spirituality. This idea is communicated by one recently qualified nurse:

> R: So you are saying subconsciously we are aware of our spirituality but we might not label it spirituality?
>
> P: Yes.
>
> R: What we are describing in this interview, you wouldn't have necessarily labelled spirituality, but you feel they are to do with spirituality?
>
> P: Yes! But I have thought about it more, because it depends on your concept doesn't it, in that, I believe that your body is your shell and your spirit is spirit, so then it has got to come into everything. *P30 (Nurse, III)*

It must be stated that some components of spirituality were readily recognised as characteristics of spirituality by many of the nurses interviewed during Phase II and some of the allied health professionals interviewed during Phase III. For example:

> R: Would you say areas such as art, reading, poetry and listening to music add anything to your life or are important to you?
>
> P: Yes.
>
> R: Again could you elaborate on that?
>
> P: Let me have a look at, what question was it sorry! Yes, all those are important, and they are spiritual as they are to do with your spirit, what feeds your spirit and what makes you happy, what makes you tick really. *P36 (Nurse, II)*

During Phase I, the property 'innate spirituality', was discussed under the category 'socialisation of the spirit'. Innate spirituality was explained in terms of those who have 'conscious awareness' and 'unconscious awareness'. The construction of this category adds to that category by providing a deeper understanding of the innate nature of spirituality. As previously suggested, by using the word 'spirituality' this acted as a trigger or stimulus resulting in the individual discussing issues that could be perceived as descriptors or precursors of spirituality despite them not recognising them as such.

This experience was observed again with many of the participants in Phase II, where I asked individuals to comment upon their perceptions of the different components of spirituality. The responses were similar, irrespective of age or life experience, suggesting that some individuals have a subconscious awareness of what constitutes spirituality, although they might not recognise it as such or possess the vocabulary to adequately articulate their perceptions of the concept. This is evident in the examples provided in this section. The following example demonstrates the subconscious association with one of the components relationships:

> R: So sharing that intimacy and closeness would you describe that as a spiritual thing?
>
> P: Yes! I have never thought of that before.
>
> R: What the closeness or the issues around relationships?
>
> P: The, closeness and relationships, thinking of that as a spiritual aspect? I never thought of that before. *P23 (Female patient, Age 18–25, II)*

This occurrence is a little like the 'Ah effect' when suddenly the penny drops and one develops insight and realisation. Yet another explanation may be social desirability: that is, the individual was aware of what was being stated and appeased the researcher by agreeing with what was being suggested. Despite this potential bias, the finding still supports the notion that people do possess innate levels of spiritual awareness, ranging from being fully conversant with the concept to having a subconscious awareness. This finding will have implications for all the allied health professions when dealing with patients' spiritual needs since it implies that the language surrounding spirituality may not be recognised. But some individuals do have a deep sense of what constitutes spirituality despite not being able to articulate the precise nature of the phenomenon.

Summary points

- Phase II explored the idea of spiritual narrative and subconscious awareness of spirituality.
- These two themes helped to explain how individuals might formulate their understanding of spirituality.
- The themes demonstrate that, while the word 'spirituality' is alien to some individuals, a number of the characteristics of spirituality are recognisable, although not consciously giving rise to the idea of subconscious awareness advancing the idea of innate spirituality.

Phase III

Phase III involved the checking out and the validation of categories generated within Phases I and II. Sampling was focused on the recruitment and inclusion of other professional groups and some members from the general public. It was not practical to include all HCPs, so a decision was made to include only those members of the health care team who were perceived as being key stakeholders in the provision of spiritual care (see Table 5.4).

Because of time and resource implication, doctors were not included. I am aware that this is an important omission, but a decision was made with my supervision team not to include them. The decision was made firstly on the basis that doctors did not really feature in participants' transcripts (emerging theory), and secondly, like nursing, it would have meant the recruitment of individuals from a wide range of different specialist areas. This would have been time-consuming, which, in turn, could have had a detrimental affect on the rest of the study.

Phase III
Duration: 14 April 2003 – 21 July 2003
Total number of interview hours: 7.8
Length of interviews: 25 minutes to 49 minutes – average 36 minutes 37 seconds

Table 5.4 Participants included in Phase III of investigation.

No.	Age	Gender	Religion	Practising	Group	Area	Date interviewed	Reason for theoretical selection
41	42–49	Female	C of E	No	Social worker	I		Explore notion of professional boundaries role of Social Worker
42	42–49	Male	Christian – Evangelical Free Church	Yes	Chaplain	I		Explore notion of professional Boundaries, role of chaplain
43	34–41	Male	Christian – Baptist	Yes	Chaplain	III		Explore notion of professional boundaries, role of chaplain
44	50–57	Male	Christian – Baptist	Yes	Chaplain	III		Explore notion of professional boundaries, role of chaplain
45	42–49	Female	Christian – C of E	Yes	Chaplain	III		Explore notion of professional boundaries, role of chaplain
46	50–57	Male	Roman Catholic – Priest	Yes	Chaplain	III		Explore notion of professional boundaries, role of chaplain
47	34–41	Female	Christian	No	Physiotherapist	III		Explore notion of professional boundaries, role of physiotherapist – acute care
48	66–73	Male	C of E	No	Patient	I		Check out patient expectation
49	26–33	Male	No	No	Public	III		Obtain a public perception

Table 5.4 (*continued*)

No.	Age	Gender	Religion	Practising	Group	Area	Date interviewed	Reason for theoretical selection
50	42–49	Female	Buddhist	Yes	Physiotherapist	I		Explore notion of professional boundaries, role of physiotherapist – palliative/ community care
51	Not given	Male	Orthodox Jewish	Yes	Rabbi	III		Obtain Jewish perspective – identified this is missing from all phases
52	58–65	Female	No	No	Patient	I		Check out patient expectation
53	74–81	Female	Quaker	Yes	Patient	I		Check out patient expectation

The principal components model for the advancement of spirituality in health care practice[2]

Final analytical decisions

This section has been termed 'final analytical decisions' because it ties together all the loose ends of the investigation. Through the use of the constant comparative method four major themes were identifiable throughout the three phases of the study and explained in the previous discussion: *individuality*, *inclusivity*, *integrated* and *inter/intra disciplinary*. These themes featured in all of the participant groups' transcripts: nurses, allied health professionals, patients and general public. I propose that these themes are the *principal components* of spirituality and I feel that they are fundamental to the management and provision of effective spiritual care. These principal components must be considered if the concept of spirituality is to be advanced within health care theory and practice.

Overview of principal components model

The four principal components model (Fig. 5.2) will help to remove some of the deficits that prevent the provision of spiritual care. Further, they provide a

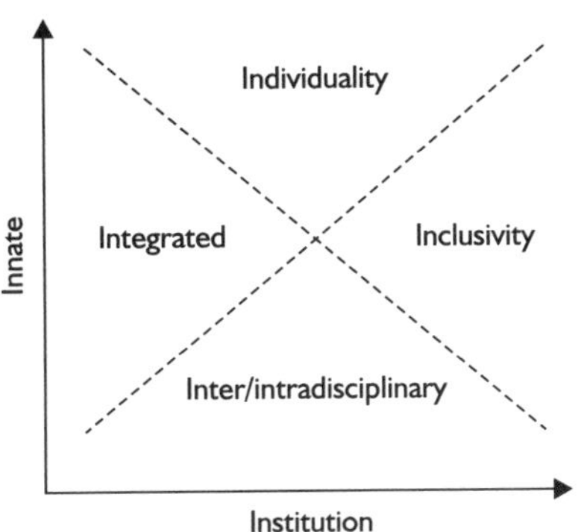

Figure 5.2 Principal components model for the advancement of spirituality and spiritual care within health care.

2 Aspects of this section are reprinted from McSherry, W. (2006) The principal components model: a model for advancing spirituality and spiritual care within nursing and health care practice. *Journal of Clinical Nursing*, **15**(7), 905–17. Copyright 2007 with permission from Blackwell.

framework for the education of all HCPs in matters pertaining to spirituality and spiritual care. The four principal components are: *individuality*, *inclusivity*, *integrated*, *inter/intradisciplinary*. These principal components depend upon two subcomponents, or axes. The vertical axis supports the theory that spirituality is *innate* and the horizontal axis stresses the importance and pivotal role that the *institution* plays in providing effective spiritual care. It has been hinted that there is a clear association between the structure of an organisation in determining how spirituality is perceived by professionals and, far more importantly, how spiritual care will be managed by practitioners.

Review of acronym-based models

The principal components described can also be summarised or represented as the *'four "I" model'*. Sampling of the technical literature revealed that acronyms have been used successfully in the area of spirituality and in advancing spiritual care. These are summarised in Table 5.5.

These acronym-based models are helpful in that they act as aids in assisting educators and practitioners to engage with some very complex issues, such as spiritual and transcultural encounters. Yet despite the proliferation of such models, the spiritual dimension is still poorly understood, remaining a neglected aspect of health care. Perhaps one reason for this is that these models fail to redress some of the inequalities that exist at an organisational and structural level. In addition, there is a need for a model that will redress the imbalance that exists between professional assumptions and service users' expectation in terms of spiritual care. Nonetheless, it must be emphasised that these models can support the integration of spirituality within nursing and health care.

However, while these models may be useful, they must not replace practitioners' intuition and common sense. To follow such models in a rigid, inflexible manner may well be more counter-productive, defeating the purpose for which they were designed. Some of these models may also be unsuitable when encountering or meeting a patient for the fist time. Yet the appropriate use of such models may well prevent the reoccurrence of the situation I experienced and recalled earlier in this book (see section on reflexivity). The correct use of such models will elicit important information surrounding an individual's religious belief and affiliation. The findings of this research suggest that practitioners are acutely aware of the need to establish a rapport and positive interaction with a patient before steamrolling ahead with any form of assessment documentation.

After formulating the idea of the principal components (Four 'I') model, I came across the work of Isaacs (1981) who, during the course of his discussion

Table 5.5 Summary of published frameworks/models used in the advancement of spiritual issues.

Highfield	1993	*Acronym PLAN:* P: Permission L: Limited information A: Activating resources N: Non-nursing assistance
Govier	2000	*Five 'Rs' of spirituality:* Reasons Reflection Religion Relationships Restoration
Ross McSherry	1996 2000	*A systematic–cyclical approach, incorporating the five phases:* Assessment Planning Implementation Evaluation Reassessment
Narayanasamy	1999c, 2001	*ASSET model (Actioning spirituality and spiritual care education and training in nursing)* ACCESS A: Assessment C: Communication C: Cultural negotiation and compromise E: Establishing respect and rapport S: Sensitivity S: Safety
Puchalski and Romer	2000	*Acronym FICA* F: Faith or Beliefs I: Importance and influence C: Community A: Address

on 'ageing and the doctor' spoke about the 'giants of geriatrics', listing these as (1) immobility', (2) instability, (3) incontinence and (4) intellectual impairment – in short, the four 'I's which are instantly recognisable as pertaining to the elderly. While the four 'I's described here may not be as memorable as Isaacs' model in so much as what they describe could be related to any aspect of care, this failure to locate spirituality within a specific context could be considered a major strength because it supports the philosophy of integration. That is, spiritual care is not fragmented and perceived as an adjunct to other essential care.

Though the 'giants of geriatrics' do not have any relevance to the area of spirituality, Isaacs does make a valid point when speaking about the implementation of the four giants. The point is extremely relevant to the discussion surrounding spirituality and spiritual care. Isaacs (1981, p. 145) writes:

> The giants are distinctive, and my case for specialization hangs on the quest for better care of those who fall victim to them. I believe that many doctors have in the past been emotionally blocked when confronted with the giants of geriatrics

This quotation has a significance in relation to the principal components model presented because it is envisaged that once the model is implemented it will assist in promoting and enhancing awareness of the individual beliefs and organisational structures that impact upon perceptions of spirituality. This focusing upon the principal components will eventually lead to the expansion of theoretical and practical knowledge, which should direct the growth of services in relation to the provision of spiritual care. By adhering to the six principal components deficits that have 'emotionally blocked' spiritual care may be broken down and removed. Nevertheless, before this can be achieved, there needs to be a comprehensive explanation of what the principal components of the model are and how they were derived.

Principal components explained

Identification of the Four 'I's

As indicated the principal components, the Four 'I's, were identified throughout data analysis. Through the use of the constant comparative method it was established that the principal components were recurrent themes featuring explicitly or implicitly within participants' transcripts. For example, the word 'individual' was used by many patients and HCPs to describe the personal nature of spirituality. This is evident in the following transcript:

> P: Spirituality, I think it is personal, it depends on what the individual believes... *P23 (Patient, II)*

Likewise, there was a realisation by participants, especially among HCPs, that the language surrounding spirituality needed to be inclusive in that it should have meaning for all people not just those with a religious belief. This is implied in the following example:

> P: ... I think it is wider than that, yes, people that don't believe in a god can still have spiritual needs or beliefs, or may believe in something else. *P26 (Nurse, III)*

Regarding the provision of spiritual care, there was awareness by patients and HCPs that spiritual care was not something separate from the caring process. On the contrary, some patients and HCPs implied that spiritual care was often hidden, provided subconsciously during the performance of seemingly routine interactions and dealings with patients. The belief that spiritual care is integrated is illustrated in the following:

> P: I think we do give a good standard of what we call care to people and spiritual care is encompassed within that care. *P1 (Nurse, I)*

Therefore spiritual care was not perceived as something separate from the caring process but integral. In addition, concern was expressed by some HCPs that there was a danger of fragmenting spirituality, seeing it as another dimension to be addressed. Almost all of the HCPs articulated that inter/intradisciplinary collaborations were central for the delivery of spiritual care:

> R: Who do you feel should be responsible for providing spiritual care?
>
> P: All of us, everybody, we have to work together as a team. Obviously, I think it is the responsibility of everybody, erm, not just the chaplain, the team, not just the social workers, I think nurses as well. *P10 (Nurse, I)*

Having explained the identification of the model, there is now a need to explore each of the principal components, and the two subcomponents in more detail.

Individuality

The findings of this investigation imply that each person had their own unique perceptions of spirituality shaped by several factors: culture, socialisation, life experiences, religious beliefs and institutions (Cawley, 1997). Therefore any attempt to define spirituality, while helpful in that it can elucidate the phenomenon, must appreciate that a definitive or authoritative definition is perhaps idealistic and unrealistic given the diversity of perceptions. It would appear that the participants involved in this inquiry had unique, individual perceptions of spirituality. The findings also reveal that for some individuals the concept of 'spirituality' in the manner in which it has been paraded in health care may be totally alien and have no significance or meaning to them.

Therefore language, metaphor and symbolism associated with spirituality will ultimately be individually determined by cultural, institutional and societal forces. This has significance and poignancy especially in relation to multicultural, intercultural and cross-cultural encounters because assumptions cannot be made regarding an individual's perceptions of spirituality. This position can be extended to include inter- and intraprofessional encounters or interactions because, while the findings suggest that the majority of professionals interviewed had a shared understanding of spirituality, a small minority of health personnel were unfamiliar and uncomfortable with the concept. The net effect is that the practitioner must be guided by the individual patient with his or her individual needs and wants whether directly or indirectly expressed. The professional discourse which makes generalisation and assumptions regarding people's understandings of spirituality and their expectation in terms of receiving spiritual care must be challenged. The professional discourse, while espousing an individualistic approach, is contradictory because spirituality is applied universally to all groups, not reflecting the diversity of opinions and views that prevail in a pluralistic society.

Central to the notion of individuality is the concept of self-awareness. Taylor (2002, p. 58) writes 'Developing spiritual self-awareness is an essential part of learning how to provide spiritual care to nursing clients'. Self-awareness is considered fundamental to the delivery of spiritual care because it enables the individual (professional or patient) to develop insights into his or her own beliefs, prejudices and feelings. It is postulated within the health care literature that self-awareness will prevent vulnerable clients from proselytising and coercion to a particular way of thinking and behaving.

Moreover, individuality must not be mistaken or confused with the notion of individualism. The findings revealed that, while understandings of spirituality are diverse and individually determined, many participants viewed spirituality not as an egocentric concept concerning self. On the contrary, many of the participants felt that their spirituality was shaped and gained expression through their association with a wider community or found meaning in the wider service to others. This was especially apparent in many of the Eastern faith traditions. It would appear that individualism for some participants does not fit comfortably with their perception of spirituality.

Inclusivity

Inclusivity in this context refers to the need to capture and reflect the perceptions and concerns of all stakeholders involved in the delivery of health care. This insight should also reflect the understandings of the wider community. The findings caution all professional groups to pay specific attention to the language and discourses that have been constructed, otherwise there is a grave risk of spiritual discrimination in that the definitions created may unknowingly alienate some religious and ethnic groups especially for individuals whose spirituality is based on unorthodox or morally deviant practices such as witchcraft and the occult.

Presently, the approach adopted, rather than being deemed inclusive could be viewed as exclusive, reflecting the views of the majority population, and therefore it has been perceived as predominantly Judeo-Christian and Anglo-American. It is my belief that this is not a deliberate attempt to exclude other ethnic and religious groups from the debate. On the contrary, as interest in spirituality within health care has grown, the debate is now reflecting the international, cultural and religious differences that exist. However, I urge caution since an inherent danger is that, if we focus specifically on the beliefs and needs of the minority ethnic and religious groups, we can inadvertently alienate or even minimise the beliefs of the majority population. What we are witnessing at present could be construed as anti-Christian because there seems to be a desire to move away from, and even eradicate, the Judeo-Christian components from the debate. Resolution to these issues is the construction and presentation of a balanced approach to spirituality that reflects the views of all groups within contemporary society.

Further, the descriptors used to define spirituality may not be universally recognised by all key stakeholders or sections of the community. This suggests that not only is there a Judeo-Christian bias but there appears to be a professional bigotry. It is a tall order, but future innovations in terms of understanding spirituality and spiritual care must address the above concerns. By redressing the above omissions in terms of reflecting the diversity of language and understanding this will ensure the creation of an inclusive definition, or what Hay and Hunt (2000, p. 42) term 'reconstruction of a common spiritual language'.

Inclusivity not only pertains to the language and discourses that have been created, but also means that all people working within health care institutions, whether these are primary, secondary or tertiary care, need to be involved in the construction of the conceptual and theoretical knowledge. Presently, the review of the technical literature reveals that there is under-representation of some professional groups contributing to the conceptual and theoretical debates. Yet the findings demonstrate that the majority of allied health professionals feel that attending to the spiritual dimension of their clients is of paramount importance. Therefore it is imperative that all of the allied health professions contribute to the dialogue so that all have a share in shaping the direction of contemporary spiritual care.

A further aspect of inclusivity is the notion of who has responsibility for providing spiritual care. It could be argued that by default this is best managed by the nursing profession. However, the findings support the proposition that all individuals, ranging from the ward house keeper to the medical director, have a collective responsibility. This inclusive model will only work if it is instituted with the principles of equality and equity, meaning that all stakeholders have an equal share and vested interest. The idea of patients undertaking a spiritual audit of all staff to identify a spiritual resource person reveals that all have a chance of being selected. Therefore, all allied health professionals, including doctors must be informed of the importance of spirituality and spiritual care for some patients. This should be extended to include volunteers, because many patients commented upon the positive contribution that such individuals make in this area.

Inter/intradisciplinary

The technical literature affirms that neither nurses nor any of the allied health professions perceived that they had a monopoly with regard to spiritual care (Stoter, 1995; McSherry, 1997; Narayanasamy, 2001; Taylor, 2002). The vast majority of the nurses and the allied health professions interviewed articulated that the key to success was to be found in inter- and intradisciplinary collaboration and working. The terms 'inter' and 'intra' in this context are defined as 'inter' – working with other professional groups – and 'intra' – working within the same professional group. Stoter (1995, p. 138) highlights the benefits of 'team working' in relation to the provision of spiritual care:

> Good teamwork will undoubtedly enhance the quality of spiritual care available for patients, clients and relatives. It will also bring added strength to the members involved as they learn from each other finding opportunities for self-development and support, sharing experiences and skills in the process.

There was an acute awareness among all the professional participants and, indeed some of the patients, of the support that can be derived from collaborating and referring to individuals with more expertise, such as chaplains, social workers and counsellors. Taylor (2002) talks in terms of the nurses being perceived as the 'generalists' in spiritual care because they do not possess any formal or advanced training in spiritual matters, while some of the other professional groups (for example chaplains, social workers and, from the non-Western religions, shamans and folk healers) may be considered the 'specialists' in spiritual care because they may have received some formal education in spiritual care, pastoral counselling and psychology.

However, I think it would be more helpful to talk in terms of partners with shared and collective responsibility rather than making such distinctions, which have connotations of inter-professional rivalry boundaries and competition. In addition, it might be more helpful to talk in terms of the generalists and the specialists having a symbiotic relationship, since each is dependent upon the other, with the desired goal of meeting the patients' spiritual needs.

This notion of dependency was clearly expressed by many of the nurses and allied health professionals who suggested that they were dependent upon each other. Chaplains indicated that they relied upon nurses, whom many perceived to be the professional group more likely to identify individuals with spiritual needs because of their continued presence and other allied health professions to make referrals and access this resource at their disposal. While many of the nurses perceived the chaplains to be an invaluable support and a point of contact when dealing with some very difficult issues. Chaplains in the acute trust and the 'psychosocial team' in the hospice were perceived by all participant groups as an integral and fundamental part of the provision of spiritual care.

Regarding intraprofessional working, many nurses spoke in terms of employing the support and skills of nurses, whom they felt to be more competent in managing spiritual issues with patients. Having interviewed such individuals it became apparent that their interest in spirituality stemmed from a strong religious belief or that they had developed their knowledge in this area either informally through personal reading, reflection or, more formally, by attending workshops or conferences. While many nurses implied that this process works well, it could still be construed as passing the buck. Besides, there is also the question of with whom the patient feels comfortable in addressing spiritual issues. These spiritual resource nurses may not be the first choice of the patient. A further dimension that warrants attention in this approach is the emotional burden placed upon such individuals in terms of depleting their own spiritual resources. This approach to intraprofessional management of spiritual issues was not specific to one care setting but was found to be operating in all.

There was a realisation that effective spiritual care could only be provided if there was good collaboration between all of the allied health professions. Many of the participants commented that there were many benefits to be derived from this approach in terms of support, sharing of resources, developing knowledge and understanding in the management of patients' spiritual needs. In essence, collaboration could lead to the nurturing of spiritual awareness increasing competence in this area.

It was commented by some nurses that it was very demanding dealing with patients' spiritual needs and, because of the emotional implications, some stated that they would avoid dealing with patients' spiritual issues. Yet, many nurses indicated that if they felt that they had insufficient knowledge or competence to support a patient then they would refer the matter on to a colleague, chaplain or a member of the psychosocial team. This mechanism of referral suggests that practitioners were recognising limitations within their own competence, but that they felt comfortable and reassured that patients' needs could be met within the wider team. This practice underlines the theory that central to the provision of spiritual care is the notion of inter- and intradisciplinary collaboration.

Integrated

In Phase I, I discussed the notion of spiritual care being integrated. This section adds to the discussion, expanding and exploring the implication of an integrated approach for the advancement of spirituality and spiritual care within health care. The dilemma that academics and HCPs face (and indeed all who have with a vested interest in the provision of spiritual care) is that they must guard against 'fragmentation'. Spirituality should not be fragmented out and be seen as another box to be filled in on an assessment/admission form. A key finding of this investigation is that nurses and some allied health professionals working within diverse care settings are already providing spiritual care, supporting patients with their spiritual needs. These professionals are providing effective spiritual care, unaware that they are doing this. Perhaps the reason for this is that they have not been affected or, you could argue, disaffected by the bureaucratic and managerial agendas. It is my firm belief that a model of integrated care is central to the future delivery of health care. Contemporary health care appears besotted with a culture of specialisation and reductionism that is very much outcome driven. Not everything about specialisation is bad. Yet it must not be allowed to infiltrate and distort the notion of individuals being viewed as holistic and integrated beings.

Consideration must also be given to the language and discourses constructed within health care that are now shrouding spirituality. Many participants see beyond the mist because they are familiar with the language and it has meaning for them. It must be remembered that, for some, spirituality and spiritual needs will not be articulated under this guise or label. Therefore we must guard against creating a terminology and paradigm that segregate spirituality from the essential care that is already provided. Should this occur, it will surely be a recipe for disaster, leading to further reduction and destruction of the concept.

Innate and institution

Constant comparative analysis of the data revealed that two further 'I's may be critical in the advancement of spiritual care, namely the innate nature of spirituality and the institution. The hypothesis that spirituality is innate within all individuals was described in Phase I of the investigation. Yet the idea of all humans possessing a conscious or subconscious spirituality supports the idea of a biological basis. The implications of this finding are that it advances and validates the principle of 'universality'. Universality means that all individuals possess the potential to experience spirituality. As one patient commented 'we all have spirituality but at very low levels'. As indicated, these levels of awareness range from those who are consciously aware and those who are subconsciously aware. If this hypothesis is correct then all individuals in need of health care will require spiritual care. However, this is not an edict to make generalisations. On the contrary, it means the area requires sensitive handling and management, thus preventing proselytising.

Sensitivity is required because individuals may not recognise the language used. This means that care and attention must be given to how such issues are broached in practice. In addition, the danger of imposing and directing individuals into an area of existence they may not have considered, or even wanted to consider, is a major ethical concern. This reinforces that practitioners must be guided by the patients (expressed need) and guard against making accusations and assumptions. If there is an indication that a patient may have a spiritual need, either directly or indirectly expressed, then the practitioner will need to manage the situation in a manner that reflects and suits the individual's understanding of the concept, which may vary dramatically.

The findings of this investigation suggest that spirituality is perceived by some patients and HCPs as a powerful resource in times of illness and hospitalisation. This supports the findings of earlier research studies that attending to the spiritual needs of patients may enhance one's sense of well-being (Hungelmann *et al.* 1985; Walton, 1999; Baldacchino, 2002). However, if this resource is to be harnessed and the quality of the patient's life enhanced, then sufficient resources should be made available by organisations to enable HCPs to achieve this goal. After all, some of the published guidelines emphasise the positive benefits of providing spiritual care (SEHD, 2002; DOH, 2003). If an organisation does not see the importance of spirituality as a powerful resource maintaining the health and well-being of patients and staff then the entire process is doomed from the outset. This recognition is of paramount importance because, if Chief Executives and Service Managers do not possess this insight, then the net effect may be that resources are targeted to other areas, with insufficient capital being devoted to, and invested in, this dimension.

The findings of this investigation suggest that management within the hospice setting was very much aware of ensuring that sufficient resources were available, in terms of staff being on duty, to meet not only the physical but also the spiritual needs of patients. In stark contrast, the acute trusts were plagued with staff shortages and underinvestment in terms of staff having time and capacity. The introduction of spiritual care guidelines (SEHD, 2002; DOH, 2003) may once again raise the profile of the spiritual dimension by placing responsibility for spiritual care provision at the feet of Chief Executives and service managers. Yet such provision should be much wider than merely addressing what Keighley (1997, p. 49) terms 'second order outcomes' that focus upon the structure and process of service delivery. It is acknowledged that it will be difficult to provide outcome measures in terms of assessing the changes in the spiritual state of an individual. However, the danger is that because of the subjectivity surrounding spirituality, that guidelines overemphasise policy and strategic measures, such as calculating sessions for chaplains, instead of engaging with practical issues, such as how best to prepare and support staff in dealing with spiritual matters.

I do not want to appear cynical, but it is now over a decade since the publication of the first version of the *Patient's Charter* (DOH, 1991) and its associated guidelines, and it would seem that very little has changed in the intervening time regarding the provision of spiritual care. I hypothesise that this will remain so until more is done to create a stronger evidence base to show the benefits of investing in this dimension for consumers and service providers. Furthermore, this evidence base should be derived from government-funded sources that invest in research studies exploring diverse aspects of spirituality. This type of investment would indicate a commitment to, and investment in, this aspect of service provision. The Department of Health should follow its counterpart, the Scottish Executive, which has commissioned such research.

Operationalisation and application of the model

Having explored the individual components there needs to be some explanation of how the model can be operationalised and applied within health care contexts. First I will provide a commentary on the schematic diagram (Fig. 5.2), explaining the relationship and dynamics of each component. The model is supported by the two solid lines or axes. The vertical axis represents the innate nature of spirituality. The direction of the arrow implies that individuals will have varying levels of spiritual awareness, ranging from a subconscious spiritual awareness at the base to those who will possess a profound conscious awareness. Furthermore, the vertical direction infers that spiritual awareness may fluctuate, either increasing or decreasing, because it is not static but dynamic across a lifespan. This axis allows application to all patients and client groups, for example individuals with learning disabilities or other organic brain diseases such as dementia. Although such individuals may not be consciously aware of a spiritual dimension, the model accommodates this via the theory of innate equating with universality in that spirituality resides in all people. In essence, the model is anti-discriminatory because it applies to all individuals, irrespective of a functioning intellect.

The horizontal axis represents the institution, referring to the context of care and the organisational structures that are responsible for providing spiritual care. Again the direction of the arrow implies the degree of importance that an organisation may attach to the spiritual dimension, ranging from perceiving it as having little importance to viewing it as having high priority and being of great importance. The more an organisation moves towards the right of the axis, the more it should correlate with improvements in service provision in this area, which will ultimately influence the quality of spiritual care in terms of strategy, structure and process. For example, if spirituality has a prominent feature within an organisation then there is every likelihood that there will be investment in staff and resources, which in turn will lead to improvements or better standards of spiritual care. In addition, these organisations may recognise a need for continuing professional development and research in the area to evaluate and advance practice. It must be stressed that an individual may possess a great innate spiritual awareness while working, or being cared for, in an institution that places little value on the spiritual dimension. In reality, the innate nature of spirituality is not dependent upon, or bound by limitations within, an organisation because it very much depends upon the individual. It is hypothesised that in this situation the individual's innate spirituality will result in his or her spiritual needs being expressed and addressed, although the emotional cost to the individual patient or HCPs may well be great in terms of not receiving adequate support.

The four principal components are represented not by solid lines but by broken lines, demonstrating an interdependence and interconnectedness with each other. If any of the components are overlooked then the model becomes ineffective. All the principal components must be addressed because they are central to understanding spirituality and in providing spiritual care. Service providers, educators and academics must focus on the individual, recognising that spirituality is uniquely defined. It must be borne in mind that language and symbolism may be diverse since it will have been shaped by many variables such as community, culture and socialisation. By focusing upon individuality and inclusivity the model will ensure that a language of spirituality is created that is culturally sensitive in that it allows for ethnic, cultural and religious variation.

The principal of inclusivity draws attention to the language and terminology used to define spirituality. By adopting this principle the proposition of a professional and public discourse can be explored and deficits remedied. Inclusivity will ensure that definitions of spirituality are shaped by all in health care and the wider community so that they have meaning and significance for them. Adhering to the principle of inclusivity will ensure that all involved in the delivery of health care have a shared and collective responsibility in determining policy and strategy in terms of meeting spiritual needs.

The concept of a shared responsibility underpins the idea of inter- and intraprofessional collaboration. Without collaboration, spiritual care provision will be only partially effective. The findings indicate that spiritual care is very much dependent upon a synergy between all allied health professions, patients and significant others. This synergistic relationship ensures that all parties feel supported and affirmed in their desire to provide effective spiritual care. Therefore any attempt to advance insight and practice in this area must ensure that all allied health professionals are consulted. Consultation will create a sense of ownership and prevent the perpetuation of spiritual care being perceived as being bureaucratically and managerially enforced.

The essential principle in the model is the theory of integration. Spiritual care is not to be seen as an additional dimension fragmented out and set apart from the essential care that allied health professionals provide. Spiritual care permeates and integrates all aspects of care provision, just as spirituality integrates and unifies all dimensions of the individual. The result in spiritual care is often a hidden, unarticulated and mysterious concept because it is fused and caught up in everyday practices, rituals and interactions with service users. Therefore any attempt to totally isolate spiritual care as a discrete area for attention, such as spiritual assessment, must be carefully planned and tested. The principle of integrated care requires creativity and ingenuity, forcing HCPs to transcend the constraints of a scientific, medical paradigm that seems to be coercing them to rationalise, reduce and compartmentalise almost every aspect of care.

By focusing upon these principal components a deeper meaning of spirituality and spiritual care will be achieved. The principal components will help to capture a language and discourse of spirituality that has significance and relevance for all working in a contemporary health care system and living in a pluralistic society. These components will provide a framework, set of guiding principles, for educating and preparing staff at all levels of organisations to meet the spiritual needs of diverse communities. The principal components model provides a structure around which spiritual care services can be formulated. It is envisaged that the principal component model will have relevance for all helping to advance spirituality and spiritual care in terms of theory, practice and education.

Activity 5.2 Relevance to practice

Spend some time reflecting on the findings of this investigation. Ask yourself how you might you implement or incorporate them within your own practice.

Conclusion

This chapter has presented and discussed the significant findings of this grounded theory investigation. First, the core category 'assumption versus expectation' was presented with its associated properties, discussing how these had relevance for all the theory created. The five subcategories constructed during Phase I were discussed, highlighting how these were expanded during Phase II to refine and validate insight into spirituality and spiritual care. Finally, the principal components model for the advancement of spirituality and spiritual care was described, indicating how this model may support future developments and insights into the spiritual dimension.

References

Allen, C. (1991) The inner light. *Nursing Standard*, **5**(20), 52–3.

Baldacchino, D. (2002) Spiritual coping of Maltese patients with first acute myocardial infarction: a longitudinal study. *Unpublished Doctor of Philosophy Thesis*, University of Hull, England.

Bash, A. (2004) Spirituality: the emperor's new clothes. *Journal of Clinical Nursing*, **13**(1), 11–16.

Bradshaw, A. (1994) *Lighting the Lamp: The Spiritual Dimension of Nursing Care*. Scutaria Press, London.

Bradshaw A. (1997) Teaching spiritual care to nurses: an alternative approach. *International Journal of Palliative Nursing*, **3**(1), 51–7.

Burkhardt, M. A. (1991) Exploring understandings of spirituality among women in Appalachia. *Doctoral Dissertation*, University of Miami, Florida.

Burnard, P. (1988a) Searching for meaning. *Nursing Times*, **84**(37), 34–6.

Burnard, P. (1988b) The spiritual needs of atheists and agnostics. *Professional Nurse*, December, 130–2.

Carroll, B. (2001) A phenomenological exploration of the nature of spirituality and spiritual care. *Morality*, **6**(1), 81–98.

Carson, V. B. (1989) *Spiritual Dimensions of Nursing Practice*. W. B. Saunders, Philadelphia.

Cawley, N. (1997) Towards defining spirituality. An exploration of the concept of spirituality, *International Journal of Palliative Nursing*, **3**(1), 31–6.

Clark, C. C., Cross, J. R., Deane, D. M. and Lowry, L. W. (1991) Spirituality: integral to quality care. *Holistic Nursing Practice*, **5**(3), 67–76.

Cobb, M. (2001) *The Dying Soul Spiritual Care at the End of Life*. Open University Press, Buckingham.

Dawson, P. J. (1997) A reply to Goddard's 'spirituality as integrative energy'. *Journal of Advanced Nursing*, **25**, 282–9.

Department of Health (1991) *Patient's Charter*. HMSO, London.

Department of Health (2003) *NHS Chaplaincy: Meeting the Religious and Spiritual Needs of Patients and Staff*. Department of Health, London.

Dobmeier, T. (1990) Professionalizing spiritual care. *Journal of Christian Nursing*, **7**(1), 32.

Donley, R. (1991) Spiritual dimensions of health care nursing's mission. *Nursing and Health Care*, **12**(4), 178–83.

Draper, P. and McSherry, W. (2002) A critical review of spirituality and spiritual assessment. *Journal of Advanced Nursing*, **39**(1), 1–2.

Elkins, D. N., Hedstrom, L. J., Hughes, L. L., Leaf, J. A. and Saunders, C. (1988) Towards a humanistic phenomenological spirituality, definition, description and measurement. *Journal of Humanistic Psychology*, **28**(4), 5–18.

Erikson, E. H. (1963) *Childhood and Society*, 2nd edn. W. W. Norton & Company, New York.

Ezzy, D. (2002) Finding life through facing death. In: *Spirituality and Palliative Care* (ed. B. Rumbold), Chapter 5. Oxford University Press, Australia.

Fawcett, T. N. and Noble, A. (2004) The challenge of spiritual care in a multi-faith society experienced as a Christian nurse. *Journal of Clinical Nursing*, **13**, 136–42.

Frankl, V. E. (1987) *Man's Search for Meaning: an Introduction to Logotherapy*. Hodder & Stoughton, London.

Fowler, J. (1981) *Stages of Faith*. Harper & Row, San Francisco.

Glaser, B. G. (1978) *Theoretical Sensitivity: Advances in the Methodology of Grounded Theory*. Sociology Press, Mill Valley.

Goddard, N. C. (1995) 'Spirituality as integrative energy': a philosophical analysis as requisite precursor to holistic nursing practice. *Journal of Advanced Nursing*, **22**, 808–15.

Govier, I. (2000) Spiritual care in nursing: a systematic approach. *Nursing Standard*, **14**(17), 32–6.

Greenstreet, W. (1999) Teaching spirituality in nursing: a literature review. *Nurse Education Today*, 19, 649–58.

Hardy, A. (1979) *The Spiritual Nature of Man: A study of Contemporary Religious Experience*, p. 131. Clarendon Press, Oxford.

Harrington, A. (1995) Spiritual care: what does it mean to RNs? *Australian Journal of Advanced Nursing*, **12**(4), 5–14.

Harrison, J. and Burnard, P. (1993) *Spirituality and Nursing Practice*. Avebury, Aldershot.

Hay, D. (1994) On the biology of God: what is the current status of Hardy's hypothesis? *International Journal for the Psychology of Religion*, **4**(1), 1–23.

Hay, D. and Hunt, K. (2000) *Understanding the Spirituality of People who Don't go to Church*. A report on the findings of the Adults' Spirituality project at the University of Nottingham.

Henley, A. and Schott, J. (1999) *Culture, Religion and Patient Care in a Multi-Ethnic Society*. Age Concern, London.

Highfield, M. E. (1993) PLAN: A spiritual care model for every nurse. *Quality of Life – A Nursing Challenge*, **2**(3), 80–4.

Hilton, C. (2002) Religious beliefs and practices in acute mental health patients. *Nursing Standard*, **16**(38), 33–6.

Hungelmann, J., Rossi, E. K., Klassen, L. and Stollenwerk, R. M. (1985) Spiritual well-being in older adults: harmonious interconnectedness. *Journal of Religion and Health*, **24**(2), 147–53.

Isaacs, B. (1981) Ageing and the doctor. In: *The Impact of Ageing* (ed. D. Hobman), Chapter 8. Croom Helm, London.

James, W. (1902) *The Varieties of Religious Experience: A Study in Human Nature*. Longmans, Green, and Co, London.

Kearney, S. (1994) Spirituality as a coping mechanism in multiple sclerosis: the patient's perspective. *Unpublished Dissertation*, Institute of Nursing Studies, University of Hull, England.

Keighley, T. (1997) Organisational structures and personal spiritual belief. *International Journal of Palliative Nursing*, **3**(1), 47–51.

Kellehear, A. (2002) Spiritual care in palliative care: whose job is it? In: *Spirituality and Palliative Care* (ed. B. Rumbold), Chapter 11. Oxford University Press, Australia.

Kirsh, B. (1996) A narrative approach to addressing spirituality in occupational therapy: exploring personal meaning and purpose. *Canadian Journal of Occupational Therapy*, **63**(1), 55–61.

Lie, A. S. J. (2001) No level playing field. In: *Spirituality in Health Care Contexts* (ed. H. Orchard), Chapter 14. Jessica Kingsley, London.

MacKinlay, E. (2001) *The Spiritual Dimension of Ageing*. Jessica Kingsley, London.

MacLaren, J. (2004) A kaleidoscope of understandings: spiritual nursing in a multi-faith society. *Journal of Advanced Nursing*, **45**(5), 457–62.

Macquarrie, J. (1972) *Existentialism*. Penguin, Harmondsworth.

Markham, I. (1998) Spirituality and the world faiths. In: *The Spiritual Challenge of Health Care* (eds. M. Cobb and V. Robshaw), Chapter 6. Churchill Livingstone, Edinburgh.

Martsolf, D. S. and Mickley, J. R. (1998) The concept of spirituality in nursing theories: differing world-views and extent of focus. *Journal of Advanced Nursing*, **27**, 294–303.

Maslow, A. H. (1970) *Religious Values and Peak Experiences*. Viking, New York.

Maslow, A. H. (1971) *The Father Reaches of Human Nature*. Penguin, New York.

Mayet, F. (2001) Diversity in care: the Islamic approach. In: *Spirituality in Health Care Contexts* (ed. H. Orchard), Chapter 13. Jessica Kingsley, London.

McSherry, W. (1997) A descriptive survey of nurses' perceptions of spirituality and spiritual care. *Unpublished MPhil Thesis*, University of Hull, England.

McSherry, W. (2000) *Making Sense of Spirituality in Nursing Practice: An Interactive Approach*. Harcourt Brace, Edinburgh.

McSherry, W. and Ross, L. (2002) Dilemmas of spiritual assessment: considerations for nursing practice. *Journal of Advanced Nursing*, **38**(5), 479–88.

Murray, R. B. and Zentner, J. B. (1989) *Nursing Concepts for Health Promotion*. Prentice Hall, London.

Narayanasamy, A. (1993) Nurses' awareness and educational preparation in meeting their patients' spiritual needs. *Nurse Education Today*, **13**(3), 196–201.

Narayanasamy, A. (1999a) Learning spiritual dimensions of care from a historical perspective. *Nurse Education Today*, **19**, 386–95.

Narayanasamy, A. (1999b) A review of spirituality as applied to nursing. *International Journal of Nursing Studies*, **36**, 117–25.

Narayanasamy, A. (1999c) ASSET: a model for actioning spirituality and spiritual care education and training in nursing. *Nurse Education Today*, **19**, 274–85.

Narayanasamy, A. (2001) *Spiritual Care: a Practical Guide for Nurses and Health Care Practitioners*, 2nd edn. Quay, Wiltshire.

Narayanasamy, A. (2004) Commentary on MacLaren, J. (2004) A kaleidoscope of understandings: spiritual nursing in a multi-faith society. *Journal of Advanced Nursing*, **45**(5), 457–62. *Journal of Advanced Nursing*, **45**(5), 462–4.

Narayanasamy, A. and Andrews, A. (2000) Cultural impact of Islam on the future directions of nurse education. *Nurse Education Today*, **20**(1), 57–64.

Narayanasamy, A. and Owens, J. (2001) A critical incident study of nurses' responses to the spiritual needs of their patients. *Journal of Advanced Nursing*, **33**(4), 446–55.

Neumann, B. (1995) *The Neuman Systems Model*, 3rd edn. Appleton & Lange, Norwalk.

Newberg, A., D'Aquili, E. and Rause, V. (2002) *Why God won't Go Away: Brain Science and the Biology of Belief.* Ballantine Books, New York.

Nursing and Midwifery Council (2002) *Code of Professional Conduct.* NMC, London.

Oldnall, A. (1996) A critical analysis of nursing: meeting the spiritual needs of patients. *Journal of Advanced Nursing*, **23**, 138–44.

Orchard, H. (ed) (2001) *Spirituality in Health Care Contexts.* Jessica Kingsley, London.

Otto, R. (1950) *The Idea of The Holy.* Oxford University Press, London.

Pattison, S. (2001) Dumbing down the spirit. In: *Spirituality in Health Care Contexts* (ed. H. Orchard), Chapter 2. Jessica Kingsley, London.

Piles, C. (1990) Providing spiritual care. *Nurse Educator*, **15**(1), 36–41.

Puchalski, C. M. and Romer, A.L. (2000) Taking a spiritual history allows clinicians to understand patients more fully. *Journal of Palliative Medicine*, **3**(1), 129–37.

Reed, P. (1992) An emerging paradigm for the investigation of spirituality in nursing. *Research in Nursing and Health*, **15**, 349–57.

Robinson, S., Kendrick, K. and Brown, A. (2003) *Spirituality and the Practice of Healthcare*. Palgrave Macmillan, Basingstoke.

Ross, L. (1996) Teaching spiritual care to nurses. *Nurse Education Today*, **16**, 38–43.

Ross, L. (1997) *Nurses' Perceptions of Spiritual Care*. Avebury, Aldershot.

Scottish Executive Health Department (2002) *Guidelines on Chaplaincy and Spiritual Care in the NHS Scotland (NHS HDL (2002) 76).* Scottish Executive, Edinburgh.

Shaffer, D. R. (1999) *Developmental Psychology: Childhood and Adolescence*, 5th edn. Brooks/Cole Publishing Company, USA.

Sheikh, A. and Gatrad, A. R. (2000) *Caring for Muslim Patients.* Radcliffe Medical Press, Oxford.

Shelly, J. A. and Fish, S. (1988) *Spiritual Care: The Nurse's Role*, 3rd edn. Inter Varsity Press, Illinois.

Shirahama, K. and Inoue E, M. (2001) Spirituality in nursing from a Japanese perspective. *Holistic Nursing Practice*, **15**(3), 63–72.

Simsen, B. (1985) Spiritual needs and resources in illness and hospitalisation. *Unpublished Masters Thesis*, University of Manchester, England.

Simsen, B. (1986) The spiritual dimension. *Nursing Times*, **82**, 41–2.

Smart, N. (1969) *The Religious Experience of Mankind.* Collins, London.

Stallwood, J. (1975) Spiritual dimensions of nursing practice. In: *Clinical Nursing* (eds. I. L. Beland and J. Y. Passos), 3rd edn. MacMillan, New York.

Stern, P. N. (1994) Eroding grounded theory. In: *Critical Issues in Qualitative Research Methods* (ed. J. M. Morse). Sage, Thousand Oaks.

Strauss, A. and Corbin, J. (1998) *Basics of Qualitative Research*, 2nd edn. Sage, Thousand Oaks.

Stoll, R. I. (1979) Guidelines for spiritual assessment. *American Journal of Nursing*, September, **79**(9), 1574–7.

Stoll, R. I. (1989) The essence of spirituality. In: *Spiritual Dimensions of Nursing Practice* (ed. V. B. Carson), Chapter 1. W. B. Saunders, Philadelphia.

Stoter, D. J. (1995) *Spiritual Aspects of Health Care*. Mosby, London.

Swinton, J. and Narayanasamy, A. (2002) Response to: A critical view of spirituality and spiritual assessment by P. Draper and W. McSherry (2002) *Journal of Advanced Nursing*, **39**, 1–2. *Journal of Advanced Nursing*, **40**(2), 158–60.

Tanyi, R. A. (2002) Towards clarification of the meaning of spirituality. *Journal of Advanced Nursing*, **39**(5), 500–9.

Taylor, E. J. (2002) *Spiritual Care, Nursing Theory, Research and Practice*. Prentice Hall, New Jersey.

Taylor, E. J. (2003) Nurses caring for the spirit: patients with cancer and family caregiver expectations. *Oncology Nursing Forum*, **30**(4), 585–90.

Walter, T. (1997) The ideology and organization of spiritual care: three approaches. *Palliative Medicine*, **11**, 21–30.

Walter, T. (2002) Spirituality in palliative care: opportunity or burden? *Palliative Medicine*, **16**, 133–9.

Walton, J. (1999) Spirituality of patients recovering from an acute myocardial infarction: a grounded theory study. *Journal of Holistic Nursing*, **17**(1), 34–53.

Waugh, L. A. (1992) Spiritual aspects of nursing: a descriptive study of nurses' perceptions. *Unpublished PhD Thesis*, Queen Margaret College, Edinburgh.

Wright, S. (2002) Out of the ashes. *Nursing Standard*, **16**(24), 24.

CHAPTER 6

Implications for the practice of spiritual care

Introduction

This chapter has two sections. The first presents the conclusion of the investigation, highlighting salient points of discovery. The second provides a set of 'propositions' for future research. These are areas that require urgent attention to apply the findings of this grounded theory investigation. It is proposed that by attending to these areas a deeper insight into how spirituality and spiritual care are understood will be gained, enhancing service provision and education.

One of the objectives of this grounded theory investigation was to test out the assumption that the concept of spirituality is universally recognisable by a range of groups within diverse care settings. The construction of the core category 'assumption versus expectation' agrees with the growing concern that we have constructed a language of spirituality, and associated terminology, that is indicative of a 'professional discourse'. This discourse is predicated on two precarious assumptions: spirituality is universally recognised; and service users require spiritual care. The identification of the 'public discourse' reveals that not all individuals are familiar with the language of spirituality and, indeed, the concept may be alien to them. In addition, the findings suggest that some patients do not have any real expectation in terms of spiritual care. The net result is the emergence of two distinct discourses based on conflicting assumptions and expectations.

The creation of the subcategories clarifies and adds to the conceptual, empirical and practical knowledge pertaining to spirituality and spiritual care. The subcategories authenticate that spirituality is a complex, multifaceted concept, possessing several layers of meaning and making it a subject rife for conjecture and misinterpretation. The findings establish that meanings and interpretations are shaped by several forces that originate from cultural, social, environmental and religious influences. The consequence of this interplay of interconnected dimensions indicates that specific inferences and generalisations about what constitutes spirituality cannot be made. This sustains the argument that there may be no such thing as an authoritative definition of spirituality that is universally recognised because individuals' perceptions of spirituality will be founded on dissimilar discourses and associations. This does not mean that spirituality is not a universal phenomenon, since the evidence implies that a vast majority of participants had a 'sense of spirituality' manifesting itself either consciously or subconsciously. This implies that spirituality is innate to the human species.

The findings of this investigation relating to definition and perception urge caution if spirituality is to be advanced and reinstated at the heart of nursing and, indeed, the whole of health care. A resolution may be that a loose definition of spirituality is constructed incorporating the descriptors presented in the taxonomy of spirituality (Table 2.2). This would mean that any definition constructed reflected the diversity of expressions and language in how spirituality is viewed within a modern multicultural society. Similarly, the definition may also embrace the commonality that may exist between some groups. To achieve this there will be a need to listen to patients and the public, as one nurse noted 'we need to listen to the voice of the patient'. It would appear that the primary concern of health care – 'the patient' – has been lost in a system that is bureaucratic and managerially driven. This has resulted in the spiritual dimension being neglected, or worse, perceived as another discrete object for attention, fragmented and isolated from the notion of integrated care.

The findings of this investigation are reassuring because the study reveals that many of the allied health professions recognise the importance of the spiritual dimension for the total health and well-being of patients. The fact that many nurses and allied health professions possess a repertoire of spiritual narratives derived from a range of sources demonstrates that they are actively engaging with patients' spiritual needs, at the same time expanding their own spiritual awareness of the concept. All this activity corroborates that nursing, and indeed health care, are still in possession of a rich spiritual/religious heritage. However, it may be that there has been an erosion of its Judeo-Christian associations which is being replaced with a more contemporary non-theistic spirituality that seeks to have significance for all in a multi-faith society. Furthermore, the findings of this investigation underline that nurses have been, and still hold, a central and instrumental role in the provision of spiritual care. Akin to these issues is a deep realisation among many of the allied health professions of the need to provide holistic care that is individualised and patient-centred in an attempt to remove some of the dehumanising aspects of a purely scientific care model. Yet the study demonstrates clearly that there is a need for reunification of the art and science of care, since both have an important role to play in advancing health care practice.

Despite the optimistic tone, there is no room for complacency. The findings indicate that there are still deficits that are impacting upon the provision of spiritual care. A potential solution to these may be found by paying specific attention to the principal components described in this investigation and by using the model as a vehicle to review and direct future service, practice and education in this area. It has been argued that dialogue between all stakeholders and user groups, in conjunction with inter/intraprofessional collaboration, may enhance service provision in this area.

Yet the above activity will be in vain if there is not some clear and firm commitment from the sources of power – political and organisational – to invest in this important yet neglected aspect of health care. Through reinvestment and in the sharing of resources and knowledge, spirituality may once again be integrated at the heart of health care.

In conclusion, this investigation supports and complements all the developments surrounding spirituality and the provision of spiritual care that have been achieved to date. Clarification is offered in that what is not being recommended is that just because some participants, from diverse ethnic, cultural and faith groups, did not recognise the concept of spirituality, we must disregard all that nursing and other allied health professionals have achieved in terms of understanding. While some individuals may not be able to articulate what spirituality means, many possess an intuitive, innate affinity with many of the descriptors associated with spirituality with which they can identify, thus supporting the theory of universality.

Swinton and Narayanasamy (2002) stated that the genie is out of the bottle and cannot be returned. These authors highlight that great advances and strides have been made in the discovery and elucidation of spirituality. This investigation acknowledges the position but urges the whole of health care to take stock and evaluate the achievements made so that such advances can be used productively along with the findings of this investigation. By reviewing and evaluating the existing knowledge base surrounding the spiritual dimension will prevent the perpetuation and widening of a professional and public discourse. My wish is that we listen to and incorporate the voice of all HCPs, but more specifically, that we listen to the voice of our patients and the public that are captured and which resonate throughout the findings of this investigation ensuring they are reflected in all future developments.

Implications

Rather than writing a long litany of suggestions that may not be totally pragmatic or achievable, it was felt that it would be more appropriate and beneficial to nursing and health care to provide six propositions under three headings: 'conceptual and theoretical propositions', 'practice propositions' and 'educational propositions'. These are propositions rather than recommendations because they represent the grounded theory methodology. The propositions highlight specific areas of investigation. It is envisaged that these can be prioritised by future researchers so that they can be achieved within the short term.

Conceptual and theoretical propositions

Proposition 1

Individuals from diverse ethnic, cultural and religious groups will have dissimilar understandings of spirituality based upon cultural and historical discourses

This investigation sought to gain the views of individuals from diverse ethnic and faith groups. It is evident that much of the research conducted to investigate several aspects of spirituality consisted of very homogeneous populations, such as White, Christian. The net effect is that there has been the perpetuation of a Western, Anglo-American and Judeo-Christian perspective of spirituality. While this investigation sought to include a heterogeneous population, this was severely limited due to several factors. The findings of this investigation reveal that there are 'diverse perceptions of spirituality' because individuals from some of the different faith communities and world religions do not identify or recognise the term as used within health care.

This type of qualitative investigation needs to be replicated on large groups of individuals from the major world religions so that a richer and deeper insight into how spirituality is perceived and developed within such cultures and religious traditions is gained. This insight may be acquired by using the 'principal components' model developed in Phase III of the investigation. The data from such an enquiry will enable cross-cultural and inter-cultural comparisons to be made, providing a richer account of how spirituality is perceived. In addition, such investigations will ensure that conceptual and theoretical understandings capture and reflect the diversity of opinions.

Proposition 2

Patients' understanding of spirituality and expectations of spiritual care will be different from those of allied health professions

The findings of this investigation support the theory that presently within health care there exists a professional discourse that is tangential to that of the general public. The professional discourse is based on a loose set of conceptual and theoretical assumptions, one being that spirituality is a universal phenomenon (a principle validated by this investigation). This investigation, through the creation of the core category 'assumption versus expectation', proposes that there are two discourses in operation: professional and public. The public discourse demonstrates that the majority of patients are not familiar with the concept of spirituality as used in health care. In addition, the findings suggest that the majority of patients have no real expectations in terms of nurses or any member of the allied health professions meeting their spiritual needs through the provision of spiritual care.

There is an urgent need for this area to be investigated formally by policy makers so that strategic developments are informed by the voice of the public. At present, it seems that policy is developed (by bureaucrats and managers) on a belief that this is what patients expect in terms of service provision. The danger with this approach is that, while it ensures that there are no omissions in service provision relating to spiritual care in terms of meeting the requirements of the *Patient's Charter* (2001), it does not reflect the voice of patients, public and HCPs. Therefore, this bureaucratic and managerial approach to spiritual care appears to be based on a false set of assumptions that do not reflect the concerns of the general public and the wider community. This finding suggests that there is a need for a multi-site, collaborative study utilising multiple methods so that regional and geographical variations in the perception of spirituality and the expectation in terms of receiving spiritual care can be sought. This type of study will establish a national picture of the public's perceptions of spirituality and their expectations of receiving spiritual care. The findings from such an investigation would prevent the perpetuation of a professional discourse.

Practice propositions

Proposition 3

> *Adopting the model of integrated care will prevent the fragmentation of spirituality within health care practice*

Focusing attention on the concept of spiritual care and presenting this as a discrete area of practice may actually be complicating and raising professionals' anxiety in terms of meeting patients' spiritual needs. The findings of this investigation demonstrate that nurses and allied health professionals are meeting patients' spiritual needs, not under the guise of spiritual care but through everyday essential care. Spiritual care in this scenario is not fragmented but integrated within the total package of care.

It is recommended that research be undertaken to investigate a representative sample from all the health care professions to explore the theory that spiritual care is provided and that patients' spiritual needs are met through the model of 'integrated care'. This type of investigation will lead to a fuller understanding of the processes and dynamics involved in the interactions between the patient and the health care professional in terms of providing spiritual care. Besides, the insights gained may help to dispel some of the fears and apprehensions surrounding the fragmentation of spiritual care.

Proposition 4

> *The idea of generic spiritual assessment tools will be ineffective within large health care organisations*

The concept of spiritual assessment was raised by many nurses, who indicated that spiritual assessment involved two stages. Firstly, there may be some inquiry into an individual's religious beliefs and affiliations. Secondly, the assessment may comprise a series of questions that are asked to establish if the patient has any spiritual needs. Both approaches use a direct method to elicit information. This method was termed as being nurse-led since it was initiated by the practitioner as opposed to the patient expressing any need in this area. Within health care, both these approaches make a valuable contribution to spiritual assessment.

It is hypothesised that spiritual assessment will not work if it is perceived by practitioners as another layer of bureaucracy, for example another set of generic assessment forms to be completed. This suggests a need for research to establish the perceptions and preferences of allied health professionals and service users in terms of spiritual assessment. The findings of this investigation imply that the key to effective spiritual assessment is contextualisation. This means that any tool created must have in mind the specific needs of the user group and the context of care in which it is being used.

Educational propositions

Proposition 5

> *Educating the allied health professions about spiritual matters will result in personal adjustment in the understanding of spirituality*

This proposition arises because it was observed that some participants may have changed or adjusted their personal views and attitudes towards the concept of spirituality as a consequence of taking part in the investigation. The finding denotes a need to explore the ethical basis of encouraging individuals to change or modify their understandings of spirituality purely on the basis that spiritual issues must be explored to fulfil competencies for registration. Ethical issues are only superficially addressed within educational or wider health care literature.

Proposition 6

> *Use of spiritual narratives in health care education will result in practitioners being better educationally prepared to meet the spiritual needs of service users*

The idea of using spiritual narratives that are derived from professional, personal and social domains will be a useful strategy for exploring spiritual issues. The use of such narratives will encourage exploration of the diverse characteristics of spirituality. This method of exploring spiritual issues will enable individuals to become more sensitised to their own spiritual nature. More importantly, these narratives will highlight the types of resources and support that may be required to address such issues within the practice arena.

Concluding remark

To return to the initial aim of this investigation: I have described how a diverse group of participants perceive spirituality and what their expectations are in relation to spiritual care. Additionally, I have provided valuable insight into the two discourses that may impact upon the provision of spiritual care.

To conclude, I feel that I have learned a great deal from conducting this investigation and hope that some of the propositions are advanced by others so that the knowledge base associated with spirituality will reflect all sections of our contemporary society.

References

Department of Health (2001) *Your Guide to the NHS*. Department of Health, London.

Swinton, J. and Narayanasamy, A. (2002) Response to: A critical view of spirituality and spiritual assessment by P. Draper and W. McSherry (2002) *Journal of Advanced Nursing*, **39**, 1–2. *Journal of Advanced Nursing*, **40**(2), 158–60.

APPENDIX 1

Sampling profiles of participants interviewed

Table A1.1 Sampling profile of nurses who were interviewed in Area 1.

	Gender	Age	Years in practice	Hours	Grade	Religious	Existential	Universal	Don't know	Religious belief	Non-religious belief	Practising	Form of religion
1	M	42–49	8	FT	CN			Yes		NA	Yes	NA	NA
2	F	42–49	9	PT	SrN			Yes		Yes		No	C of E
3	F	34–41		PT	EN		Yes			Yes		No	C of E
4	F	34–41	4	FT	CN		Yes			Yes		No	C of E
5	F	50–57	8	PT	SN		Yes	Yes		NA	Yes	NA	NA
6	F	50–57	5	FT	SN			Yes		Yes		Yes	Methodist
7	F	34–41	3:3 months	PT	SN			Yes		Yes		Yes	C of E
8	F	34–41	3:6 months	PT	SN			Yes		Yes		No	C of E

Table A1.2 Sampling profile of nurses who were interviewed Area II.

	Gender	Age	Years in practice	Hours	Grade	Religious	Existential	Universal	Don't know	Religious belief	Non-religious belief	Practising	Form of religion
1	M	34–41	13	FT	Man			Yes		Yes	NA	Yes	Quaker
2	F	50–57	33	PT	Man		Yes			Yes	NA	Yes	RC
3	F	42–49	26	FT	SrN		Yes	Yes		Yes	NA	Yes	C of E
4	F	34–41	17	FT	CN		Yes			Yes	NA	Yes	C of E
5	F	42–49	23	FT	Spec Nurse		Yes			Yes	NA	Not formally	C of E
6	F	42–49	23	FT	EN			Yes		Yes	NA	Yes	Born again Christian
7	M	34–41	11	Ft	SN		Yes			NA	Yes	NA	NA
8	M	26–33	7 months	FT	SN			Yes		Yes	NA	yes	RC
9	F	26–33	6 months	FT	SN		Yes			Yes	NA	No	C of E

Table A1.3 Sampling profile of nurses who were interviewed Area III.

	Gender	Age	Years in practice	Hours	Grade	Religious	Existential	Universal	Don't know	Religious belief	Non-religious belief	Practising	Form of religion
1	M	34–41	0.794	FT	CN			Yes		Yes	NA	Yes	Bahai
2	M	34–41	5	FT	SN			Yes		Yes	NA	Yes	Christian
3	F	42–49	23	FT	CN		Yes			Yes	NA	No	C of E
4	F	26–33	10	FT	SN		Yes			NA	Yes	NA	NA
5	F	18–25	2	FT	SN			Yes		Yes	NA	Yes	Methodist
6	F	26–33	3.4	FT	SN			Yes		Yes	NA	No	C of E
7	F	42–49	5.3	FT	SrN		Yes	Yes		Yes	NA	Yes	C of E

Key:

FT	Full Time
PT	Part Time
CN	Charge Nurse
SrN	Senior Nurse
SN	Staff Nurse
EN	Enrolled Nurse
M	Male
Man	Manager
F	Female
C of E	Church of England
RC	Roman Catholic
NA	Not applicable

Table A1.4 Sampling profile of patients who were interviewed.

	Gender	Age	Day per week or days in hospital	Religious	Existential	Universal	Don't know	Religious belief	Non-religious belief	Practising	Form of religion	Area
1	F	> 82	1	Yes				Yes	NA	Yes	C of E	I
2	M	66–73	1				Yes	NA	Yes	NA	NA	I
3	M	66–73	1		Yes			Yes	NA	Yes	Pagan	I
4	M	> 82	1	None selected				NA	Yes	NA	NA	I
5	F	74–81	Blank	None selected				Blank	Blank	Blank	Blank	III
6	F	18–25	21 days		Yes			NA	Yes	NA	NA	II
7	F	26–33	5		Yes			Yes	NA	Yes	Jehovah's Witness	II
8	M	58–65	2			Yes		NA	Yes	NA	NA	I
9	M	50–57	2		? against this		yes	NA	Yes	NA	NA	I
10	M	58–65	2		Yes			Yes	NA	Yes	Christianity	I
11	M	66–73	1			Yes		Yes	NA	Yes	C of E	I
12	M	66–73	1		Yes			Yes	NA	No	C of E	I
13	F	58–65	1		Yes			NA	Yes	NA	NA	I
14	F	74–81	1			Yes		Yes	NA	Yes	Quaker	I

Table A1.5 Sampling profile of individuals from main world religions who were interviewed.

	Gender	Age	Religious	Existential	Universal	Don't know	Religious belief	Non-religious belief	Practising	Form of religion	Area
1	Male	26–33			Yes		Yes	NA	Yes	Islam	II
2	Female	26–33		Yes			Yes	NA	Yes	Islam	II
3	Male	Not known	Not known				Yes	NA	Yes	Hindu	II
4	Male	Not known	Not known				Yes	NA	Yes	Sikh	II
5	Male	42–49		Yes			Yes	NA	Yes	Buddhist	II
6	Male	Not known					Yes	NA	Yes	Orthodox Jewish	III

Table A1.6 Sampling profile of allied health professionals who were interviewed.

	Gender	Age	Religious	Existential	Universal	Don't know	Religious belief	Non-religious belief	Practising	Form of religion	Profession	Area
1	F	42–49		Yes			Yes	NA	No	C of E	Social worker	I
2	M	42–49			Yes		Yes	NA	Yes	Christian	Chaplain	I
3	M	34–41			Yes		Yes	NA	Yes	Baptist	Chaplain	III
4	M	50–57		Yes			Yes	NA	Yes	Baptist	Chaplain	III
5	F	42–49		Yes				NA	Yes	C of E	Chaplain	III
6	M	50–57			Yes		Yes	NA	Yes	R C	Chaplain	III
7	F	34–41			Yes		Yes	NA	No	Christian	Physio	III
8	F	42–49		Yes			Yes	NA	Yes	Buddhist	Physio	I

APPENDIX 2

Correspondence with areas and ethics committees

Table A2.1 Summarising activity with all areas and LRECs – Letters outlining specific details enclosed in chronological order.

Area I	Researcher Initial contact 3/8/00	Area I Responded 9/8/00	Researcher Replied 11/08/00	Researcher Further reply 3/12/00	Acceptance/ approval 19/12/00	→
Area II LREC	Researcher Submits forms for LREC 18/10/00	LREC respond with request to attend 26/10/00	Researcher attends meeting on 7/11/00	LREC area II respond with feedback from attending the meeting 9/11/00	Researcher responds to request for amendments by LREC 17/11/01	→
Area II	Researcher contacts Deputy Chief Nurse 31/7/00	Researcher responds to a request for more information 10/08/00	Deputy Chief Nurse responds forwarding LREC documentation and identifying a link person 30/8/00	Researcher writes to approximately 25 consultant working in area II – 25/08/00	Researcher contacts Area II R&D Liaison Officer for advice by email 30/8/00	→
Area III LREC	Researcher LREC forms completed sent 31/7/00	LREC responded 29/8/00 raising concerns	Researcher attended LREC – 16/10/00	LREC Respond 20/10/00 – ethical approval deferred awaiting response	Researcher responds to LREC requests 17/11/00	→
Area III Trust	Researcher writes to Assistant chief Nurse 12/12/00	Area III respond 20/12/00 – information passed on to RDF	Area III respond 5/01/02 – invitation to meeting	Researcher attends meeting 16/01/01	Researcher Responds to requests from meeting 15/02/01	→

Note: table extends across three pages

Table A2.1 *(continued)*

Area I	Visit discuss research	Amendments 29/01/01			→
Area II LREC	LREC area II contact giving approval and undertake outstanding modification 25/01/01	Researcher responds to contact from LREC area II 31/01/01	Researcher request 6/03/01 to use a questionnaire	LREC area II respond to request to use a questionnaire – 3/4/01	→
Area II	R&D Liaison Officer Area II replies with advice by email 31/08/00	Area II Finance Manager writes to chair of Research and Development copy to researcher 20/09/00	Area II Director of research and Development Trusts approval granted 15/11/00	Researcher contacts all speciality managers to visit and to attend meetings	→
Area III LREC	LREC respond – study was approved with the addition of a caveat	Researcher responds 12/12/00 fulfilling request			→
Area III Trust	Area III RDF responds asking for form to be completed	Researcher after speaking to all nurse managers – completes form 12/7/01	Area III RDF responds 12/07/02	Area III respond formally approving study, now can proceed 31/7/01	→

Table A2.1 *(continued)*

Area I				
Area II LREC	Researcher responds again in light of previous letter going missing 5/4/01	Researcher responds to LREC 3/5/01	LREC area II acknowledge amendments 5/6/01	LREC area II respond 18/09/01 giving approval
Area II				
Area III LREC				
Area III Trust				

APPENDIX 3

Consent forms

INFORMED CONSENT FORM
(A COPY OF THE SUBJECT INFORMATION SHEET IS ATTACHED)

Full Title of Study
Meaning of spirituality: an investigation into how nurses and patients understand the terms spirituality and spiritual care

PLEASE TICK

- I have been given a complete explanation of the Research Study in which I am being invited to take part, including details of how I will be involved, and what this will entail.
  Yes
  No
- I have had the opportunity to ask questions.
  Yes
  No
- I have received the information sheet on the study, which I have read and will keep safe.
  Yes
  No
- I know that there is no obligation to take part in the study and that I need not give any reason if I do not wish to take part.
  Yes
  No
- I am aware that I may withdraw from the study at any time without the need to give a reason knowing this will have no effect upon my care.
  Yes
  No
- I agree to the interview being tape-recorded and that I understand that the tape will be erased after the Study has been completed.
  Yes
  No

Consent
I .... (name in block capitals)

Agree to take part in this research project, the nature, purpose and possible consequences of which have been described to me

Subject signature
.... dated.........................

Researcher signature
.... dated.........................

Signature of Witness .... dated.........................

Top copy to be retained by Investigator
Second copy to be retained by subject

INFORMED CONSENT FORM
(A COPY OF THE SUBJECT INFORMATION SHEET IS ATTACHED)

Full Title of Study
Meaning of spirituality: an investigation into how nurses and patients understand the terms spirituality and spiritual care

PLEASE INITIAL BOX

- I have been given a complete explanation of the Research Study in which I am being invited to take part, including details of how I will be involved, and what this will entail. ☐
- I have had the opportunity to ask questions. ☐
- I have received the information sheet on the study, which I have read and will keep safe. ☐
- I know that there is no obligation to take part in the study and that I need not give any reason if I do not wish to take part. ☐
- I am aware that I may withdraw from the study at any time without the need to give a reason knowing this will have no effect upon my care. ☐
- I agree to the interview being tape-recorded and that I understand that the tape will be erased after the Study has been completed. ☐

Consent
I .... (name in block capitals)

Agree to take part in this research project, the nature, purpose and possible consequences of which have been described to me

Subject signature
.... dated........................

Researcher signature
.... dated........................

Signature of Witness .... dated........................

Top copy to be retained by Investigator
Second copy to be retained by subject

APPENDIX 4

Questionnaires

RESEARCH ADDRESSING NURSES AND PATIENTS UNDERSTANDING OF THE TERMS SPIRITUALITY AND SPIRITUAL CARE

My name is Wilfred McSherry and I am Lecturer in Acute Care of the Adult working at The University of Hull, Faculty of Health, School of Nursing. I am currently conducting some research (for a higher degree – PhD) into how nurses and patients understand the terms spirituality and spiritual care. The purpose of this research is to gain a better understanding of how nurses (working in different clinical areas from different world faiths) and patients (with a range of physical conditions from different world faiths) understand the word spirituality. This understanding is necessary if nurses indeed all health care professionals are going to be able to offer patients support with this aspect of their lives. It is hoped that the findings of this research will be used to develop nurse education and practice. Therefore I would be grateful if you could complete the small questionnaire and indicate if you would be willing to participate further in my research. In order to maintain your anonymity and confidentiality I have asked the Charge Nurse to distribute this questionnaire. However, if you would require more information then this can be obtained by contacting me on 01482 ...

May I thank you in advance for your support!

PLEASE CAN YOU GIVE THE NECESSARY INFORMATION ABOUT *YOURSELF*?

The questionnaire will take approximately five minutes to complete *(Please place a tick in the appropriate box.)*

1) Are you Male ☐
Female ☐

2) To which age group do you belong?

18–25 ☐ 26–33 ☐ 34–41 ☐
42–49 ☐ 50–57 ☐ 58–65 ☐
66–above ☐

3) How long have you been Qualified?
(Please state number of months/years) I have been Qualified .... months/years

3a) Do you work Full Time ☐
Part Time ☐

3b) Are You? Charge Nurse ☐
Senior Nurse ☐
Staff Nurse ☐
Enrolled Nurse ☐
Other (*please specify*) ....

4) PLEASE COULD YOU TICK THE STATEMENT WHICH YOU FEEL BEST DESCRIBES YOUR UNDERSTANDING OF THE WORD SPIRITUALITY? IT IS IMPORTANT THAT YOU TICK ONLY ONE BOX.

Spirituality involves only religion ☐
Spirituality is concerned with finding meaning, purpose and fulfilment in life ☐
Spirituality applies to all people even those who are unsure or do not believe in any god ☐
I do not know what is meant by the term spirituality ☐

AS IT IS POSSIBLE THAT CONNECTIONS MAY EXIST BETWEEN RELIGIOUS AFFILIATION AND THE RESPONSE YOU HAVE GIVEN, I WOULD APPRECIATE IF YOU WOULD ANSWER THE FOLLOWING QUESTIONS

5) Do you have a religion?
Yes ☐ No ☐
(If yes can you please state your religion)?
....

6) Are you practising your religion?
Yes ☐ No ☐

The nature of my research means that I would like to talk to some nurses about the responses that they have give.

Would you be willing to participate in an interview?
Yes ☐ No ☐

If Yes can you please provide the following contact details

Name: ....
Address: ....
.... Tel No: ....
Signature: .... Date: ....

May I thank you again for taking the time to complete this questionnaire? Can you please hand the questionnaire in to your Charge Nurse!

Wilfred McSherry
Lecturer in Acute Care of the Adult
The University of Hull

RESEARCH ADDRESSING NURSES AND PATIENTS UNDERSTANDING OF THE TERMS SPIRITUALITY AND SPIRITUAL CARE

My name is Wilfred McSherry and I am Lecturer in Acute Care of the Adult working at The University of Hull, Faculty of Health, School of Nursing. I am currently conducting some research (for a higher degree – PhD) into how nurses and patients understand the terms spirituality and spiritual care. The purpose of this research is to gain a better understanding of how nurses (working in different clinical areas from different world faiths) and patients (with a range of physical illnesses from different world faiths) understand the word spirituality. This understanding is necessary if nurses indeed all health care professionals are going to be able to offer patients support with this aspect of their lives. It is hoped that the findings of this research will be used to develop nurse education and practice. Therefore I would be grateful if you could complete the small questionnaire and indicate if you would be willing to participate further in my research. In order to maintain your anonymity and confidentiality I have asked the nurses to distribute this questionnaire. However, if you would require more information then this can be obtained by contacting me on 01482 ...

May I thank you in advance for your support!

PLEASE CAN YOU GIVE THE NECESSARY INFORMATION ABOUT *YOURSELF*?

The questionnaire will take approximately five minutes to complete *(Please place a tick in the appropriate box.)*

1) Are You Male ☐
Female ☐

2) To which age group do you belong?

18–25	☐	26–33	☐	34–41	☐
42–49	☐	50–57	☐	58–65	☐
66–73	☐	74–81	☐	82 and above	☐

3) How long have you been in hospital?
(Please state no of days) I have been in hospital .... Days

4) PLEASE COULD YOU TICK THE STATEMENT WHICH YOU FEEL BEST DESCRIBES YOUR UNDERSTANDING OF THE WORD SPIRITUALITY? IT IS IMPORTANT THAT YOU TICK ONLY ONE BOX.

Spirituality involves only religion ☐
Spirituality is concerned with finding meaning, purpose and fulfilment in life ☐
Spirituality applies to all people even those who are unsure or do not believe in any god ☐
I do not know what is meant by the term spirituality ☐

AS IT IS POSSIBLE THAT CONNECTIONS MAY EXIST BETWEEN RELIGIOUS AFFILIATION AND THE RESPONSE YOU HAVE GIVEN, I WOULD APPRECIATE IF YOU WOULD ANSWER THE FOLLOWING QUESTIONS.

5) Do you have a religion?
Yes ☐ No ☐
(If yes can you please state your religion)?
....

6) Are you practising your religion?
Yes ☐ No ☐

The nature of my research means that I would like to talk to some patients about the responses that they have give.

Would you be willing to participate in an interview?
Yes ☐ No ☐

If Yes can you please provide the following contact details
Name: ....
Address: ....
.... Tel No: ....
Signature: .... Date: ....

May I thank you again for taking the time to complete this questionnaire? Can you please hand the questionnaire in to the nurse responsible for your care?

Wilfred McSherry
Lecturer in Acute Care of the Adult
The University of Hull

APPENDIX 5

Covering letter to participants

Date

Dear

Re: Participation in Research Study

Thank you for agreeing to participate in my research study titled – *The Meaning of Spirituality: A Grounded Theory investigation into nurses and patients' understanding of the term's spirituality and spiritual care.*

I would be grateful if you could read the enclosed information sheet. The reason for my asking you to read the information sheet is to provide you with an understanding of the research. Should you have any questions then do not hesitate to contact me on 01482 – (work) or (Home) 01482 –

I will contact you next week to arrange a date and time when it will be convenient to come and speak to you.

May I take this opportunity to thank you again for your support and assistance with my research?

Yours sincerely

Wilf McSherry
Lecturer in Acute Care of the Adult

Enc.
Information Sheet

APPENDIX 6

Information sheet

INFORMATION SHEET

TITLE OF PROJECT

Meaning of spirituality: an investigation into how nurses and patients understand the terms spirituality and spiritual care

Dear

Thank you for volunteering to take part in my research study. Before we proceed it is important that you understand why this research is being done and what it will involve. What follows are a series of questions you might have about the study. Please take time to read the following information carefully and discuss it with friends, relatives, or the nurse looking after you. You may also contact me Wilfred McSherry if there is anything that is not clear or if you would like more information.

Thank you for reading this.

What is the purpose of this study?
The purpose of this research is to gain a better understanding of how people with a range of physical illnesses, and from different world faiths understand the word spirituality. This understanding is necessary if nurses and indeed all health care professionals are going to be able to offer patients support with this aspect of their lives. This type of information will hopefully be of use to all nurses, and health professionals.

Why have I been chosen?
The consultant directly responsible for your care is aware that this research is being conducted. The nurse responsible for your care has forwarded me your completed questionnaire on which you indicated that you would be willing to assist me further with this research. I will contact you and arrange to visit you at home, or a venue which you prefer.

Do I have to take part?
Before proceeding with the interview you will be asked to sign a consent form, a copy of which you will be given to keep. You are free to withdraw at any time without giving a reason. It is important to note that your participation or non-participation in the study will not affect the standard of care you receive.

What will happen to me if I take part?
This study will involve interviewing you on one occasion for not more than one hour. I will ask you to reflect upon your understanding of the word spirituality and how nurses have attended to your spiritual/religious needs while in hospital. With your permission the interview will be tape recorded to allow me to study our discussion later. This is important as it allows for a more detailed and careful investigation of what you have told me.

Will my taking part in this study be kept confidential?
Apart from myself no one else will know your identity and all the interviews, both taped and written, will not at any time carry your name or address and will be destroyed at the end of the research. Your identity will not be revealed at any time during or following this study and all information will be treated in the strictest confidence.

What are the risks of taking part?
There are no obvious risks involved in this research study. It is possible, however, that discussing some circumstances may cause anxiety if you recall sad events or memories. If this proves to be the case you can terminate the discussion at any point and if you wish to you can withdraw from the study. The researcher will be on hand to offer immediate support and will answer any questions or queries. If required the researcher can access other support if requested.

If after the research you feel you would like to talk over any issue that may have come to light during the conversation then you can contact Mr ___ at the University of York Tel ___ Monday to Friday – 09.00 – 16.00

What are the benefits of taking part?
Participating in this research will not bring you any direct benefit. By agreeing to take part, however, you will help to improve the understanding of how people from different world faiths define spirituality. This understanding could greatly help in the future education of all nurses and health professionals, which in turn will enhance the quality of spiritual care provided within health care settings.

What will happen to the results of the study?

I am carrying out this research for a Ph.D. degree at Leeds Metropolitan University. At no time will your identity be revealed in the research report or any published work.

Contact for further information?

If you require any further information on this research study please contact myself Wilfred McSherry (Lecturer in Acute Adult Care – Department of Nursing and Applied Health Studies, The University of Hull) directly on 01482 – any weekday between 9am and 5pm.

Once again thank you for taking the time to read this information sheet.

Index